10·52   Ł2·49

WHAT'S UP WITH ROS?

Me, myself and Tommy Sheridan

A true story by

ROS NASH

Published by Potential Publishing
Copyright © 2015 Ros Nash
All rights reserved.
ISBN: 978-0-9932179-0-6

For Rob

ACKNOWLEDGEMENTS

Many thanks to Kirsty Moore and Alistair Mooney for their help, advice and encouragement.

Day 1 — 22nd December 2010

Even though it's only a five-minute walk from our flat to the GPs' surgery, Rob decides to drive me. It's treacherously icy, as it has been for weeks. And anyway, I'm not too steady on my feet. When we get in the car Rob has to put the seatbelt on for me and even shifts my legs into the foot well. As we get close to the traffic lights at the bottom of our street and Rob starts indicating right, I grab the steering wheel towards me, as if I want to go left instead. The car swerves but there aren't any other cars around so luckily I don't cause an accident. Rob shouts at me not to do it again, as if I'm a child. I can't explain why I did it, what was going through my head, but I do feel bad for a second, because I've been scolded. Then I instantly forget that I've done it.

Rob comes in with me when it's time to see Dr Crichton. As always when I hear that name, I think of the Crichton in Dumfries, which is now a university campus and events venue, but was once a psychiatric institution. Dumfries is the Scottish town where I grew up.

Rob explains to the doc that I haven't been sleeping very well for the last week or so. I notice that Rob looks really concerned and this surprises me. I'll be totally fine once I get a few decent sleeps. Dr Crichton is frowning at me. In fact it's such a heavy frown that it's almost unreal, a comedy frown. It makes me think that we're not really in the doctor's room at all; are we all actors in some 'Monty Python'-style sketch? Is Dr Crichton the straight man? He asks me some questions but I can't concentrate on what he's saying. I feel agitated and can't sit still, so I get up and walk over to his window. It strikes me what a lovely big office he has. For some reason I decide to pick up some of the ornaments from Dr Crichton's windowsill. Some part of me must recognise that this is unusual behaviour, because I sit back down and try to concentrate, but I'm struggling to stay with the situation. I feel spaced and can't work out why we're here.

I'm surprised to find myself back in the car and get the feeling I've just missed something. Rob tells me to wait there and goes back inside. I still don't understand what's going on. It's nearly Christmas so we should be heading to my Mum's, but something isn't right. It feels like Rob's been in the doctors for a really long time, but when I look back at the clock on the dashboard I'm shocked to see that he's only been gone a couple of minutes.

I turn the dial on the radio and a brilliant track comes on, 'You And Me' by Nero. I turn it up and enjoy the bass. A few bars in I get a strong feeling that it's not actually the radio that's playing, that somehow Rob is controlling what's being played from inside the surgery; I imagine he's surreptitiously looking out

1

the window watching my reaction. Perhaps he's made me a special Christmas mixtape? I look in the surgery windows but only see strangers. Nero keeps asking, are you ready? I wish I knew what I was supposed to be ready for. Work? Christmas? A Christmas surprise? I hope it's not a Scrooge sort of surprise.

I wonder whether the strangers I can see through the window are actors who have parts to play in this, this elaborate joke Rob's playing on me. I've had that feeling several times over the last week, that things aren't quite what they seem.

Now Fearne Cotton is talking on the radio. I feel pretty sure that what she's saying has a special significance for just me, that she's talking specifically to me rather than generally to everyone listening. I imagine that Rob has done a kind of Cassetteboy job on Fearne; he's listened to loads of her shows, then cut her voice up and edited various segments to make her say stuff that's only relevant to me.

I wonder what's going to happen next. I can't decide but I'm hoping we'll head off to Dumfries as planned, to be with my family for Christmas. Maybe the doc will give Rob some pills to help me sleep over the holidays. As long as I don't have to go to work.

But when Rob comes out he doesn't look like he's been busy playing a trick, or a treat, on me. He looks angry. Or maybe it's concern, worry I see etched on to the face next to me. I'm not sure. Either way, his face isn't saying anything good.

On some level, I think I'm aware that some fairly important part of my brain isn't working any more. There are some important details that I don't remember at all. I don't remember Rob having to help me shower and dress earlier on. Or that my period started this morning but I couldn't figure out what exactly to do about it. Poor Rob came back to the flat to find blood everywhere. God knows what must have gone through his mind. I don't recall any of these things at the moment, but I do know something very strange is happening to me.

I keep getting tearful but when people show concern I'm unable to explain what's upsetting me. I ask whether we're going home now but Rob says we're going to the hospital. I still don't get what's going on here. But I love and trust Rob more than anyone in the world so I go along with this hospital idea. At times during the drive I remember we're going to the hospital. Then I start to think this is part of a big joke someone is playing on me. Perhaps it is a bit like Scrooge; is someone trying to teach me a lesson about what Christmas means? Time isn't moving at a normal pace. We seem to go in slow motion, spending years waiting for the lights to change, then suddenly we're speeding along. I feel spaced out and get mesmerised by each set of traffic lights.

2

I glance over at Rob and think, not for the first time, how much I love this man. Our histories are so closely intertwined. Like elements in a well-whisked cake mixture, it's impossible to separate us. There are so many things I love about him. He'll help anyone, without thinking twice. He'll talk to anyone too, he's the friendliest person I know. He's always smart, creative and practical, calm, level-headed and kind. But he's fun, adventurous, funny and cheeky as well. One of the best things about Rob is his huge range of laughs; he never cries but he'll whip out the right laugh for every occasion. One of my favourites sounds just like Boycie's from 'Only Fools And Horses'. When we're out together in a large group, I'll often stop and smile because I can hear him laughing from the other side of the room. Sometimes he laughs silently, and you only know he's doing it because you can see his shoulders shaking. Of course, he's not perfect. He has some very annoying habits too.

People might not notice how nice-looking Rob is straight away, but when you look properly you see big intelligent friendly blue eyes and the sweetest most inviting smile, two clear clues to his golden soul. But he's not smiling now. And his eyes have red rings round them. I can't work out what I've done wrong but I feel horribly guilty that it's me who's made him sad.

We get to Shawpark, a mental health centre in Glasgow's poverty-stricken Maryhill area. Our time there — it seems to me — mostly consists of waiting around. Me and Rob are taken into various rooms, where we wait to see various doctors or health professionals, who all try to talk to me and then start frowning the way Dr Crichton did. I wish they'd stop doing that, it's not making me feel better at all. Mostly they ask how I'm feeling, I say fine and they leave, unconvinced.

When Rob and I are left alone to wait for the next frowner, I feel that he's being a bit short-tempered, but I'm sure it's my fault if he is. Without realising I'm becoming repetitive, I ask several times whether it's time for us to go home yet. He keeps saying, 'No, we've just got to wait here for Dr so-and-so'. But he says it as if he's talking to a child, as if he's frustrated he has to keep explaining the most obvious things. He's probably just knackered. It must be pretty tiring, living with an insomniac.

I feel guilty for putting him through the last week, which has been hellish for me and probably just as bad for him. I wonder if he's sorry he married me.

While we're talking to one of the doctors, whose name I can't remember, she asks about my appearance on the Fred MacAulay show on Radio Scotland last month. They were doing a feature on whether you should change your name or not when you get married, whether you should double-barrel, that sort of thing. And because I'm the editor of a wedding magazine, I had to go on as a wedding expert. At least I *think* the doc was asking me about that, although what that's got to do with me not sleeping properly is a mystery to me. To be honest it's quite possible she said nothing of the sort; communication is difficult today. Maybe she didn't mention it at all. It's strange that holding a conversation should be so tricky, because it's something I'm normally not too bad at. I probably just need a few good sleeps and then I'll be fine. Mind you, I've been saying that for a while. It feels like my brain is refusing to go into shutdown, like an ancient computer that needs a new hard drive. Or maybe some more RAM.

In one of the rooms at Shawpark I see a little snowman that lights up. It's pink and made of plastic with little white tinselly strands coming off it. It makes me think of my sister Sylvia, who loves anything Christmassy and pink. She would love this snowman. For some reason I can't bear to let go of the little thing. I ask the doctor if I can hold on to him. It doesn't occur to me how mad this sounds; there isn't room in my head for this kind of thought. I can only hold one thought down at a time and at this point, the most important thing is keeping hold of the little snowman.

When Rob and I are left alone in another room, I try to stuff a jar of coffee into my handbag. It's one of those huge industrial-size jars. Rob looks appalled and amused at the same time.

"Ros, what are you doing? You can't take that, it's not yours. What made you think you'd get away with stealing something that big? There's no way it would fit in your bag!"

I look down and realise he's right. I put it back on the shelf sheepishly. Not long after that, I try to pinch part of a skeleton that shows how all the bones in the human body are connected. I'm not sure why I want these things. Maybe it's to help me remember what's happening, since my memory seems to have gone a bit sketchy. At one point I try to steal a sellotape dispenser. Of all the things I could have picked... I try to think when exactly I became a kleptomaniac.

In another room, probably with another doctor frowning at me, I spot a hobby horse in the corner. It makes me think of my friend Jo. When me and a couple of mates were on her Hen Party Committee (Jo is extremely organised so we thought we'd better be too) she requested a gymkhana as part of the fun activities. I remember having to look up the word 'gymkhana' in the dictionary. Just like the snowman, I feel compelled to hold on to the hobby horse. I am severely lacking in self-awareness today; it's not that I don't care how strange it appears to hang on to kids' toys, it doesn't even occur to me. Likewise I don't notice Rob's look of surprise when he sees what I've got.

I can't help sniggering when one of the nurses tells me I'm about to meet a Dr Sowerbutts (pronounced sourbutts).

"I know, an unfortunate name," she says.

The next time I ask Rob if we're going home now, he says we're going to hospital. This confuses me because I thought we were already in one, but (I learn later) Shawpark is more of a drop in day centre type of facility, it doesn't have wards or anything like that.

When we're nearly ready to go, Dr Denver says we need a few more minutes while we wait on the taxi so Rob and I are just to wait here. That's when I decide to make a run for it. It's not something I planned on doing, I just find myself running over to the door and trying to open it by pressing the big white button. But it won't open, because it's a secure room. No escape. Everyone looks a bit shocked afterwards. I'm a bit embarrassed.

When we're all in the waiting area watching out the window for the taxi, which seems to take absolutely ages to arrive, I see a toy on the coffee table and, even though my back is only half-turned away from the medical people, I try to snatch it.

"Ros, what are you doing? You can't take that," Rob says wearily. I put it back sheepishly, a naughty child again.

It's weird that instead of going to the Western or the Infirmary, the two Glasgow hospitals I would go to if I'd broken my leg or got run over, we are going to Stobhill. Later on I understand that this is because they have psychiatric units at Stobhill. At the time this would have scared me, so it's lucky I don't get where we're going.

Rather than going with Rob in his car, I am put in a taxi with several of the staff from Shawpark. I'm on the back seat in the middle and across from me to the right is Dr Denver, the senior psychiatrist. She's attractive, in her early forties with long dark hair and nice even features. She looks a tiny wee bit like a friend of my big brother's, a guy I went out with, only once, a long time ago. His name is Richard Denver and he's from Dumfries. I wonder if they are related or not. On my left is a plump lady in her fifties with a friendly face and silvery grey bob. Opposite and to the left is a blonde pretty doctor I remember speaking to earlier in the day.

They make conversation about things like the cold weather, but I find it difficult to follow the flow of what's being said. I'm not at my most perceptive at this point, but I can tell the blonde one is worried. There's that frown again! She has a really grim look on her pretty face and I feel a bit sad that I've put it there. At one point I look down and notice that my arms are linked with the people on either side of me. I don't know whose idea this was.

I see tower blocks but I've no idea which part of Glasgow we're currently in. South? East? One of the care assistants asks me where I work and I tell her I'm the editor of a wedding magazine.

"Oh, whereabouts are you based? Is it near here?"

I'm unable to give a proper answer, but totally lacking a sense of direction is not unusual for me. I imagine her writing notes on how unbalanced I must be not even to be able to describe where my workplace is in relation to my current location. She isn't to know I couldn't do this on a good day.

I feel really confused about what's going on. I'm not even sure whether I'm in Glasgow or Dumfries. Where's Rob? Perhaps because of the two coincidences with the doctors' names, I start to believe I'm in Dumfries. I try to slip down in my seat so that I'm not seen by anyone on the way. The care assistants encourage me to sit up properly.

That's it, I think I've figured out what's happening. As I sit here in a taxi on the way to get checked in to a mental ward, I am utterly convinced that I'm about to take part in a nativity play. That's what this must be about, I decide. Finally, I understand: I'm playing the part of the Virgin Mary.

The next thing I remember is being in a hospital but still not properly understanding why. My mind is flipping about a lot. One minute it's clear to me that I'm here because I'm not well, because the insomnia that's always been a part of me has got worse, much worse, than ever before. That it's gone too far this time. The next moment I'm back to being convinced that this is all some kind of joke, a sort of Christmas jest or prank that someone's playing on me. Any minute now my family and friends will jump out from behind a curtain and shout,

"Surprise! Ha, we really got you this time!"

I keep thinking it's a 'Doctors and nurses'-style hen party trick. Though why I would be on my hen night three years after I got married is not clear. At other times I think maybe the whole thing is a test and my prize, if I get the right answer, is being allowed to go home.

I feel a compulsion to hold on to my lip balm. This seems unbelievably important. This isn't in itself particularly unusual behaviour for me; I'm a Carmex addict and keep it by my side at all times. But today – is it tonight yet? – it feels like a matter of life and death.

I seem to be spending quite a lot of time in what they call The Interview Room, which is more like a big cupboard than an actual room, with tonnes of box files, a computer that looks so old it reminds me of the 1980s, and a massive filing cabinet. I feel preoccupied and keep looking around and picking up random things; a pen, a piece of paper, a plastic cup. They all seem to symbolise important parts of my life, rather than just being ordinary everyday objects.

I feel easily distracted. A nurse called Claire, with a friendly face and mischievous brown eyes, is trying to make me take a pill. I refuse, because I think it's part of a plot to try to make me believe in God. I'm so focused on Claire's nice brown eyes and not giving in to her request that I'm surprised when I notice Rob is here too. How can someone forget that their own husband is in the room? And such a small room too!

"Honestly nurse, you wouldn't believe what Ros is normally like," Rob says, with that concerned look on his face again. They both try to reason with me and I eventually agree to the pill. But when it arrives it's blue and I want to know why. Why is it blue? It reminds me of a film — 'Labyrinth' maybe? Or 'The Matrix'? — where the central character has to make a crucial decision about whether to take a red pill or a blue one. Actually it's two different doors the Matrix guy has to choose between, isn't it? Or am I thinking of 'Alice In Wonderland'? I ask Claire why it's blue.

"That's just the colour they make them," she says. But I'm convinced it's not right, so I refuse to swallow it.

"Would you feel better if it was a white one?" Claire asks.

"Maybe..."

People continue asking me how I feel and I continue saying fine, which nobody believes, not even me. I keep wandering around, picking things up as if something lying around might give me some clues as to what the hell I'm doing in this place. I keep wondering where Rob is. When one of the nurses tells me he's gone home, I get upset and start crying.

My thoughts aren't working. I can't concentrate and keep mumbling things about 'Adam and Steve', about messages coming from the TV. People ask me questions I can't understand. Have I ever thought about suicide? Have I had any thoughts about harming myself or others? I don't know what to say.

A nurse appears beside me as I'm wandering aimlessly.

"Nurse, can I go home now? I've answered all the doctor's quiz questions." But she doesn't seem to think this is a good idea. I'm given pills. Diazepam and bromazepam at first, then lorazepam later on, though I don't know any of this at the time.

When I'm in the frame of mind where everything I'm experiencing is part of a big test, I always think the answer should be Rob. Some of the nurses are trying to trick me into giving the wrong answer. So when Dr Ali starts to examine me I don't want him to, because I think I should wait to see Rob. I nearly let him look me over at one point, but only because I'm distracted by the big scar on his left cheek. Dr Ali is young and handsome and I start to think about Al Pacino in 'Scarface'. I actually shout Scarface at him at one point. Usually I'm very sensitive to how other people feel, but right now it doesn't occur to me that this isn't very polite or that it might hurt his feelings. I'm not sure if I dreamt this later on or if it actually happened, but I have a memory of him letting me touch his face where the scar is. Sounds like quite a strange thing for a doctor to do. Then again, everyone knows head doctors (psychiatrists I mean, not the ones in charge) are mostly madder than the patients.

I soon remember this is all part of the test. I don't want Al Pacino or this Dr Ali Pacino guy, however good-looking he is. I just want Rob! You know what though? I'm tired of this trick or test or whatever the hell it is. If it is a joke, I don't see the funny side.

I walk up and down the ward corridor a lot with the nurses, but I don't know why I'm doing this. Maybe they're trying to tire me out. Maybe I'm looking for Rob. I see a tall thin male nurse with reddish hair. He smiles.

"Hey," I say to the nurse I'm with. "That man's got a nice smile. Where's he going?"

I try to follow him. Maybe he knows where Rob is. But the nurse makes me go the other way, towards the beds. I see a few other patients as I'm pacing up and down. They all seem to be looking for someone too.

The nurses try to give me some more pills but I refuse at first as I'm not sure they're real. I'm a bit suspicious of these nurses to be quite honest. Are they real nurses? I'm not even sure this is a real hospital. The nurses keep asking where I think I am, but I don't know. A prison maybe? After quite some time they convince me the pills will help me feel less distressed, so I take them. One of the nurses tells me I had an acute stress reaction to sleep deprivation and that I have a perfectionist personality. She is trying to help me understand what's going on in my brain. But unfortunately I seem to have no capacity to retain information; apparently I've been told this explanation for being here at least six times today.

Day 2 — 23rd December 2010

6.30am Feel like I slept pretty well last night. I'm still very confused but feel better than I did. I knew I just needed a good night's sleep. I have a shower.

10am I have a meeting with Dr Denver plus a nurse I don't recognise. They ask me lots of questions and I manage to sound quite normal. I think. Except for one time when I forget what I'm doing and drift off into a little daydream. They advise me to think about going for some CBT (Cognitive Behavioural Therapy) to tackle my perfectionist personality. I am up for this.

12pm I ask the nurses for a pregnancy test today, and thank fuck it is negative. That's been really worrying me the last few days. I know they probably all think I'm mad (madder than I really am) because I've got my period, but you do hear of women who bleed while they're pregnant, don't you.

2pm I talk to Nurse James for a while. He's the tall thin one with the nice smile. I explain that my workload has increased my sleep deprivation over the past month.

4.30pm I suppose I should make a few notes. Seeing as I've just been sectioned under the Mental Health Act. Or to be more precise, the Mental Health (Care and Treatment) (Scotland) Act 2003. And for once in my life I'm not eggzadd.... eggzadd... weirdly I can't seem to think how to spell the word I'm looking for — hmmm, not a good sign, especially not in my line of work. OK, let's go phonetic crazy — as well as just crazy crazy — and call it eggzaddurating for now, as there's no spell check function on this damn e-reader I'm typing into.

As I say, the fact that I can't think how to spell that word is a *tad* worrying. I'm a magazine editor, which means I'm supposed to be good at, you know, spelling and stuff. But everything's going reeeeal slooow right now. Must be all the drugs they've given to quell me. Quell, is that the right word? Well it's certainly a good one and will do for the moment.

Definitely getting a 'sleep has come to get me' vibe, there's no way to stop him now. Mmm, it's nice though, so relaxed. I'll explain everything later.

One final thought before I go (not in a Jerry Springer style though, I'm in no fit state for such wisdom). I keep wondering, what about... yeah, what about poor Tommy?

8.30pm I feel scared, *really* fucking scared and totally fragile, like I might physically snap in two at any moment. I still don't really understand what's happening. Every time I see a nurse I ask whether I'm in a real hospital, which they assure me I am. I don't trust them though.

At one point in the evening — it feels late but I have no idea whether it really is or not — I stand at the front door smoking a cigarette with a girl called Nikki. There are some nurses (guards? bouncers?) making sure we don't make a run for it. I definitely think if I'm guilty of freaking out any one person in particular during my stay at the hospital, it's Nikki. She bears the brunt of my craziness. She has brown eyes and long frizzy curly hair. It's impossible to tell what her figure is like as she always wears big baggy jumpers. Tonight we have a ridiculous conversation where I am trying to work out why she is here without appearing too nosy.

"Are you with the police?" she asks me.

I laugh.

"No, I'm definitely nothing to do with the police."

She says something about not being sure about marrying the guy she is seeing because he is older than her. I think I then say something completely inane along the lines of, 'But if you love him why don't you just marry him?'

She still seems a bit worried that I am something to do with the police. I repeatedly assure her that whatever else I might be, I am 100% nothing to do with the authorities. She seems wary though.

It seems like we're having a very intimate private conversation but then I turn round and notice a young red-haired nurse sitting with us. Weird, I didn't even know she was in the room that whole time but I guess someone has to keep an eye on us.

Even more weirdly, I then notice a bloke sitting there too. Where did he come from? So I start to chat to him, for some reason asking him whether he supports Rangers or Celtic. He just lifts his fist up and shows me a gold ring, in a gesture that implies 'this should answer your question'. Only I can't really seem to see the ring properly for any clues as to the answer, so I end up walking over to him, going really close up to see what's written on it. I think I can sort of make out some letters, perhaps RFC?

But I must get a bit too close because he suddenly shouts, "Don't *touch* me!" I jump away in fright. Wow, he's a bit scary.

From then on I think of him as Angry Man.

Day 3 — Christmas Eve 2010

Jesus, I have *horrific* memories of acting like a complete and utter lunatic last night. I remember trying to get up on to the top of the wardrobe next to my bed, though I can't remember why. Jeez, even the other mental patients must think I'm a complete nutter! I'm fairly sure I was quite disruptive last night. In fact I was such a nuisance that they sat me in the waiting room with the night staff, so that I couldn't annoy the other patients any more. I also very vaguely remember protesting noisily when I saw a needle coming towards my right arm. Bloody hell.

My sister Sylvia and her husband Mark come to see me this afternoon. I didn't know they were coming so I am pretty shocked to see them. Freaked out actually. As soon as Sylv sees me she starts crying and leaves the room. When she comes back I keep asking her what's wrong, but she just says she has a bit of a cold. I don't know why she's so upset but I don't think it's a cold. I think maybe my Dad has died and they're all too scared to tell me.

I say to Sylv, "Three out of four, three out of four..." and she just looks blankly at me. "Remember, one used to be missing?"

Eventually she gets it.

"Oh, you're talking about the Christmas tree, aren't you?"

I nod (though I'm not really sure what I was on about to be honest) and she turns to Mark and Rob to explain.

"We used to have this Christmas tree and it only had three legs instead of four, so we had to prop it up every year."

That's how I feel, like somebody needs to prop me up and if they don't I'll fall. Sylv is really concerned that I'm not warm enough, but I don't feel hot or cold or anything really.

As we sit in the visiting room, I see a tabloid newspaper headline. Just one word: PREDATOR. It could have been about anyone, but I assume they are accusing Tommy Sheridan, the disgraced Scottish Socialist Party MSP, of being a predator. I'm sure it's my fault he's in all this trouble.

I am so disturbed by thoughts of what I've done, getting Tommy into trouble and acting like a weirdo last night, that I can't concentrate on what I'm supposed to be doing in the present. Even the simplest things — cleaning my teeth, getting dressed — are beyond me at the moment. I start off OK then get absorbed by horrendous flashbacks. I also have a horrible feeling that Rob's Dad died two months ago and that I was working so hard I didn't even notice. I must be a really nasty, selfish person to be feeling this way.

Being constantly watched makes me even more anxious.

I have a meeting with Dr Denver and another lady today. I'm feeling OK at the time and think it goes all right, in that I manage to sound quite normal. Except for one point when I go off into a bit of a daydream and forget where I am.

Sylv and Mark come to visit again tonight. I notice that we all have our hands on the table, then remember that I've asked to hold their hands and that's why.

"This feels like a séance," I say.

They nod and smile, like you do when you're talking to a mad person.

I notice that Sylv hasn't got any make-up on, which isn't like her.

"Are you all right?" I ask. She says she is totally fine, but I'm not so sure. I feel like they're keeping something from me, that there's a big family secret and I'm the only one who doesn't know yet. At first I think someone, maybe one of my brothers, is gay. I think about my older brother Clive and wonder whether he and his girlfriend Andrea are in actual fact the same sex. Maybe Andrea is actually a boy called Andy? Then I start to think something bad has happened, something really terrible. I keep asking them if Mum and Dad are all right and even though they tell me they are fine, I can't shake the feeling that someone has died. That something awful has happened that they're not telling me because they don't think I'm strong enough to handle the truth.

Sylv is so insistent that everything's fine, she even writes it down on a heart-shaped piece of paper for me: 'We are all fine! Believe us! From all of us x x x x x'.

I am so focused on discovering the awful secret that I know I keep forgetting to do really obvious stuff, like eating and drinking. I go off into little daydreams, except they're more like day-nightmares.

I notice that Nikki is in the visiting room too, with her boyfriend. She always seems to be here when I am. I keep thinking we're linked in some way. Perhaps we both have something to do with the Tommy Sheridan trial?

That Adele song, 'Rolling In The Deep', seems to be constantly on the radio. I feel sad every time I hear it. When she sings 'We almost had it aaallllll', I keep thinking of me and Rob; we *did* almost have it all! Until I went mental and ended up in here. The other tune that's always on is Katy Perry's 'Firework'. Angry Man seems to like that one on at full blast.

If I had to choose a word to describe how I feel at the moment, it would be confused. Or, even better, perplexed. That's it, perplexed.

The nurses take my engagement and wedding rings off me today, because I keep leaving them lying around and they didn't want them to get nicked or lost. Apparently I keep putting them in my mouth too, and they were worried I would swallow them. I know that sounds like a crazy thing to do. But I think I was just trying to keep close to the things that are important to me, that make me feel safe. I just took the idea a bit too far. I'm pretty sure I wasn't actually trying to eat them. My hand looks horribly naked now.

I have an urgent feeling that I should be writing some Christmas cards. I really was going to get round to doing them this year. At some point today, I find some traditional-looking cards in my e-reader case. I've absolutely no idea how I got them or where they came from and when I show them to Sylv and Rob, they are equally surprised. I must have borrowed them from another patient. I hope I didn't steal them.

I sometimes wonder if I'm in here because I have a secret that I haven't told Rob, a little health problem. This is nothing to do with the secret that my family is keeping from me. But I remember telling my Mum my health secret just before Christmas, and telling her I hadn't told Rob.

"How is Rob supposed to know why you're acting like a bear with a sore head if you don't tell him?" she said. Maybe if I admitted it they would let me go home? Perhaps I'll tell him tomorrow.

I think back to an incident that happened when I was about eleven. I was in the Littlewoods cafe with my Mum and sister. Me and Sylv go to the ladies but while we're waiting in the queue a woman says to me, "This is the ladies' toilet, you should be next door in the men's."

I blush a deep crimson and am too embarrassed to explain that I am actually a girl, it's just that I have short hair and a boyish figure.

I know the nurses are watching me all the time, because I'm under 'constant observations'. I tell one of them that this makes me even more anxious.

Day 4 — Christmas Day 2010

I have a day pass. I feel very emotional, tearful and fearful. I am so eager to get out of the hospital that it doesn't occur to me to put a jacket and hat on, even though it's obviously freezing outside. Rob has to remind me. I am annoyed at myself when I notice that the nurses notice this. I imagine a note being written about it.

Rob takes me home and thank goodness we don't bump into any neighbours on the way in. I just couldn't handle that. What would I say? Anyway, we make it inside OK. Rob has bought me a poinsettia plant in a pretty dark gold pot. This reminds me of our wedding almost three years ago, when we had poinsettias as table centrepieces. It's so lovely that it makes me cry. I feel bad that I haven't got him anything.

I open my Not So Secret Santa gift that my family organises every year (we can never keep quiet about who is buying for who, or should that be whom?). It's a Waterstones voucher that I can buy e-books with. Brilliant. It's literally just what I wanted. Seeing my Mum's nice curly handwriting on the card makes me cry too.

I see that Rob has made us lots of lovely food and for the millionth time I think how good he always is to me, how lucky I am to have him as a husband. This also makes me cry. Quite clearly I'm not going to get through much of today without crying.

Rob is doing his utmost to keep the atmosphere light and happy and to chat to me like I'm not a weirdo. But to me Christmas is a noisy frenetic time with all the hustle and bustle that goes hand in hand with having your whole family around you. It makes me feel so sad that it's just the two of us. It doesn't feel right. I feel guilty too, because if it wasn't for me losing the plot we would be with my family and everything would be just the way it's supposed to be on Christmas Day. I also feel bad that once Rob takes me back to the hospital he'll be spending the evening alone.

It feels like Rob is keeping a very close eye on me. I am sure he is trying to keep sharp things away from me in case I stash them away and do myself in while no one's watching. If I'm in the bathroom for more than approximately one minute he shouts up, "Ros, are you OK?" in a 'concerned but trying to sound bright and breezy' voice.

I also feel like there are people watching me from the block of flats opposite. I imagine our neighbour Sarah (who's a social worker rather than a nurse, but there you go) over there with a pair of binoculars in one hand and a mobile phone on the line to the hospital in the other, keeping tabs on me. I feel like Rob is signalling to them when he thinks I'm not watching. When he pulls the curtains closed, I think this is him giving the watchers a pre-arranged signal, that it means something like, everything is OK. I don't particularly mind this though, it makes sense in my warped head.

Despite feeling very sad about putting Rob through all this, being at home feels amazing. I've never appreciated Rob or our cat Jay (who barely raises an eyebrow when I reappear) or our beautiful flat as much as I do now. Every now and then, for just a minute or two, me and Rob are chatting away just as we always do; it all feels lovely and normal and for just a second I completely forget that I'm only out for the day. When I remember again it's devastating, like realising you've just been punched on the nose. A horrible sinking feeling in the pit of my stomach. When it really is time to go back, I feel absolutely awful.

I see Nikki when we get back. I still don't understand how we're linked but I notice now that she looks a bit like my old mate from uni, Irina. Irina and I both interviewed Tommy Sheridan when we were students. I wonder if Nikki is Irina in disguise? It's possible. Or maybe she's Irina's daughter and Tommy is the father! No, she's only a few years younger than Irina, she can't be her daughter. Can she? Maybe I'll ask her if she knows Irina.

When it's time to take my final meds of the day, at 10pm, I try to slope back to my room without anyone noticing, but the nurse encourages me to eat something. Which means interacting with the other crazy people. There's some kind of tragic Christmas spread laid out in the dining room. A few of the patients are in there, enthusiastically eating sandwiches and Christmas cake and other festive food, which seems totally inappropriate to me, considering where we are. I mean, what have any of us got to celebrate tonight?

Dawn (an older, rather refined lady who stays in the room next to me) is there, so is Angry Man, plus Mina and a few others. Mina is the only Asian woman on the ward. As usual she is buzzing round at a million miles an hour. I half-heartedly pick up a sarnie to see if it's veggie. It's not. I put it back and choose another safer-looking one. But Mina spots this manoeuvre. She is standing within an inch of my face now, talking about God doesn't even know what.

"You've got to be really really careful with food you know? Because food carries germs and germs can spread disease," she says, as if I might have somehow reached the age of 34 without any inkling of this.

"Yeah I know," I mumble. "Think I'll be OK."

"No you won't be! You don't understand! Germs are dirty, DIRTY!" she shouts, getting upset now. I try to ignore her without being rude but she's really intense. She carries on for a bit before a nurse gently leads her away. I sigh and escape to the safety of my own room.

I still haven't told anyone my other secret. Maybe tomorrow. There's another thing that worries me. I'm afraid that the nurses think I'm a boy. I think they've put me on the male side of the ward. Which I know sounds silly, but my boobs aren't exactly massive so it is *possible*. The other thought that seems to loop round and round my head is, perhaps I've *always* been like this. Mad, I mean.

Perhaps people have always covered for me in the past, made allowances, humoured me. But now, it's just got too much for everyone; maybe they can't bear the pretence any longer, can't bear *me* any longer?

Day 5 — Boxing Day 2010

I dream that Rob pops his head round my door and looks at me pleadingly. He is saying, "Come on Ros, you've got to get up. We've got to leave *now* or we'll miss the ferry!" It must be the day of my brother Adam's wedding. His fiancée Catriona is from Islay so they must be having the wedding there. But I'm so tired I just turn over and go back to sleep. In my mind's eye I see him walk away, disheartened that he'll need to go by himself and slightly disgusted that I can't be bothered getting out of bed for my own brother's wedding.

When I wake up, the dream fades but I am left with a haunting feeling that I've overslept and missed something really important. I run down the corridor of the ward, desperate to find someone who will tell me what it is I've missed. The dream starts coming back to me and I think I must have missed Adam's wedding to Catriona. In reality, they split up last year. But when I realise this, I have a nasty feeling that it might have been my fault they split up. Or they got back together and didn't tell me in case I ruined it again. It all makes sense now. They've put me in this place so that they can have the wedding without me ruining it. The nurse assures me I've missed nothing at all, but I can picture Adam and Catriona coming to visit me in hospital after the wedding, which is probably secretly organised for tomorrow or the next day.

"We would have invited you," they'll say, "but you've turned into such a drama queen and we didn't want to risk you taking over, like you always do. You're a complete control freak."

When I ask the nurses questions, they tell me I've already asked them several times, but I don't seem able to retain any information. I still don't trust them. Every time they try to give me pills I check whether it's my real medicine.

A nurse encourages me to get ready for Rob picking me up at 10am but I don't seem able to concentrate on the task in hand. Instead I wander around the ward picking up random things and leaving them lying around in different places. I don't know why. I can't even get dressed without help this morning.

When Rob comes to visit me with Sylv he says we have another day pass, but I don't feel like going anywhere. I just don't really feel up to it. I keep thinking about the other patients. I mean, it's all very well for me with my day pass, but what about them? I'd feel guilty about them being stuck in here while I went out.

And anyway, I'd still have to come back here, so what's the point? Sylv is very concerned that I'm cold. It is pretty draughty in the visiting room but I don't notice being cold or hot or much at all about how I feel physically. She keeps bringing me lip balms because I keep losing mine and forgetting to put it on even when I don't. I used to be such a Carmex addict and now I don't even notice that my lips are chapped until Sylv points it out.

I ask them why I can't just come home but they say I have to stay in here. I keep thinking about the family circle of trust. I must be outside it now. I can't even be trusted with my wedding and engagement rings any more. Rob is keeping them safe for me.

Whenever I get a visitor I feel that it's important for me to hold their hand all the time they're there. I feel safer that way, as if maintaining a physical link with someone who's not mental gives me a better chance of being less so myself. I also feel like the nurses will think I'm doing something suspicious or demonic if I don't keep my hands above the table. Sometimes I forget that they're nurses and think of them more like prison guards.

Because I'm frightened I look to make sense of the things I see around me. But I keep looking for meaning where there is none. The young pretty but chunky female nurse, for example, wears a sweatshirt with the number 79 embossed on the back and I ask her why it says that.

"That's just my age," she says, deadpan.

"I'm not that daft," I tell her, and even in my messed up, drugged-to-the-eyeballs state, I find this a little bit funny. Ironically, as well as trying to find meaning where there isn't any, on some level I'm aware that I'm oblivious to some really obvious things. I'm so concerned with what everything means and its symbolism and working out how I got here, that people still have to prompt me to do the simplest things, like eating and drinking and showering in the morning.

I'm convinced that some of the people on the ward, both nurses and patients, are people I know in disguise. Sometimes I think the nurses are just members of my family, pretending to be working here. In fact because of the time of year I ask quite a few of the larger nurses if they are Father Christmas. Not that he's in my family of course. I'm still suspicious of my medication too, unsure whether it's real or not.

There is a male nurse who looks a little bit like my half-brother, Joe. I tell him he reminds me of Joe and he says, "Oh be honest though – I'm much more handsome aren't I?"

Although people keep denying it, I feel like I'm on this ward because I'm guilty of some terrible crime. I'm not sure what crime I've committed, I just know that I must have done something really bad. This is where Tommy comes into it. It can't be a coincidence that at the same time I go into hospital the ex-MSP Tommy Sheridan is standing trial for perjury, can it? I'm absolutely convinced that it's somehow my fault he's going to prison. I see a policeman or two in the ward every now and then (do I really or is this my imagination?) and this makes me even more sure that I'm here as a prisoner, not a patient. I decide to mention this to Sylv and Rob during the visit today.

"I know I interviewed him when I was studying journalism, but I honestly don't remember going to any sex parties with him… Maybe I've blanked it out?" I don't think they hear the last bit though, because they're both pissing themselves laughing.

"Yeah, in your dreams Ros, in your dreams!" Sylv says. "Ros, just let it go," she insists, as if we've discussed this dozens of times before. Maybe we have?

"We keep telling you you've got nothing to do with Tommy Sheridan. He's famous. You've just got these thoughts in your head because you fancy him and he's one of your obsessions."

Even Rob's laughing, so I suppose I should believe them.

When Sylv stops laughing she says, "You keep trying to work out how you got here and why you're in here, but you're too tired to put these things together at the moment. You just need to focus on getting better."

The ward is organised with all the patient rooms and dorms at one end, then further up towards the exit are the communal areas, the dining/visiting room, the activities room and the sitting rooms. Then right at the top of the corridor, near the revolving doors, is the office or nurses' station. At the moment there's a huge Christmas tree opposite the nurses' station, and you can see its lights twinkling all the way down the corridor. It's decorated with blue and pink baubles and ribbons.

Today I find myself admiring the tree with Mina. Every time I see her she tries to tell me that she understands me, but I don't really see how that could be true. "I've been here before, remember," she says now. "I know how you feel. I know what it's like, you see this doctor and that doctor and your family don't understand you. I'm trying to tell you how to get out of here…"
I'm aware that the nurses in the office can see us having this strange conversation. Mina points at the ribbons and baubles and moves around me so fast I can't keep track of her.

"Blue is for a boy, pink is for a girl," she sings. I am mesmerised by the sparkly tree, but I'm confused by what Mina is trying to tell me. She seems so intent that I get the message and now her hands are gesturing wildly at different parts of the tree, as if the tree itself holds the answers to our troubles.

"But I still don't understand what the answer is, Mina," I say as I remember for the second time that the nurses are watching. I start to walk away. I take a blue ribbon with me and keep it on my bedside table as a reminder of my ridiculous behaviour.

When I get back to my room I remember I've left my e-reader in the waiting room, again. What an idiot. I can't seem to hold a single thought in my head for any length of time and it's incredibly frustrating.

During the second visit today, Sylv and Rob are both there. One of the other patients is also in the room, with a few visitors.

"He's called Rab," I whisper.

Sylv and Rob exchange a look and Sylv says, "Is he really though? You seem to think all the men here are called Rab, Ros."

Well I'm pretty sure I got it right but maybe I imagined it. They both find it quite funny that I think everyone is called Rab. It makes even less sense since, although just about everyone we know refers to my husband as Rab, I still call him Rob. I can see why it's amusing but don't actually laugh. I seem to be getting quite a lot wrong these days. I ask them whether it was my fault Adam and Catriona split up.

"No Ros," Sylv says. "We've told you this already, that was nothing to do with you. How could it have been?"

I can't explain, I just had a feeling that I was here because I was being punished for something, and maybe I wasn't friendly enough to her when they came to visit last year.

The shutter that separates the dining room from the kitchen keeps rattling and I shudder every time I notice it.

"I think that means it's time to go now, or that someone else wants to come in," I tell them.

"No Ros, that noise doesn't mean anything. Don't worry about it," Rob says.

Rather than having proper thoughts, my mind flits from one phrase or riddle to another. 'Home is where the heart is', for example, is one of my favourites. The words are like shopping trolleys in a river; they have no business being there but get wedged and refuse to budge.

19

I spoke to Dad on the phone today, just for a minute, during the last visit. It was good to hear his voice.

When I came back to the visiting room Sylv says, "You see Ros, we told you Dad was fine, didn't we?"

But I don't feel reassured at all. I start breathing a bit heavily, because there's lots going on inside that I can't express. I'm full of nasty thoughts trying to fight their way out.

I turn to Rob and say quietly, "So is it your Dad who's died then?"
He says his Dad is fine, but I don't really believe him. I can't shake the idea that everyone is lying to me and that someone I love has died.

I finally tell Sylv and Rob my secret.

"Sylv," I say it quietly when Rob's busy talking to one of the nurses. "I've got piles... and I haven't told Rob about it."
She just laughs.

"Yeah Ros, you already told me that loads of times, and Rob knows. Look, to be honest, if that's your big secret, there's not much to worry about, is there?"
I suppose not. Then why do I feel so anxious?

Day 6 — 27th December 2010

I notice a couple of knots in my pyjamas this morning. Actually I remember making them myself, only I don't know why, what they mean. They're supposed to remind me of something ('please remember, to tie a knot in your pyjamas'), I just don't know what.

I am agitated, confused and perplexed. Has my brain exploded? I keep wandering around the ward picking up things that aren't mine, as if one of the objects might hold some clue as to why I feel like this. I also keep grabbing people as they walk past. But when the nurses ask me why I'm doing it, I can't explain myself. Sometimes I find myself walking backwards or in little circles. Again, I don't know why. That makes no sense because I *know* I have to follow the yellow brick road. I constantly ask the nurses for Rob and they keep telling me I'm in hospital, but it just doesn't sink in. I want to stay in my room on my own as much as possible but the nurses keep trying to encourage me to mix.

I don't seem to have proper thoughts any more, at least not meaningful ones. It's more like riddles or phrases or babyish rhymes going round and round instead. All in all, I'm not doing very well.

I try to leave the ward this morning, to look for Rob. I'm sure something is going on. Either I'm now a boy (or I've always been a boy but have been deluding myself for years that I'm actually a girl), or someone in my family has died. Something major is definitely happening.

I notice that my name is written in red pen, on the little piece of whiteboard outside my room. I look around and see that some of the other inmates have their names written in black. When Rob comes in with my Mum, who has come up from Dumfries to visit me today, I tell them that my name is in red because I had a particularly bad day yesterday.

"It's like a red alert," I say confidently. "It was in black yesterday but because I had a red letter day they've put me in red today. It means they're worried about me because I was crying a lot."

I get a bit annoyed when Rob doesn't believe this. He goes to see the nurses to verify my story.

"I've just checked and the colour of the pen means nothing," he says. "They have a red pen, a blue pen and a black one and just happened to have a red pen on them that day. If it makes you feel better you can have your name in another colour."

I apologise to Mum for looking such a state.

"I wish I'd had time to get my eyebrows and my hair done before I'd come in here," I say.

Mum tells me I am very brave to see visitors at all. I ask about Dad. She says he's fine and coming to see me in a couple of days.

"So I don't have to choose between you then?"

"No, of course not," she says.

That's weird, I really thought I had to.

Mum brings me lots of nice things, including a beautiful bunch of flowers, cotton buds and some lovely toffee bonbons. Later on I share them round the female waiting room (the bonbons that is, not the other things). I feel like I'm being a bit naughty doing this; I'm sure some of the patients aren't allowed sweet things — aren't a few of them diabetic? But nobody tells me off.

During the second visit Sylv and Rob are there. Weirdly, Nikki is there too, but she's on her own as her Mum turned up and then immediately left again, to get a McDonalds I think. I feel really uncomfortable as she is just sitting looking at us and it feels like she's listening in. She comes over and asks if I know where her hairdryer is. I say sorry, no I don't. But she keeps going on about it.

"Look Ros, I know you're not well but it's not fair, it's my hairdryer," she says. I don't remember stealing a hairdryer, but maybe I did. Rob goes to check with the nurse, who says that I don't have it, but I still feel guilty. I feel really uncomfortable and after a while I ask Rob and Sylv, "Do I have an apology to make?"

"No, sit down Ros," Sylv says quite emphatically, so I do, but I still feel bad. Nikki is obviously not convinced either because Rob has to go and get the nurse again. She comes in and tells Nikki I don't have it and that it is the ward hairdryer anyway, not hers.

When Nikki has gone, Sylv says, "Look Ros, remember that Nikki's in here too, so she isn't well either. You don't have to believe anything she says to you, OK? If she starts bullying you again just tell the nurses." But I can't help feeling I'm at fault somehow. I have a memory of Nikki pulling my hair, as if we are little kids in primary school, and asking for the hairdryer quite aggressively. I don't know if this is a dream or it really happened.

I notice how superstitious I've become, then instantly forget. Like someone who won't tread on the cracks in the pavement, I avoid standing on all the grey plastic separators that are spaced every couple of metres down the corridor. I'm not sure why but every time I walk down the corridor I hear this phrase in my head: 'You'll be out of here as quick as a hop, a skip and a jump'. I don't know who said this to me, maybe I just dreamt it. But a part of me believes that if my feet land on the grey separators, it'll take me longer to get home.

I imagine Sylv and Rob sadly watching me walk down the corridor like an old person, which is how I feel as I shuffle away. Sometimes I forget where I'm going and a nurse has to help me back to my room. Other times I'll forget that I've already said goodbye and when I see them waving at me I think they're waving me back, and I'll have to go over and go through the whole hugging routine again.

Later on, I don't know whether I'm still awake because I haven't been to sleep yet or I've woken up in the middle of the night, but for some reason I find myself awake and in the waiting room. It feels late at night. There are lots of nurses here but I seem to be the only patient. Actually I think Mina is up, but somebody takes her off to bed before they deal with me. Like many of the patients/prisoners, Mina often displays a total lack of ability to concentrate on anything, even for quite short time periods. The words pot, kettle and black possibly apply here, but I'm *fairly* sure I'm not quite as cuckoo crazy as Mina. Rob saw Mina having a whole conversation with herself, acting out the two sides by physically moving into position to play each role.

I was in the bed next to her for my first couple of nights, before the nurses gave me my own room. With Pakistani heritage, Mina speaks with a broad Glaswegian accent. Mina is a nice girl but she's starting to drive me even more mental. She follows me around at meal times and she's always trying to look after me in a way that doesn't actually help.

Mina often talks about her family and is clearly worried sick about how they're coping without her. She has lots of visits from her husband and kids, but the saddest thing is she seems too away with the fairies to notice when they're around. Something else that makes me sad about Mina is her shoes. She wears a traditional-looking sari but when I glanced down at her feet I saw men's shoes. Not just mannish ladies' shoes, actual men's shoes.

Mina can be tiresome but some of the other patients here really scare me. Carol in particular scared the bejesus out of me. She was here for a night or two when I first came in but thankfully she's gone now. She was young, around eighteen, quite short and looked more like a boy than a girl. She looked like she'd had a hard life and had one permanently half-closed eye. Now I know this sounds strange, but at one point I was convinced that this person was 'Ros of Christmas past'. Although I don't think I've ever behaved as badly as Carol.

I wonder what happened to her. Did she go up the scale to a scarier psych ward or did someone in her family manage to get her back on track? It's hard to imagine her getting better, but who am I to say? She was quite aggressive at times — Rob remembers her spitting at a nurse — and I worried that she was going to steal my stuff.

Other patients seem rather nice, surprisingly so. Take Dawn for example. She's the older lady who's in the room next to me. I can't understand how someone who seems so wise and in control could be in a place like this. So I ask her why she's here. She tells me she was in a serious car crash and has a very sore back. She seems perfectly sane to me. Her obvious problems are more to do with physical pain than mental instability, but again, what do I know? She is always very nice to me. She has a little machine that attaches to her waist and has headphones. She *says* this little gadget gives her pain relief, but I keep thinking it's actually a recording device, that she reports every word of what I've said to her back to the nurses. I share this idea with Rob and he says (in a kind voice) that I am just being paranoid. But he doesn't know everything, does he?

Before they give me something to make me sleep, I turn to Nurse Paul, a chubby guy with glasses, a moustache and a fatherly way about him that makes you feel like you should do what he says.

"Why am I the only one who's up all night?" I ask him.

He shushes me and assures me I'm not the only one. But I don't believe him. I tell them I need Rob.

One of the other nurses says, "Rob brought you here because he couldn't live with you any more, remember?"

Couldn't live with me any more? This momentarily upsets me. Then I start to feel quite angry with Rob for abandoning me to this terrible place. Soon I sink back into anger with myself.

What am I doing here? Is this a prison or a hospital? Is this my punishment for being a stoner in my twenties? Or have I done something much worse, something evil? I can't concentrate long enough to work it out. My mind is racing and I keep running up and down the corridor.

I feel guilty that I get so many visitors and many of the other patients don't. I also feel like, if Rob and Sylv come to see me, the other patients might feel like they can't come into the dining room, as if they don't have a right because we were there first. Again Rob says I'm just being daft.

I can't find my zigzag ring. I know my important ones have been taken off me, but where is the other one I wear? Nobody seems to know. I can't even remember what it means, that other ring. Is it something to do with Seamus, our cat who died last year?

I feel like I've forgotten who I am. I think about my best friend, Charlotte, and wonder if actually I don't exist at all, if I'm just her alter ego. Like in 'Fight Club'. She's always been more outgoing, more extrovert than me. People often get us mixed up, calling me by her name and vice versa. I could never understand why, we don't even look alike. Is it because we're two sides of the same coin, two halves that make a whole? In the past, when Charlotte got really drunk and stayed up all night, maybe it was me doing those things. Maybe Charlotte is the carefree uninhibited version of Ros. Charlotte did once tell me there were seventeen versions of her. Maybe there is no Ros! Maybe there is only Charlotte in control — the person I thought was me — and Charlotte out of control; the wild Charlotte, who is actually just another side to Ros. Is wild Charlotte the part of myself I can't accept? Does that make sense? Probably not.

Day 7 — 28th December 2010

I sit in my room trying to read, but it's really difficult to concentrate. I'm on 'Around The World In 80 Days' at the moment. It's about this dude who bets his mate £20,000 he can make the journey in time, only it's set in the old days when £20,000 was a much bigger deal. And of course getting round the globe in 80 days was a lot harder then too. It's a good story but I have to reread the same paragraph over and over before I can take it in. I get through about a page but then have no idea what I've just read and have to start again. I worry that I've done my brain permanent damage. I worry that my memory is never going to recover. I even worry about my eyesight. I find it easier to read and write with one eye closed at the moment, which sounds strange but does work best.

At some point today I am wandering aimlessly up and down the corridor and I spot Nikki sitting on her bed. I still suspect that a lot of the characters on this ward are people I know, but in disguise, despite everyone (including the so-called patients themselves) assuring me this is most definitely not true. I decide to ask Nikki about Irina — maybe she's her sister or something — and the Tommy Sheridan connection. She is looking at an Indian takeaway menu. I think it's strange that a person would consider ordering a takeaway while they're a patient on a psychiatric ward. It's such a *normal* thing to do. She looks up at me.

"I'm not trying to freak you out, [always a good conversation starter, I find] but we weren't at uni together were we?" I say.

"I've never been to uni," she says, confused.

"Oh. So your last name's not Nelson is it? It's just you really look like my friend Irina Nelson, who I was at uni with. I thought maybe you were her sister…"

She says no, she just wants to know what happened to her hairdryer. I tell her again I honestly don't know where it is.

"You can come in my room and check if you want but I've looked and it's not in the cupboard or anything."

I notice her holdall bag, which says Tommy, as in Tommy Hilfiger. But it makes me think I'm right about me and Nikki and the Tommy connection. I see it as a sign.

I tell Rob about the 'I scream van,' which has all sorts of nurses' equipment on it, stimulants to wake you up, sedatives to calm you down, anything really. He doesn't really believe me and I get annoyed that he won't take my word for it.

"You don't know what it's like in here," I say testily. "You're only here a few hours a day, remember."

Which — although it doesn't occur to me at the time — is pretty unfair because he is here every single visiting time, even though the nurses told him the point of having two visiting slots each day was that you could come to one or the other, not both. He laughs and says he's glad I'm feeling feisty enough to argue with him again, even though I'm "completely wrong". Eventually I laugh a bit too as I remember that my recent track record on truth, reality etc hasn't been exactly spotless.

My newly formed klepto habit strikes again today. Unfortunately I'm not very good at it. Sylv and Rob are standing talking to Nurse Claire about something (she's the one with the nice brown mischievous eyes) and I'm standing by her right shoulder. She looks straight at me and (Sylv told me afterwards) I look really shifty. Then I just reach into her pocket and take her glasses. I don't know why I did it really, in fact I didn't even remember doing it until Sylv reminded me later. I just saw the case, which has a pink tartan pattern, and took it.

"Is that you trying to steal my glasses? I'll have those back, thank you," Claire says calmly. I don't get into trouble for some reason. It's such a blatant and bad attempt at thieving that everybody just laughs at me.

I'm still trying to figure out why I'm here. Perhaps I'm wrong about the terrible crime I thought I'd committed. Maybe I'm not on trial at all. And everyone completely denies that someone I love has died. My mind keeps wandering back to my wedding day. Is it something to do with my relationship with Rob? I wonder whether I've been keeping a secret from myself all these years... lately I've been starting to wonder whether I'm actually a boy and Rob and I are a gay couple. Maybe I've just chosen to *act* like a girl rather than physically being one. I distinctly remember Rob's auntie having a fit during our wedding. That could have been because she's a Christian and disapproved of our same-sex marriage.

Now I'm starting to think I'm here because of a big family secret. I think about growing up in Seaford, a tiny town near Brighton on the south coast of England. Then there was the Brighton bombing, which happened in... 1984 was it? It was definitely round about then, just before we left. And we'd only been living in Dumfries for about a year when there was *another* bomb, this time in Lockerbie. That was right before Christmas 1988, wasn't it? Our first year in Dumfries. Both locations were only around ten miles from where we lived. Now, is that really just a coincidence? Or could my Dad have had something to do with both incidents? Maybe that's why I'm in here.

During the evening visiting slot, Rob comes to my room with a takeaway from our favourite Chinese restaurant. It's our third wedding anniversary. I struggle to eat anything. I find the situation weird because I know that Rob is not meant to be in my room. There's a sign at the other end of the corridor that says 'Inpatients only beyond this point', and my room is right at the end of the corridor, way beyond that point. I don't understand why Rob is allowed in here. I keep ducking my head down in case any of the other patients see us through the window. At one point I look up and Rob is waving at me.

"Ros, I've been trying to get your attention for about five minutes. You've just been staring into space," he says, not accusingly, just with that worried look on his face that's become pretty much permanent. I'm amazed that I've just been ignoring him for ages.

"I'm sorry, I can't do this," I tell him.

I can't explain it to him properly, but it feels like we're pretending everything is OK when it's not. I'm not. I feel like a zombie. I'm just going through the motions. I'm trying to act normally so they let me go home but I just feel numb. Uncomfortably numb.

One of the nurses has bought me an anniversary card to give Rob, but I'm so spaced out I can't really think how to deal with it. I end up putting an 'X' at the bottom. How ironic. I used to churn out thousands of words every week and now I can't even sign my own name. And I'm so out of it I won't even remember this tomorrow.

I have a nightmare that reminds me of the bit in 'Trainspotting' when Renton takes some heroin and you see him falling down through the carpet. I'm in the house where I grew up in Dumfries and because of something I've done the house is falling apart, it's falling away from underneath me and all the rooms are caving in on themselves. Mum is looking at me disapprovingly, massively disappointed, the way parents do when you're little and you've been naughty, as if to say, 'Look what you've done, Rosalind'. I wake up feeling panicky and the dream stays with me, leaving me unsettled.

Still can't find my zigzag ring and none of the nurses know where it might be.

Day 8 — 29th December 2010

A couple of nurses drag me into the shower this morning. I'm not sure if this is because I've been given so many drugs that they have to revive me with cool water, or if I'm just so out of it that I've been neglecting my daily ablutions and they're inflicting some kind of forced cleanliness routine on me. Either way, it's not pleasant. I'm embarrassed to be naked in front of them but don't feel self-aware enough to be humiliated by someone deciding I'm incapable of washing myself. I constantly rub the area between my shoulder blade and my backbone.

One of the nurses says, "Why do you keep doing that? You're going to hurt yourself if you carry on like that."

I tell her it's because it hurts but I think it's also an excuse to keep my arm in a position that will cover up my boobs, as well as giving me something to concentrate on, a distraction from the pathetic situation I'm in.

My Dad comes up from Dumfries to visit today. I feel a bit like crying when I see him standing in the corridor with Rob. He is lifting his arms up and down like a penguin, something he often does to try to make me laugh. I wonder whether he's going to admit to the bombings today. He looks quite emotional too but gives me a smile.

It's just the three of us in the visiting room so we can talk freely. He asks about the other patients and I say I find them very off-putting at meal times. I say that I can see in others traits that remind me of people in my family. He points out that the other patients have no connection to me and that whatever their behaviour, I shouldn't let them get to me, that I don't need to take any notice of them. It makes sense.

"One thing you definitely don't have a problem with is other people, Rosal," he says. I'm glad he says this because I'd managed to convince myself that the nurses thought I was a racist. Which I'm really not.

We go out for a walk, even though it's still cold and icy as hell outdoors. On the way out Dad pops his head round the nurses' office door, where Nurse James and Nurse Suzanne, a young red-haired girl, are sitting.

"She hasn't been any trouble, I hope?" he says. They fix him with a steely, wary look, as if to let him know they're ready for troublesome parents.

"*Dad!* He's just trying to be funny," I say hurriedly, pulling him away before he can embarrass me any more.

Later (it may be earlier, time plays lots of tricks on me) I wander into the staff room, which is right next to Room 101, where the medicines are handed out. Obviously I'm not allowed in the staff room and one of the nurses tells me so as she ushers me out. A small TV is on in the corner. They're watching 'Coronation Street'. I get deja vu and realise this isn't the first time I've done this.

"But I feel like I've lost..." I tail off as words fail me. I don't really know what or who I'm looking for, I just know I need something, maybe someone to talk to.

The nurse suggests "Your other half?" and smiles as she says, "Rab will be here at visiting time, Ros."

Another day I wander in and the same nurse says, "That really was right in the middle of 'EastEnders' that time..." before gently guiding me out and into the waiting room.

Some of the patients really scare me, including Scott. Now I *think* his name is Scott. Although I must admit, for a long time I thought all the men in the ward were called Rab. Then I thought (I'm still not sure about this) that the nurses had a kind of code that meant they referred to all the men as 'johns' and all the women as 'dames', as in madams. I thought I heard them say things like, 'We've got a John down', as in he needs medicine to bring him back to normality.

Anyway this Scott guy is pretty stocky and not very smiley and gets very short-tempered if his meds are not handed out at just the right time. He wears a lot of Bench clothes. For quite some time I'm utterly convinced that this guy was not a patient at all but a nurse posing as one, a kind of undercover nurse. Rob is quite worried when I tell him this. He spends lots of time convincing me Scott isn't a nurse.

"Don't tell him anything you'd tell a nurse, and don't think you have to listen to him or do what he says," he says.

Scott scares me less and less as it sinks in that he isn't an undercover nurse at all. He's just a guy with some problems of his own. I wonder why he's in here. He smokes a lot of cigarettes; he always seems to be outside smoking when I get back from a walk. One day when he'd seen me with Rob and Adam, he asks me whether they were my brothers.

"One's my brother and the other one is my husband," I tell him.

"They're some size int they? Look like undercover cops. Thought they were gonna interrogate me."

I laugh uneasily. Scott quite often comments on the number of visitors I get.

"It's more than the rest of us get," he has said a couple of times. I feel a bit bad for him that he doesn't seem to get any visitors. And I'm a bit defensive about it too; I get the feeling he thinks I don't appreciate all these people who care about me.

I'm in my room when a nurse brings my e-reader in.

"Ros, you left this in the dining room. You need to take good care of it; there are some sticky fingers in here, you know."

I thank her, feeling stupid as I know I've left it lying around a few times. Why is it so hard to remember things?

I stay seated at the dining table after I've finished my tea tonight, since Helen, one of the older patients, is still eating. There's no one else here and I don't want her to eat alone. She asks about my food and I lie. Yes it was very nice, I really enjoyed it. Helen is quite large and has trouble moving around. I think only one of her eyes works.

"I've not had a good life," she tells me now.

"Really? Oh dear. I'm sorry to hear that..." I say lamely.

"No, it's been hard. I've been through a lot and my family don't care."

Outwardly I sympathise, but I don't think this can be entirely true because I've seen two blokes, about the right age to be her sons, visiting her plenty of times.

Day 9 — 30th December 2010

They keep saying I need to rest. The word respite has been mentioned a few times. I *think* it means if I rest for a while I will stop talking shite.

Rob and I have a meeting with Dr Ali (Scarface) this morning. There are a few other people there, a nurse I recognise, and a guy that nobody bothers to introduce. I didn't notice but Rob says afterwards he had the feeling this guy might be assessing Dr Ali, as he seemed a wee bit edgy.

Dr Ali asks how I've been over the last week. Instead of answering the question I say that everyone in the hospital reminds me of someone in my family.

"In what way?" he says.

"Well, just in that they're all someone's brothers or sisters."

Even I wonder where I'm going with this. I fail to explain what I'm on about and afterwards I wish I'd said something that would make them believe I was getting better. Rob thinks the drugs from the night before hadn't worn off by the time of the meeting, which could explain why I was talking so much utter bosh. I can't remember much more about it now, to be honest.

I am tearful and agitated today. I tell the nurse I know I have to follow the yellow brick road, but she doesn't understand. I also mention that I think Carol is the ghost of Christmas past. Which probably won't get me released any quicker, now that I think about it.

Mostly I am very upset and sad that I've let everyone in my family down by being this way. I'm extremely confused and can't focus on what people are saying to me. I still don't even think to do things like eat or drink without being prompted. I have small moments of clarity when I understand what's happening but then it goes again, like a TV with poor reception. Every time I can't understand why I'm here I get very distressed.

When Rob comes to visit again later on, I try to explain how important the cups are in this ward.

"Honestly, I know you don't believe me, but it's all about the cups in here."

He looks at me like I'm talking rubbish.

"It's to do with the cup of friendship. You share everything in here, including the cups."

He still looks doubtful. There is nobody else in the visiting room, which doubles up as a dining room. I can't explain it but I *know* that if I just behaved properly with the cups, if I just got that right, the nurses would know that I was getting better. For a while I feel really angry that he doesn't believe it, and say as much.

As usual during visiting times, the metal concertina thingy is pulled down to cover the hatch where you come up and get your food. I see a spoon lying on this side of the hatch and tell Rob that the staff have left it there on purpose. He frowns but I carry on.

"The spoon is all about timings and family..." I babble on, convinced of the secret but significant symbolism of the humble spoon. In as nice a way as he can, Rob tells me I'm talking rubbish. I get angry again, because I know I'm right but he doesn't believe me.

I'm getting used to the routine in the hospital now. I'm still on a lot of drugs to keep me right. I can't keep up with them all but Rob seems to have a handle on it. What amazes me is the way that sleep is so different with all this medication in my system. People talk about falling asleep, but at the moment it's not like that for me. There's nothing gentle about it. I don't drift off to sleep, I'm grabbed and thrown headfirst down a tunnel of unconsciousness. But I like that. I no longer worry about being able to get to sleep. Which is amazing. The promise of sleep is hardly ever broken in this drug-regulated place.

There is lots of talking and activity while Rob, Sylv and Mark are here and I get frustrated at one point because nobody is listening to me. But when I get everyone's attention I lose the thread of what I'm trying to say.

"No offence Ros," Sylv says, "but we've listened to quite a lot of rubbish coming out of your mouth recently."

I know she's right but I'm sure there was something vital I needed to tell them. It feels as if Sylv and Rob are here all the time so I imagine they must be staying here round the clock. They must be staying in one of the little interview rooms. I worry about this, because it must be really noisy and uncomfortable. I imagine them trying to sleep while some of the madder patients bang on the door, trying to get in. It must be awful for them.

I still don't know what I'm doing here. Maybe I've failed to comply with the terms and conditions of my marriage? Rob and I promised to understand the importance of making each other lots of cups of tea during our wedding vows. Perhaps I've been neglecting my kettle duties?

Nikki and her boyfriend are in the visiting room again tonight. They seem to argue quite a lot. From what I can make out it's over silly, trivial stuff, like what to order from the Chinese. He's always on the phone, which makes me think he's up to something dodgy. It is strange to come to visit her and then not really communicate at all while he's here. And if he is dodgy, it's a more likely reason for her not wanting to marry him, rather than him just being a bit older. In fact, it would explain why she kept asking me whether I was anything to do with the police during that strange conversation on my first night here.

I don't really argue with Rob. We just get a bit nippy with each other now and then, if one of us is tired or stressed or hungry.

I never see Nikki do anything overtly crazy, but maybe she's just better at hiding it than I am. Or she's further along the 'getting better' path.

The weirdest thing happens today. I've been missing my zigzag ring for ages and suddenly it appears in the corridor. As if someone had just thrown it down towards me, like a clue in a treasure hunt. Here, take a little piece of your life back, see if you can figure out the rest. Having said that, it might have just fallen out of the pocket of the jeans I was wearing today. I'm glad to have it back but I still don't know what the ring *means*.

Day 10 — 31st December 2010

Today is the day Rob persuades the doctors to stop giving me haloperidol, a powerful antipsychotic drug he is convinced makes me worse.

"I know you're the experts here," he tells them, "but I know Ros, I've known her for sixteen years. I can see it looks like the haloperidol has calmed her down but she's like a zombie now; she's not expressing anything. But I can see the fear in her eyes. All that drug is doing is masking everything, bottling her emotions up. It's not helping."

I have no clue this is going on at the time of course, and perhaps the docs would eventually have taken me off it of their own accord, but if I had known I'd have been very thankful Rob was fighting my corner. This is a turning point for me; I start to get better quite quickly when the haloperidol works its way out of my system.

But for now, I am still only dimly aware that rather than proper thoughts going through my mind, a few silly sayings have taken over instead. I repeat them, quite possibly out loud. Follow the yellow brick road is one of my favourites. At night it's usually 'clothes, wee, teeth, pyjamas and into bed', which my Mum used to say when I was little. I think the reason I'm obsessed with this particular one is that I'm scared of doing things in the wrong order. I worry that I'll be punished for it. Sometimes I get flustered trying to do simple tasks. I feel stuck, unable to make a decision over something silly, like which top to wear. I am frozen in fear because they could be watching. When they realise I can't even decide something as insignificant as this, of course it will be seen as proof that I'm still out of my mind.

The phrase 'she's gone gaga' keeps going through my head. This is how my Mum describes people who have lost the plot. I keep thinking Jesus, it's happened to *me* now, I've gone gaga. Which always reminds me of Lady Gaga and the Queen song 'Radio Ga Ga'. That Kelly MacDonald line from 'Trainspotting' often goes through my head too: '… a little bit mad, a little bit crazy'.

Yet another thing that keeps popping into my head is a variation of a line from 'Last Christmas' by Wham! Whenever I see Rob I look at him and think, 'Last Christmas you gave me your heart', but I really don't remember giving it away the very next day. Did I do that?

I wonder for the umpteenth time if I've always been like this, but was too mad to realise I was mad. To back up this theory, a memory comes back from my student days. I once called the police because there was a really annoying drilling sound coming from outside our flat in the middle of the night. All my flatmates were getting stoned in the living room. I hadn't joined in because I didn't smoke at the time. The buzzer went ten minutes after I'd made the call. My flatmate Al answered hello.

"It's the police here," a deep voice said.

There was (I was told later) a pause as Al's eyes widened. Either we were getting raided or Sting had called round.

He eventually managed a weak, "OK, hi there."

"Someone at the residence phoned about the drilling sound so it was just to let you know that there's some emergency work going on because of a gas leak."

"OK, well, thank you for… letting us know."

I poked my head round my bedroom door and Al, now white as a sheet, said, "Ros, did you phone the police?"

"Oh, yeah, sorry. I should have said shouldn't I?"

"Bloody hell Ros, we nearly had a heart attack!"

"Sorry, Al. I didn't think."

We all laughed about it at the time. It was especially funny because when one of us came back to the flat we'd quite often ring the buzzer and say 'Strathclyde Police' in a scary voice, just for a laugh. It never really worked, because we recognised each other's voices, but we enjoyed the joke all the same. There was always a split-second pause as the person who answered hesitated, just in case it really was the police.

But now, as I think back to that, I wonder whether this is really what happened. Perhaps there never was a drilling sound? Perhaps my friends had to make that up to stop the police doing me for wasting their time? My memory plays tricks on me these days. It can take a solid memory and warp it so that I don't know what's real and what's imagined. It's disturbing, because what is a person without their memories, their history?

Sylv was here again today with Rob during visiting hours.

"I just want to go home," I tell her. "I don't understand why I can't."
Sylv tells me that I'm here to get better so that I'll be able to come home.

"I know, this is about the circle of trust," I tell them. They look at me blankly, but I can't explain. I just know that I'm outside it now, because I've done something really bad.

I ask Sylv about Mark's parents, if they're both OK. I still have an overwhelming feeling that somebody has died and I know that Mark's Dad was quite ill last year. She said they were fine.

"Ros, you seem to be focusing on other people a lot, you know, worrying about Dad and then about Rob's Dad, but it's *you* who isn't well, it's you everybody else is worried about."

At one point I say, "Look, you two can go now if you like. I don't want to keep you."

I only say it because I'm aware how precious people's time is and I don't want to be a burden. Sylv laughs and says they've only been here five minutes.

"We've come to see you Ros, and now you're dismissing us when we've only just arrived!"
She's laughing and so is Rob. I kind of find it funny too but can't quite manage to laugh properly.

I feel like what I'm doing in here affects everybody, as if when I'm eating nobody else can, or when I'm getting visitors, they won't be able to have any. I don't know what makes me think I'm important enough to control everything.

I keep looking at my wedding photo, which is sitting in a frame on my bedside table. I think Rob's given it to me as a message, a coded message about the future: this is how happy we can be again if you manage to get better.

I'm so out of it that when I go to bed at 10pm-ish (that's when the lights go out), it doesn't even occur to me that it's New Year's Eve and I'm spending it in a mental ward. Or that I'm going to miss the bells for the first time in my life. Well, the first time since I was about eight.

I only sleep for around four hours tonight. When I'm up I wander around the ward aimlessly. I really miss Rob. I wish he was here.

Day 11 — New Year's Day 2011

Rob gets me a day pass and drives me home. It's still annoyingly icy. When we get in the building, once again I'm really glad we don't bump into any neighbours.

My younger brother Adam, Sylv and her husband Mark are lazing about in the flat. They are all a bit hungover, snacking on Pringles and watching trashy telly. The scene looks so fantastically normal that I could cry.

I'm hopelessly fragile, emotions all over the place. I feel self-conscious, very aware of what I'm saying and doing and whether any of it will appear normal or not.

We watch some of the Banksy film 'Exit Through The Gift Shop'. It's less about Banksy and more about some French guy who seems to film absolutely everything that happens to him. With surround sound and a 50-inch TV screen, it all feels very intense. Although I'm quite into it, we have to stop watching about halfway through because it gets too much for me. It's hard to explain but I had a strong feeling about the story having some special significance for me. I knew it was Banksy's story, not mine, but I felt that I was just like him, hiding behind my work, anonymous.

My sister gives me a Christmas present. It's a fluffy white monkey, a brand new version of Lee, my all-time favourite teddy when I was a kid.

"I couldn't believe it when I saw him in the shop," Sylv says.

At first I think this is lovely but then I start to think back and I remember that Adam used to have a brown monkey just like Lee. His was called Coco. I start thinking that maybe this monkey is Sylv's way of telling me that big family secret I was worried about. What if she's trying to tell me that Adam is my son, not my brother? Could that be true? I don't *remember* giving birth to him but maybe I've blanked it out. Maybe that time I went to hospital with a sprained wrist it wasn't really a sprained wrist at all.

Maybe it's an even bigger secret than that. Maybe I'm guilty of something much, much worse... perhaps I was really evil to Adam when we were kids, maybe I was abusive in some way? And a new Lee symbolises a new beginning. It's my family's way of telling me it's OK now, they've forgiven me and we can make a fresh start.

It doesn't occur to me that I'm looking for hidden meanings and ulterior motives where there are none. That my sister just bought me a present because she thought I'd like it.

Adam starts to get his things together to go back to Edinburgh and that's it for me, it's all the evidence I need. I'm 100% sure now that he's leaving because of something awful I've done to him in the past. Was I some kind of terrible abuser? Was Adam my *victim*?

"Are you going because of me? I feel like you're leaving because you don't want an argument with me," I say to him, my voice pathetically weak.

"No no, it's nothing to do with you Rosal, I'm just going to see a man about a dog. Ros, honestly, no one wants to argue with you. We're all thinking nothing but positive thoughts about you."

Although this is good to hear, it's not enough to steer me away from the weird train of thought I've jumped on. I'm sure it's my fault he's leaving.

I ask for a word with Nurse James in the Interview Room when I get back. James has twinkly blue eyes and a kind, longish face, the sort of face that makes you instantly trust him. He is maybe mid-forties and might look a bit soft if he didn't have several tattoos on his arms.

"I've been thinking about what's happened to me," I tell him.

"That's good," he says, looking slightly wary as to what rubbish I might come out with next.

"And the question I keep asking myself is why; why did this happen?"

James gives me a look that says he's heard all this before.

"Well if you figure it out you just come and find me and let me know," he says, standing up to let me know our little chat is finished. He doesn't say so, but he's sure none of us is ever going to work out why this kind of thing happens, to me or to anyone else.

I still feel massively confused and my thoughts are often muddled up, but I think I'm starting to at least understand what I'm doing here. Perhaps I'm getting better.

Day 12 — 2nd January 2011

I keep seeing rabbits outside my window. They remind me of Rob, who I sometimes call Rabbit. I also think I'm seeing them because it's the Chinese Year of the Rabbit. Even though it's freezing out there, I envy them because they're free.

I look in the mirror and am surprised to see someone who only looks about 34 looking back at me. I feel more like 74.

I see Scott during the last meal slot today. He's the one I used to think was an undercover nurse. I don't think that any more. He clearly has his own problems. He comments on my day pass yesterday.

"What did you do? And don't say greetin'," he says, giving me a hard look.

"I wasn't going to. I just saw my family," I tell him, slightly intimidated.

Without actually saying anything, he gives me the impression he reckons I've got nothing to cry about, that I'm ungrateful, having so many friends and family who care about me and not appreciating them. Maybe he's right, or maybe he doesn't think anything of the sort. Anyway, who is he to judge? I've never seen him being nasty to anyone, but I get the feeling he could be pretty aggressive if you pissed him off. I've seen him in the 'ladies only' waiting area a few times, pacing up and down impatiently before getting his meds. Which must be against the rules?

Some of the flowers that Mum gave me have wilted a bit, so one of the nursing assistants helps me sort them out in the laundry room. Once we're in there, I get deja vu. I definitely remember being in this room before, with Nurse Claire I think. What was I doing in here though? I have a feeling I was looking for Rob... yes, that's right! Oh God, I was checking for him in the washing machines! Jesus. That must have been at the height of my 'episode'. The thought makes me blush. That was when I still thought it was all a big game, that I was part of a huge game of hide and seek.

What a fruit loop. Well, at least I realise now how mad that was. That's progress, surely! I have an image of Claire trying to put some washing on and me getting in her way. I remember her saying, "Now you're really not helping me, Ros..."

I sweep the room's old memories away so I can try to concentrate on the task at hand, getting rid of the dead flowers. I notice the assistant has a heavy-duty pair of scissors in her hand. Well, she can't think I'm too much of a danger to society if she'll let me anywhere near those.

Day 13 — 3rd January 2011

I feel like putting some make-up on today but I just can't remember what to put on first. Perhaps I'm overthinking it. Being watched all the time makes me nervous about doing things properly.

At certain times of the day the rooms and dorms are locked, so you're forced to interact with the other patients. The better I feel, the more I dislike these periods of the day, or the more I notice them. The more of it I endure, the more I want to get home and be normal.

When Sylv comes in with Mark, I ask why I can't come home yet. Sylv says I'll only be allowed to go home once I'm definitely better. I try to believe her, but it feels like I've been in here for years.

I'm restless again tonight, wandering the ward aimlessly. I think I only get a few hours' sleep. It's the first time for a while this has happened.

Day 14 — 4th January 2011

There's a TV in the female waiting room, where people congregate before and after getting their medication. When I first got into hospital I didn't even notice what was on. Now I realise I must be on the mend, because I'm getting increasingly irritated by the trash that most people want on. I like documentaries, or quiz shows like 'QI' and 'Have I Got News For You', programmes you might learn from or at least get a laugh from. I do remember watching an episode of QI in here. The subject was hypnotics, which was just a bit close to the bone at the time. But mostly the patients like watching 'EastEnders', which, surely, can only make people more depressed. Or, even worse, 'Britain's Biggest Loser', a programme designed to humiliate fat people by stripping them down to their undies before weighing them. The point and snigger school of entertainment. Horrible.

To distract myself from the TV, I pick up a newspaper, even though it's the Scottish Mail On Sunday. Normally I'd rather boil my own head than read this tosh. I spot the column written by my neighbour Cat, who's a breakfast show DJ on Real Radio. She'd written about the New Year party at Trinity. I start to laugh as I read it: "My normally reserved neighbour Rab was seen space hopping down the stairs at 4am..."

That's *my* Rab she's talking about! I'm so surprised I show the nurse who's in charge of the TV room. She reacts as if she believes me, but probably assumes it's another delusion.

I am reading in my room this afternoon (or trying to, I still struggle to concentrate) when Mina comes right up to the window, knocks loudly and starts waving maniacally. I feel sorry for her, but I'm irritated by her sometimes. On the other hand, she's starting to make me feel relatively sane.

When Rob comes in later, I tell him about the article.

"Sounds like you had a good night?"

"It was all right," he shrugs. "I wasn't there for the bells though..."

"What do you mean? Where were you?"

"I went up to the flat just before twelve and sat there for a little while."

"On your own?"

My eyes fill as I picture him, all alone, seeing in the New Year.

"Oh Rob, I'm so sorry."

He takes my hand.

"It's OK, it's absolutely fine. There was just no way I was going to stand there cheering while you were in hospital."

When Rob and Sylv come in for the second visit, I say, "So is that why I'm in here?" and they both just look at me.

"Is what why you're in here?" Sylv replies.

Then I realise that I only said the thing I was thinking of in my head, not out loud. But I decide to keep quiet after all. I still think I'm right about the Tommy Sheridan connection, but nobody else agrees. Sylv says I need to concentrate on the future, on getting better, rather than working out what happened in the past.

One of the other patients, a guy called John, nearly breaks my heart tonight. To be honest, I'm not really sure his name is John, but he's John to me. He looks homeless, like someone who's had all the life battered out of him, someone who's almost given up. There's a defeated look. Also, he always wears the same clothes and smells of booze and stale tobacco. He walks slowly, with a stick.

Tonight he's writing a letter and asks me to help. It's to his parents and although I don't read it, he checks a couple of spellings with me. He says something about wanting to make amends, and that he was writing because his brother had died. I am torn between wanting to help him and not wanting to patronise him or stick my nose in where it isn't wanted. I draw a love heart at the bottom of the page, as he requests.

Whether he's well enough, or has the wherewithal, to post that letter, I'm not sure. Maybe the act of writing it made him feel better. A few days later someone tells me John has gone home. I really hope so.

Day 15 — 5th January 2011

At 10am, 2pm, 6pm and 10pm each day, all the patients get their medication. The timings are designed to coincide with mealtimes, so you get the first lot after breakfast, the second after lunch, the third after tea (or dinner, if you prefer) and the last batch with your late evening snack. They call it supper here but that word makes me shiver.

The medicines are given out in the treatment room, also known as Room 101. It really is called that by the way, I'm not making it up. And it's not just that people have started to call it Room 101, there's actually a sign on the door.

The atmosphere in the ward changes when one of the nurses shouts, 'That's the meds going out'. I suppose it's the biggest reminder of where you are and why. Some people queue up immediately, others hang around in the waiting area until the line goes down a bit. I don't know if my reaction is typical, but I find the queuing aspect distasteful, almost humiliating. It reminds me of heroin addicts waiting for methadone in the chemists. So undignified.

When you get into the treatment room and it's your turn, one nurse dishes out your pills into a little clear plastic cup (see, just like heroin addicts), after another nurse consults a sheet and tells them what you're supposed to get. When you've got your pills they offer you another cup, with your choice of water or orange juice to wash it down with. Once you're done, you dump the two empty cups in the sink and it's someone else's turn.

There's a third nurse sitting on a chair. This one doesn't actually do anything. I don't think I even noticed them for the first couple of weeks. I think they're mainly there to watch out for trouble. The nurses all look a little on edge as the meds are handed out, hyper-alert in case someone tries to nick a big batch of pills while the cabinet's open. I suppose it's also the time when patients are most likely to show signs of aggression or distress.

Although people keep telling me I'm improving, I'm not always sure if that's true. Having said that, we have a meeting with Dr Ali today and I think I make sense for at least a portion of it. But I still find it hard to stay in the moment, to stop myself drifting off. I slip very easily from 'here and now' into another time or place. I am still disconcerted when I see Dr Ali. I keep thinking back to shouting 'Scarface' at him when I first came in. So embarrassing!

I wonder whether the nurses who witnessed that went home and told their other halves about it; "God, you should have seen the state of this woman today..." Or whether that sort of thing is so common they don't bat an eyelid.

When I get my 6pm meds tonight, Nurse Paul tells me I've got the whole pill-drink-throw-cup-away routine just right now. I wonder if he's praising me because I was so resistant to taking anything when I first got here.

"Thank you," I say, feeling pleased, today's star pupil.

"You're welcome. And what do we not do, Ros?"

I pause for a second.

"Ah, we don't say sorry," I say. Last week I kept apologising whenever it was meds time, a hangover from my suspicious 'Are these real?' days.

"That's right. See, you're living proof that we do have some success stories."

"I still feel embarrassed..." I start to say, but Paul cuts me off.

"Ros, don't be. What you've experienced, just think of it as a bump in the road. We've all had them."

While I'm taking this advice in, I'm also taking it far too literally. I think of the tiny bumps along the ward corridor. They're not even bumps really, more like ridges, perhaps with cables hidden underneath. I am always careful not to tread on them, not that I'm usually superstitious. I imagine the yellow cones that cleaners put up to warn you the floor's wet. I'm like the guy illustrated on the side of the cone, mid-slip at 45 degrees because of a hazard whose warning signs I ignored. A bump in the road I didn't see. I was probably going too fast or not paying due care and attention.

I'm still thinking this through when one of the nurses speaks.

"Yeah, too right we've all had them. You should have seen the state of him last Christmas," she says, using her thumb to point at Paul. He gives her a really serious look and for a second I feel my old friend, Mr Guilt, sidle up to me with a sneer on his face. But then Paul softens, smiles a bit. Maybe it was a mock-indignant look all along.

"Ah, but that was alcohol related," he says. "That doesn't count."

I think I see what they're trying to do here. Even though I perceive them as authority figures, they're pointing out that they're just people, human beings with weak spots and frailties just like me. Well, they might object to the 'just like me' label right at this moment, but you get the point.

Day 16 — 6th January 2011

I'm attempting to read in my room when Nikki appears in the doorway. I tell her I've got a day pass tomorrow and that if it goes well, I should be going home for good soon.

"Wow," she says. "Lucky you. That's great isn't it."

She sounds genuinely pleased for me, but I detect just a touch of something negative. Envy perhaps, or disbelief.

I am really pleased to look down and see my wedding and engagement rings back where they should be. And I have absolutely no urge to take them off and put them in my mouth, so that's progress.

By the time Rob comes in, I've got some make-up on. I even remember what order it all goes on in, which feels like a giant leap forward.

When a nurse asks how I am today, I tell her I feel much better, although I'm still embarrassed about what I was like when I came in.

"Don't worry Ros, we've seen it all before, and worse," she says with a smile.

"I still get confused when I think about how I could have got into this situation..."

"Best to look forward rather than backwards."

"Yeah. I do feel a lot less anxious, a bit more like my normal self. But I know I still look disorganised... or vague at times. I honestly think that has something to do with being watched all the time though."

"Well, I can understand that."

"I'm just looking forward to going home for good and getting my life back to normal."

"That's good. But please remember to take things slowly, one day at a time. Because if you try to get better too quickly there's a risk that you could be back here. And we don't want that do we?"

"No. I understand."

When I get freaked out, which still happens occasionally, one of the nurses usually comes to calm me down. That's the point when I'll ask the same questions of them that I've been asking since I got here. These less than lucid outbursts are happening less often. But during the quasi-counselling sessions that follow, a few things have come up. Am I autistic? Is it OCD that's caused my condition? Or good old-fashioned perfectionism? We didn't have any of those things when I was at school, so maybe I have them all. I don't honestly know which, if any, of these ideas are in my head and which have actually been suggested by medical people.

I remember someone saying perfectionism is a trait seen in many people who become mentally ill. The snooker player Ronnie O'Sullivan is one example. I always felt secretly proud that I cared enough to want to get things exactly right every time. I knew other people viewed it as being fussy, pernickety etc. I just thought they had low standards, to be honest. That they weren't as good, as dedicated as I was. My attitude was, I wouldn't have to insist on controlling everything, if only other people would do things properly! But maybe there's something to be said for the slapdash slacker approach after all. Maybe I'll try being a bit lazier when all this is over.

The nurses do a great job of helping you get better, helping you feel like your old self again, whilst doing their utmost not to make you feel like a weirdo. But as I recover, being constantly observed unnerves me more and more. I look up at the light on the ceiling in my room and see its little green sensor blinking at me. Does it have a camera inside that someone in the staff room can see me with? Surely not. Nevertheless, it feels as if someone's always watching.

After lights out at 10pm, I have to leave my curtains open just a fraction, so that the nurses can shine a torch into the room to check on me once an hour. By now, I understand they're only keeping their beady eyes on me for my own good. And perhaps being aware of them watching me is a good sign; at my lowest points I barely noticed who else was in the same room, never mind whether they were looking at me.

Day 17 — 7th January 2011

Today when I am in the queue to get my meds, I notice the lady I think of as Paddington Bear looking distressed. I call her that (not to her face) because she looks like a gone-wrong version of my friend from school, whose surname was Paddington. She comes running back into the treatment room after taking her pills.

"I can't breathe, I can't breathe," she shouts, looking very upset.

A few of us get out the way so the nurses can deal with her. I usher a couple of the new arrivals away from the scene; they look as if they're just going to stand there staring if I don't. I'm not sure if she's having a panic attack or actually choking on her pills, but the nurses soon calm her down.

Rob and I have a meeting with Dr Patience today. When Nurse James comes into the dining room to tell me this, I think it's some kind of test, that he's giving me a silly fake doctor name to see if I notice he's talking nonsense. Or is it a word association game? He says 'doctor, patients' so I should respond with 'nurses, visitors'? But no, that's really the guy's name. When I tell Nurse Claire I think this is a funny name for a doctor, she says, "Yeah, it's even funnier for him because he hasn't got much!" She laughs at her own joke and I manage a smile. I wonder how many times she's made that joke.

When we get to the meeting there's Dr Patience, a serious-looking dark-haired guy with a deep authoritative voice, plus two nurses, me and Rob. The doctor asks me how I'm feeling.

"Much better now. Although I do feel embarrassed about the state I was in when I came in here..." I say, the pink blush of shame reaching my cheeks.

"In what way?"

"Well, I was all over the place, a mess," I reply, trying not to think about the details too much. That would just put me off. The doctor asks a few more questions, mostly about my background, and makes encouraging noises about how much progress I've made and how I should try to concentrate on the future rather than the past. I've heard this more than a few times by now. He asks about the nature of my sleep problems and when they started.

"I've always been a poor sleeper. My Mum says even as a baby I didn't sleep well. Apparently I used to just lie there with my eyes open."

Which sounds pretty damn freaky to me. It took me many years to think of the obvious follow-up question: how did you know I wasn't just awake? "You weren't!" was the not-completely-helpful response to this inquiry. My Mum does admit that her and my Dad had "difficulty" making me go to sleep when I was very young. Apparently I would shout out for them once I'd been put to bed. It was probably caused by all the cups of tea I was drinking. Because, well, parents in the 1970s didn't know about the power of caffeine.

"And is the problem waking up too early or getting to sleep in the first place?" Dr Patience asked.

"Getting to sleep in the first place. I find it hard to switch my brain off."

I thought about my sleep problems. It's not as if they had blighted my whole life. It's more sporadic than that. However, I distinctly remember sitting on the stairs when I was quite a young kid. I knew I should have been asleep at the time, but for whatever reason, I was awake. I also knew that if I went downstairs to the living room, where my parents were, I would be swiftly but gently encouraged back to bed. So I sat silently and very still on the stairs. I don't remember how long I sat there, or what I was thinking about or how many times it happened. I do remember scooting back into bed pretty quickly if I heard my Mum or Dad on the move.

Sometimes when I've almost dropped off, the feeling of being pleased that I'm about to get to sleep, that excitement, actually wakes me up again. Which is really annoying. Apparently there is an actual scientific name for this. When I've had a bad night, I wonder why I couldn't have been born with narcolepsy instead.

It sounds delightful to someone with the opposite problem. I know it's a very serious, sometimes dangerous disorder, and certainly wouldn't be much fun if I really had it. But I'd settle for hypersomnia, getting too much sleep.

Visualisations can help me sleep. Sometimes. But sometimes they just don't work. Take one of the most obvious relaxing scenes, a walk on the beach. If I try to imagine this, as a sleep-inducing strategy, I just know something will start bothering me. For example, am I wearing the right footwear for the beach? If we're in Scotland it's not likely to be very warm, but if I'm wearing boots maybe my feet are too hot. Or if we're too close to the sea, they're getting wet. Why not simply imagine you're wearing sandals, you say? Well, yes, but that could possibly be even worse. I might be distracted by the prospect of stinging jellyfish or nasty insects, ones that might crawl up my leg. The insects, that is, not the jellyfish. It's not just about shoes, of course. If I'm walking along the beach I'm likely to be with Rob, who will probably be taking photos of the lovely scene. And why not? Maybe there is a beautiful sunset or he'll catch the waves crashing. But I imagine after a while I might get annoyed, because rather than just enjoying this pleasant experience, he will spend all his beach time trying to frame the perfect shot. I might even go in a huff because he's pretty much forgotten I'm even there, trying to enjoy this relaxing flipping beach with him. None of these thoughts help me sleep. I suppose that's why people often call them 'positive visualisations'. You're not supposed to imagine things that irritate you.

Anyway, I must do a good job of sounding normal because Dr Patience listens for a bit and then says, "Well, I think it's time we revoked Ros's STDC."
I realise after a second that this is a Short Term Detention something or other. Wow, this means I'm officially no longer mental! I think.

I am really happy about this but two minutes after the meeting finishes, I start to worry that I've only imagined it.

"Do you think that went OK?" I ask Rob when the rest have gone.

"Yeah of course, it went brilliantly! Didn't you hear what he said?"

He has a huge smile on his face. Not seen that for a while.

"But... are you sure Rob?"

"Yes! Ros, this is really good news."

Phew, I didn't imagine it then.

Rob leaves me to it as it's lunchtime. When I get to the front of the queue I see the black guy serving, the guy I couldn't even look at when I first got here. I was paranoid that people thought I was a racist. I thought he was there as a test. Not sure where that came from. Today I look him right in the eye. Oh well done

Ros, I inwardly tut at myself. You're actually pleased that you've managed to look another human being in the eye. Big deal! But it was in a way.

One of the options today is sausage and mash and I ask him whether there are any veggie sausages.

"Oh man! That's the one thing I forgot," he says, turning to the assistant next to him and slapping his forehead in mock self-reproach. I can't work out if he's taking the piss, in a friendly way, because he knows I've been so forgetful recently. Or because all patients are forgetful. Maybe this is a good sign, the staff can tell I'm now strong enough to take a joke? I smile and say that's OK, no problem. But one of the nurses jumps in and says she'll get some from another ward. A few minutes later, I'm tucking into my veggie sausages. They're quite nice. I wonder how much meat I've accidentally eaten over the last few weeks and immediately push the thought away, like a plate of unappetising food.

More good news today. Rob has been to meet my boss, Lorna, and she's been really understanding about the whole thing.

"She said you can do whatever you want. You can come back part-time, or just go freelance but have a guaranteed amount of work each month," Rob says.

"Wow, that's amazing."

This is music to my ears. Going freelance would be amazing. I would get to do all the best parts of the job, without having to worry about the rubbish bits, the admin and the office politics. I actually feel lighter.

I end up sitting next to Angry Man at dinner tonight. He mumbles something in my direction.

"Sorry?" I say, still a bit scared of him.

"I said you're looking a lot better," he says, louder and slightly irritated now, annoyed I didn't hear him the first time.

"Oh, yeah, thanks. I'm feeling better too."

That's about as far as our conversation goes. I consider asking how he's feeling, but keep quiet. It's such an obvious question. And he might have said, "Still very angry actually".

I make an amazing discovery about the 'I scream van' today. Every so often one of the nurses shouts 'I scream van'. At least that's what I thought they said. Until today I believed that it was a nurses' code, that he or she was alerting the other nurses, telling them one of the patients had had a funny turn and they needed assistance in quelling them.

I also thought the 'I scream van' was constantly going up and down the ward. The van had everything you could possibly need to help you either get up in the morning or go to bed at night. It was a kind of mobile treatment room. So it had sugary foods for those whose blood sugar was low and needed a glucose hit. It (of course) had ice to cool down patients with a temperature. And, needless to say, it had a great array of uppers and downers; the nurses needed these to control the patients' moods.

This all made even more sense when Rob informed me that 80% of patients on the ward have some kind of sleep problem. It must be a delicate balancing act for doctors on the ward, deciding on just the right amount of medicine for each person as they improve or deteriorate. With the knowledge that if you get it wrong, all kinds of hell can break loose. I imagine one unruly patient setting off another, a domino effect. Oh there goes Mina again, pacing up and down the ward talking to herself... bugger, she's woken Ros up, who was sound asleep. That kind of thing. Not that I recall being disturbed by anyone else, I just imagine it's a potential hazard.

But back to the van. Imagine my surprise when I saw with my own two eyes the actual *ice cream van*. Well, OK, ice cream trolley. It's full of sweets, fizzy drinks and chocolate bars and wheeled by a sweet though understandably wary-looking old man. I didn't see any actual ice creams but I'm imagining tubs rather than cones, to minimise mess. Well what do you know, I thought, there really is an ice cream van! It's nothing to do with screaming. Rob tells me later that money and other valuables are kept in a safe in the office and patients have to ask the nurses for cash when they want to buy stuff.

Maybe I didn't get the 'I scream/ice cream' thing *totally* right, but the staff must have some kind of code word system in a ward like this. Otherwise how do they deal with people without setting all the other mental people off? Is it a worry that I still think there's something in this?

Day 18 — 8th January 2011

I have a day pass today and our good friends Charlotte and Mikey are up for a visit. Rob picks me up from the hospital and when we get home they are at the flat with my little brother Adam. I feel shy when I see them, not quite sure how to act. They are both being very nice but look not quite sure how to act around me either.

Rob reminds me to take my pill before we go out for the afternoon and, although nobody asks for an explanation, I try to appear lighthearted by describing it as my happy pill.

"Oh, can I have one of those too?" Charlotte jokes.

We drive to the Braehead Shopping Centre to have a look around and get some food. This is the first time I've been anywhere other than the flat during a day pass. I'm slightly dazed and confused as we wander; it feels so weird to be in a place with this many people in it. I get sensory overload, but only in that I'm super-aware of it all, not in a panicky way. There are lots of neon signs and bright lights and kids running around. We stop to watch children working their way up one of those indoor climbing walls. The ones at the top look incredibly high. Some of them are just little kids. I'm impressed by their bravery. But they're so young, fear doesn't even occur to them.

I feel like I've forgotten how to shop and mostly just follow Charlotte around each place, trying not to be too obviously clingy. I look at all the stuff blankly and think, do I want any of it? No, not really. Buying stuff would mean making decisions, and I may be nearly normal, but I'm not yet ready for that.

We have lunch in Frankie & Benny's and it tastes amazing to me after all the bland dishes I've been eating in the hospital. Wow. Although I enjoy the food, I feel awkward over lunch, self-conscious, like the others are keeping a really close eye on me, which would be understandable in the circumstances. Conversation isn't exactly stilted but I let the others take the lead. After all, my experiences over the last few weeks don't really make for great anecdotal material. Oh, you should have seen the queue at lunch the other day! Or, well I think I'm definitely less mental now, how do I seem to you?

It feels strange to have metal cutlery put in front of me rather than having to take plastic knives and forks from a hatch. Despite my awkwardness, lunch is a positive experience for me.

When we get home we watch the darts final. It's between Martin 'Wolfie' Adams and Dean 'Over The Top' Winstanley. Even for a darts player, I'm not sure about your nickname, Winstanley.

I love the darts and everything about it. I love how they describe it as sport but the players are famously un-athletic. I love the silly costumes and signs in the audience at the Lakeside. I love the walk-on songs and the way they strut on to the stage as if they're boxers or something. I love the simplicity of the game. It's not like cricket or rugby, which bore me because I have no idea what's going on and no inclination to find out. I love the twists and turns of an exciting game. I love how quickly one player can lose it psychologically, failing to hit the double needed to finish a game. One person can be way in front, then something rattles them and before you know it their opponent exploits the weakness and takes the lead. I love how it's a sport Rob and I can properly enjoy together.

I notice the Robinsons are a bit quiet. I look round and both Mikey and Charlotte are fast asleep on the sofa. People look so innocent and peaceful when they're asleep, like children. As long as they're not snoring.

It's a great game. Rob phones the hospital to check it's OK to drop me off a bit later than planned, so we don't miss the end of the darts. No problem, they say. They probably think it's healthy I'm 'taking an interest' in something. We laugh, wondering if a patient has ever come back late because of the darts before.

Mikey and Charlotte offer to give Adam a lift back to Edinburgh when evening takes over from afternoon. Is it my imagination or does Adam pop back and forth like a yo-yo? I can't keep up with him.

When I get back I see that three new patients have come in today. I find it a lot easier to remember the names of the ones who came in after me. Linda is a petite blonde in her fifties and says that she and her husband run a cleaning business. She seems so non-crazy that I assume she must be a visitor at first. She's very friendly and smiley and asks lots of questions. But soon I spot that inability to concentrate on anything, just like I had when I first got here. I think she might have OCD as she is continually cleaning up after people. Or maybe that goes with the territory in her line of work. During the late meal slot, Linda asks the catering assistant for a particular type of bread and makes a couple of other quite specific food requests.

"You're not at the Ritz you know," the lady laughs, not unkindly.

Then there's Julie, a thin plain-faced lesbian from Dundee around the age of twenty, who tells me I remind her of a clever girl she used to be friends with at school. Another smoker. Like many people on the ward, she seems both intelligent and completely clueless at the same time. She loves reading and tells me on her first morning that she stayed up all night with a book the first night she was here. I notice her jittery legs; they are almost constantly moving, fidgeting. That's a sign of agitation or nerves isn't it? She keeps saying she fancies a walk, but doesn't appear to realise that she would need someone to accompany her if she goes outside – perhaps she doesn't know where she is.

She doesn't notice any irony in her choice of college courses; she's aiming to become a psychiatric nurse. Her partner comes in to visit one night. She seems like a nice person, doing her best to comfort and reassure her girlfriend.

Julie immediately begins a friendship with Sarah, a heavy woman with a soft kind face, who's 23. She lives on her own and tells me her Dad brought her in. She is really worried about whether he would be looking after her cats properly.

She's quite tearful when she first comes in, then cheers up when she and Julie start chatting. I think they're both using the friendship as a distraction from where they are and what they're doing here. Listen to me... oh what amazing insights I can offer these poor newly captured nutters! Maybe I should wait until I check out before I start analysing other people.

Day 19 — 9th January 2011

Today I attempt a game of Scrabble with Mina, Linda and Julie. It works out OK actually. Well, OK considering all the players are mental.

I am shocked to hear that neither Mina nor Linda have ever played Scrabble before. Is that even possible? Or have they just forgotten? I try to explain the rules without patronising them. Neither really gets it though. They keep trying to put two words down together, or different bits of the word on different areas of the board. Or they put an actual word down, but it's not attached to anything else. At first I try to keep them right, in the nicest possible way, but soon I give up and let them do what they want.

Not long into the game, two players drop out. Linda, so enthusiastic about the idea at the outset, says whatever the doctors have given her (Valium, she thinks) is starting to kick in and she needs a lie down. Mina, after muttering something about not being able to spell in English, wanders off somewhere and never comes back.

Julie and I plough on. It was never going to be the most scintillating game of Scrabble in the world, not helped by the absence of the little rack gizmos you put your letters on. No hiding your letters round here! Well, it killed some time I suppose. I let Julie win.

Day 22 — 12th January 2011

I was on another day pass today. But Rob's just been on the phone to the hospital and they've decided I'm doing well enough to be allowed home. As in, permanently! I listened as Rob spoke to one of the nurses; he was obviously getting good news. He gave me the thumbs up while he was talking but I couldn't quite believe what that might mean. So I was quite shocked when he told me the amazing news. It's incredible, knowing that I won't have to go back to that place.

It felt weird to get the news so informally. One minute I was just out for the day and the next I was deemed normal enough to be launched back into society.

No big meetings or tests or interviews, no waiting around to be signed off by three different doctors... just a quick call and I'm free!

As a kind of thank you to all the people who'd looked after me, we decided to buy a new set of table tennis bats and balls, plus a net, for the seldom-used table in the Activities Room. I'd walked past that room many times and seen a sorry-looking table, but I'd never seen anyone play on it. The nurses explained that the bats and balls had been nicked a long time ago. No doubt it wouldn't be long before the new set went the same way, but still.

After a quick trip to Argos, we took the new equipment in and picked up my belongings at the same time. Rob got his tool kit out and spent some time adjusting the table so that the two sides fit together properly. It looked much better when we left.

I stayed in the interview room while Rob worked away. It would have been awkward to bump into the other patients now that I've got a permanent pass. The nurses gave me a little stash of pills to take away. Normally I'm only to take the mirtazapine from now on. Although it's an antidepressant, I take it to help me sleep. I'll probably be on it for another six months or so. But they also handed over a couple of diazepams, in case I get anxious, plus a few temazepams, in case I can't sleep even with the mirtazapine. These extra ones are for emergencies only, they said. The little bag reminds me of those wee presents you used to take home from kids' birthday parties.

We were given my belongings in a black bin bag — the staff nurse said it would be a bit more subtle than the clear plastic ones with NHS stamped all over them — and headed home for the last time.

Before we left, Rob suggested I went down the corridor to my old room to see if my plant was still there, but I decided not to in case I bumped into anyone.

We hit traffic on the way back and Rob got irritated, but I didn't mind. I was just happy to be out in the real world again.

I found it ridiculously fantastic to be shopping in Lidl on the way home. Wow, just look at all this choice! There was so much food. Not bland-looking industrial-scale gunge in big metal containers, as I'd become used to, but lots and lots of lovely colourful tempting things. I'd missed all these shiny vegetables, and look at all the beautiful cakes and sweets and chocolates!

This was so different from my usual state of boredom during a food shopping trip. Sometimes I would just stay in the car while Rob went inside and did the business. Now I was just so thankful to be free again. Wouldn't it be amazing if I could make this feeling last? I knew that was unrealistic, but vowed to keep it going as long as possible.

When we got home I regretted not asking about my plant. Never mind.

After we'd put the shopping away (I even enjoyed that bit), I went upstairs and sat for a minute on the end of our bed, looking out the window. The sun was shining and I closed my eyes to enjoy the heat on my face for a second.

Our wee black cat Jay jumped up on the bed and mewed at me. I looked at her cute little face as I stroked her chin, remembering how, when I was descending into madness I'd got it into my head that Jay was trying to manipulate me. I even thought I could see something inherently evil lurking behind her big amber eyes. She always seemed to be staring at me and it had started to freak me out. Whenever I was awake, she was too; this had made me think she was in some way *causing* my insomnia.

How could I have believed that?! She was such a sweet little thing. It almost seemed funny now. I stroked the cat and vowed never to take her or my home for granted again.

I just sat there, appreciating the peace, our lovely flat, the incredible view across Glasgow's skyline. How beautifully normal it all looked.

Day 23 — 13th January 2011

I could tell that Rob was trying to keep me busy so that I didn't have time to dwell on my stay in the loony bin. He was careful not to leave me alone for too long either, which was understandable. In fact, I was grateful. I might get The Fear if he did leave me to my own devices.

Going to the cinema is one of my favourite things to do. Normally Rob is more reluctant and I have to badger him for ages to get him to go with me. After I got home from the hospital though, we went to the cinema quite a bit, at Rob's suggestion. It's such a brilliant way of escaping your own life for a little while.

Every time I had to interact with a stranger, the guy selling the tickets for example, I thought it was odd that only a short time ago I was being held by the state; the stranger had no idea. You took my money and gave me the tickets just like you would with any other person, as if you were dealing with a normal person. I wondered what they would think if they knew. It's strange to think that people go mental and then just slip subtly back into society, as if nothing happened.

Today we went to see 'The King's Speech' with Colin Firth, which was excellent. On the way home Rob suggested calling in at the Chinese takeaway.

When we got there he left me to order while he went off to the cash machine down the road.

I noticed that my hand was shaking as I gave the guy our order. I couldn't understand what I was so nervous about. Then I realised this was the first time I'd been out in public without Rob since it all happened. An unnerving feeling. Nothing bad happened, of course, but I was glad when he got back. I felt safer.

Day 25 — 15th January 2011

I felt a bit down today. I think I'm still coming to terms with spending three weeks in a psychiatric ward. I was thinking about all the different words for mad people and madness. Mental, crazy, insane, demented, deranged, crackers, lost it, lost the plot, off your head, fruit loop, nutter, nutjob, weirdo, loony, wacko, whack job, unhinged, unbalanced, psycho, bananas... So many words to describe something that most people are totally ignorant of.

I felt unsure of everything, and very self-conscious. I thought I would be so happy just to be out of the hospital, but I don't know how to just *be* any more. I looked around at all the get well cards and flowers and plants people have sent. I know I should thank people for their kind gestures but I just can't face it at the moment. Everyone has sent best wishes but I feel anything but best. I've got an empty feeling that keeps resurfacing.

Rob's Mum is coming up tomorrow.

Day 26 — 16th January 2011

I still get a nasty surprise every time I realise what's just happened to me. Getting sectioned, that's something you never expect. What if it happens again? What if it keeps happening, every couple of years?

I've been signed off work until February 10th but I'm lacking a sense of purpose at the moment. I was really awkward around people too, as if I'd lost the ability to communicate. Actually that's not right. It's more that I'd nothing to offer, nothing interesting to say. My instinct was to avoid people but clearly that wasn't the answer. I felt like curling up into a ball and hiding away from the world. The weather was awful, which wasn't helping. A run would probably have done me good but it was pouring down and looked like it would never stop.

It also felt like everything was up in the air. Before I got sectioned we'd put our flat on the market. We had grand plans to sell up, move to the highlands and buy a piece of land where we could set up a wigwam-style campsite. The idea was to completely change our lives; set up home in a beautiful place in the sticks, be our own bosses, make some dough for ourselves instead of someone else for a change. I wasn't naïve enough to think any of this would be easy, but I believed putting ourselves in control would create less stress, at least in the long term. But it might take several months to find a buyer. I felt as if we were living in limbo, stuck between our old lives and some imaginary unknown new one.

I didn't know what to do about work. Should I hand my notice in? It was good that Lorna was flexible but I didn't feel capable of making any decisions.

I don't know what to do with myself, hour to hour, day to day. I haven't remembered who I am yet. People talk about emotional roller coasters. Mine must have been dreamt up by Salvador Dali. Or Tim Burton. It's warped in places and goes down when it should go up.

My major worries now are to do with managing my exit from the magazine. Without jeopardising a mortgage for our new place. I also had worries about moving to the countryside. I wanted to change our lives, feel less like a hamster on a pointless wheel, but I'm scared I'll be lonely and isolated in the sticks. That the only new friends I'll make will be chickens, sheep... That I won't be happy, that I'll miss the city and desperately want to come back.

More than one medical person advised me on the importance of expressing myself appropriately and honestly, not burying my worries and keeping things bottled up. All fairly obvious yet surprisingly easy to forget, even in the cold bright light of a newly restored, more balanced mind.

Practising my new strategy of openness, I've just outed my 'moving to the country' worries to Rob. I said it all quickly before I could stop myself. He didn't seem at all surprised by the revelations I'd built up in my head.

"It's only natural," he said, in his even, reasonable way. "And don't forget, it doesn't have to be forever does it? If we try it and we don't like it, we just move again."

True. So wise.

Rob's Mum came up from Somerset to see us today. She's staying at a B&B down the road so as not to disturb me or my fragile ability to sleep through the night. When we see her, she is just as friendly and warm as ever. But quiet. Unnaturally quiet. Usually she's a real talker, barely stopping to breathe between sentences, but I'm touched (if I was feeling better, I might even be mildly amused) to see her acting this way just for me, so silent that I manage a little old-person-afternoon-snooze on the sofa while she reads a book.

Day 28 — 18th January 2011

2.30am. I haven't slept very well for the last few nights and tonight I couldn't seem to fall asleep at all. Flashbacks were suffocating me.

3.30am. Still not asleep. I couldn't believe I was about to have a relapse. I was scared they'd take me back to that place if I couldn't sleep soon. I tried not to disturb Rob but the stupid bloody squeaky floorboards gave me away.

"What's wrong, baby?" he said, all groggy.

"I can't sleep and I'm scared."

He hugged me for a while, which took the edge off the fear.

"What are you scared of?"

"I'm scared that I still can't sleep even though I've taken a pill that's supposed to help me sleep. And I'm scared that I'll end up back in that place!"

I probably said that a bit aggressively; to me it was so obvious what was worrying. Quite unreasonably, I felt that Rob should have realised why I was scared.

"Don't be daft Ros..."

"*Daft*? Look Rob, you don't know what it was like in there! What those other people were like. I don't want to end up like that."

"But that's not going to happen-"

"How do *you* know it's not going to happen?"

Then it was his turn to sound a bit harsh.

"Because you're not anything like most of the people in there. Most of those people have serious mental health issues; you just had a nervous breakdown because you were working too hard. It's completely different."

The way he said it was as if every word was *so* obvious. At first I was ready to be annoyed that he'd dismissed the worst three weeks of my life as '*just* a nervous breakdown'. As if I'd sprained my wrist or got the shits or something! Only a wee breakdown, no biggie. But, I suppose, compared to being a schizophrenic or having multiple personalities, it really isn't a big deal.

It's strange though, I'd never considered that I was different from the other maniacs on the ward. Obviously I *hoped* I wasn't as deeply disturbed as some of them, but I never allowed myself to believe that I really wasn't. So this was news to me, good news. It definitely made me feel better.

Rob encouraged me to take a diazepam to help with the anxiety (that's what it's for, he said with his usual common sense) and although I still couldn't sleep, I felt loads less worried. My brain continued ticking over, but thanks to the chemicals sweeping through me, instead of fretting over things, now every path my mind took me down ended with the same sentiment; *it'll be fine*. Whatever happened, whether we moved up north or not, whether I went back to work or not, *it'll all be fine*. Even still being awake at 5am didn't worry me any more.

Eventually, inevitably, the drug wore off. I was still awake and The Fear sloped back into bed beside me. Poking me and nudging me with nasty images. Rob told me to take a temazepam. These had been given out strictly 'for emergencies only'. Again the pill made me feel better, but didn't deliver sleep. Or maybe I did drift off for a little while, I'm not sure.

Day 29 — 19th January 2011

Rob's Mum went home today. Much as I love Rosie, and get on well with her, and appreciate her kind gesture, coming all this way to see me, I'm not sure spending four days with your mother-in-law is the best way to recover from anything.

Our friend Ronnie dropped by for dinner tonight. We chatted for a little while and then he asked how I was.

"I'm OK. It's just weird when everyone's being so nice to you," I said, gesturing to all the plants, flowers and get well cards.

"Oh fuck off!" he said.

"See that's more like it. That's normal."

Later Ronnie asked what it was like, what happened to me.

"I'm not sure I can explain it really... but you know when you're really tired and not on the ball? It's like that but multiplied by 1000."

I started rambling for a bit then, failing to explain or describe it in any coherent way.

"I think I can understand how strange it must have been," he said. "I mean, just before you fall asleep you get really weird thoughts going through your head, so maybe it was as if your brain started believing them."

Maybe. But it's probably a bit like getting married or giving birth; impossible to understand unless you've actually experienced it yourself.

Day 30 — 20th January 2011

I was back to sleeping OK but it disturbed me that I couldn't sleep at all the other night. I think it's partly to do with a lack of routine since I came home. While I was in there, there was a strict timetable, which undoubtedly helped my body recover. Since coming out, I'd been sleeping in late and consequently finding it increasingly difficult to drop off again each night.

And as I recovered more fully at home, I'd started to think about work again, which sometimes made me anxious. A lot of the current anxiety is to do with worrying about money, worrying about the future, worrying about dealing with future stresses.

Maybe another reason for my mini-setback is that in hospital I was on a lot of different drugs four times a day; diazepam, temazepam, whatever else. Once I was discharged, suddenly I was relying on one little mirtazapine each night. I must have been on a huge comedown while I physically adjusted to coming off all those addictive chemicals.

Day 33 — 23rd January 2011

I feel a lot better than even just a few days ago. I've definitely improved and feel more like my usual self. I'm still slightly awkward around people, friends and family I mean. Strangers are OK. That's getting easier. But last night, for example, we had dinner with Sylv and Mark and our friends Al and Elaine. I was a bit apprehensive about seeing Elaine, only because I hadn't spoken to her since being in hospital. It turned out OK though.

What really annoys me about my recent experience is that I didn't see it coming. One minute I was a normal person with a normal, seemingly happy life. The next thing I knew I was on a mental health ward thinking how the hell did that happen?

It's all so fuzzy, looking back, but Rob reckons it wasn't just the drugs and lack of sleep that affected my memory.

"The brain has its own way of... protecting itself; a mechanism that must have kicked in to stop you remembering the really bad bits. It has to, doesn't it."

So my own brain didn't want me to remember the very worst of the worst. Memories that could bring back The Fear. Clever really. Although it's disconcerting too, the idea of self-imposed mental black outs.

I still believe there is some dubiety about the tablets I'm on. I know the doctors know what they're doing, generally, but I'm on antidepressants now and surely my problem is more anxiety-related than depressive? When I mentioned this at my follow-up appointment with Dr Ali last week, he said I was an "abnormal presentation". I suppose that's doctor-speak for an unusual case. I like to think that was his way of agreeing with me. He also said I displayed some signs of depression in the hospital. I felt like saying, well of course I did! Who wouldn't be depressed to come to her senses and find herself locked up in a psych ward with a load of crazy people? Surely it would be more worrying if I *didn't* find that depressing. He also said depression and anxiety were inextricably linked. I thought that was quite a good answer.

Day 34 — 24th January 2011

We went to see the Peter Mullan film 'Neds' at the GFT, Glasgow's brilliant indie cinema. It's all about this clever Weegie kid and whether he can escape the whole gang culture problem his shitty family gets him mixed up in. The film was fantastic but brutally violent. I felt slightly cheated by its darkness, because there were lighthearted, you might even say funny, parts, but these were mostly restricted to the first half hour. I was a bit jumpy when we got outside afterwards. I saw a figure in the dingy street light coming towards us fairly fast, and gripped Rob's hand harder, imagining it was someone with a knife coming to jump us.

Day 35 — 25th January 2011

I've just been to an appointment with Dr Ali. My GP Dr Ali that is, not to be confused with good-looking Dr Ali the psychiatrist (AKA Scarface) who's based at Shawpark, the mental health place. I like GP Dr Ali, she's funny. She's from Iran so has a great accent, making everything she says sound just slightly comical. She gave me some very basic but sound advice today: "Whatever you feel, just say it. Don't keep it inside. If you feel like crying, just do eet. Don't try to be strong."
I promised I wouldn't.

Dr Ali signed me off work for another two weeks but agreed that I'm doing much better. She said something called a 'phased return to work' would be a good idea. It means I would initially go back part-time and gradually build up to my usual role.

After the doctors, I phoned Lorna to give her an update. Rob was right to encourage me to make the call; I'd been tempted to send an email. It sounds pathetic but I was a bit nervous before ringing her. It was a slightly awkward conversation because she was in the car and I couldn't really hear her properly. Anyway she was very nice and said she was glad to hear from me. I explained about the phased return idea and we agreed I would give her an email or call at the office next week, to arrange a catch up meeting for the following week. Then hopefully the week after that, I can go back three days a week for a few weeks and finally go full time again.

Afterwards, replaying the conversation in my head, I remembered that Lorna said it had been so strange for her not seeing me for such a long time, almost like not speaking to a member of her family. What a nice thing to say. I feel slightly bad that I'm planning to abscond from the magazine family and Lorna doesn't have a clue. Hopefully by the time of the meeting, we'll have sold the flat and bought a place Up North. If not then I'll just need to keep quiet about our plans.

Day 36 — 26th January 2011

I've said it already, more than once I'm sure, but I felt the need to tell Rob yet again just how sorry I was to have put him through such a horrible experience.

"In some ways, it was probably worse for you than it was for me," I said. "At least I was on loads of drugs, I know I don't remember the worst bits. Whereas you..."

"Oh don't worry. I was self-medicating, you know," Rob turned round from the computer to smile as he said this. I knew he meant red wine.

"But still, I am sorry you know. I'm conscious I must have said some really weird things."

"Mmm. You did say some strange stuff to the nurses."

"Oh no. Like what?"

"Well, at one point you told them I was gay."

I burst out laughing.

"Oh my God! Honestly? Did I really say that?"

I had a vague memory of thinking someone in the family was gay, but I have no recollection of thinking my own husband was! I couldn't stop laughing.

"God, how embarrassing for you! Ohhhh, I wonder if that was when I thought I was a boy. That would sort of make sense, you know if I thought I was a boy, and we were married, that would make you gay."

"And when you stopped saying that, you told the nurses you were having an affair."

"Nooo, seriously? Well, you know there's no truth in that, don't you?"

Rob was upstairs on the mezzanine floor with his back towards me during most of this conversation, so I couldn't actually see his face.

"Yeah well, I told Sylv about it and she said, 'Look Rob, you can't pick and choose what you decide to believe'. And that made sense."

Thank goodness my sensible sister was around. I got a sarky text from Sylv today: "I see Tommy [Sheridan] got 3 years, hope ur not too upset!"

Of course, I realise *now* that Tommy Sheridan's court case had absolutely nothing to do with me. Thank goodness. But I still felt sorry for him. OK, he was found guilty, but I just couldn't bring myself to believe he was anything other than a good man. I don't claim to be bias-free when it comes to Tommy Sheridan. He was my first proper interviewee as a journalism student, so I'll always have a soft spot for him.

"Not too soft, I hope," Rob said, when I mentioned this.

Day 41 — 31st January 2011

I was still sleeping OK with the aid of a mirtazapine each night. I need to arrange a meeting with Lorna next week to discuss coming back the following week. It feels like going back to school after the holidays. Except I'd been off a month longer than anyone else. And I'd gone mental during the holidays. Apart from that it was just the same. I know I'll be fine once I get back into it. I'm just dreading that first potentially awkward set of conversations with colleagues.

Day 42 — 1st February 2011

I've got an appointment with the GP this afternoon and have just heard back from Lorna, so now have a meeting next Wednesday to discuss my 'phased return to work'. I'm sure I'm going to be nervous before going back into work, I just hope I'm not so nervous that I don't sleep properly the night before. I suppose I shouldn't build it up in my head too much — after all, what's the worst that can happen? It's just a meeting! It's really the thought of facing people for the first time that's making me nervous. It feels like years since I was last in the office. It's certainly not the work itself, that's the easy bit.

Day 43 — 2nd February 2011

Finally got round to reading the small print on my tablets. There is the usual list of side effects, many of which sound a whole lot worse than the reason you're taking the medication. Then it hits you with the killer; the side effects include *increased appetite* and *weight gain*. Well that's just bloody brilliant – an antidepressant that makes you fat! Honestly.

Day 47 — 6th February 2011

Rob and I were driving around the highlands together, looking at properties we could buy where we could start our own wigwam-style campsite. Nothing seemed quite right though; for one reason or another I just couldn't see myself living in any of these places. At the same time, I'm trying to follow Rob's lead because I don't feel completely capable of making big decisions yet.

While we were on the road, Rob took a call from our solicitors. A lady called Christina had put in an offer on our flat. We decided to reject it and let her know what we would accept. A couple of hours later, it was done. We told the lawyer to officially accept her new improved offer. Wow.

Day 48 — 7th February 2011

We're back in Glasgow now, having not found any suitable properties. I felt like I was in limbo: stuck between my old life and my new one.

Rob and I went to meet Mum and Dad for lunch in Betty's Tea Room, their favourite Glasgow haunt. I tried to appear as happy and normal as I could manage, but I was aware of how close an eye they were keeping on me. I felt slightly self-conscious, especially about how much I was eating. But for all that, generally I was OK.

We apologised that, because we'd been away, this was the first time we'd seen them, even though they'd been in Glasgow a couple of days. But they didn't mind, they'd been having a whale of a time, going round all the museums and art galleries.

It wasn't long before Mum said, "So how are you feeling, Rosalind?"

"I'm OK," I said, trying to smile. "I'm still coming to terms with it all really."

"Well, that's only natural," Mum said softly. "It's going to take some time..."

"You seem like you're missing... something," Dad chipped in. "Like you wouldn't be able to stick up for yourself properly."

"How do you mean? I don't need to stick up for myself at the moment do I?"

"Well no, not with us, of course you don't. I don't know, you're just not... it's that fire in your belly, I suppose."

Maybe he's right.

That evening Rob found a house advertised online. It was on Scoraig, a peninsula south of Ullapool. He seemed pretty excited about it. The community there lives off-grid, and are mostly powered by wind turbines. There seems to be a bit of an alternative lifestyle going on. The place looked pretty cool, and the house prices were appealing, but the remoteness scared me a bit. It's only accessible by boat or a five-mile walk.

We talked to Mum and Dad about Scoraig and they were surprisingly positive, given how far away it is. When we happened to be on our own for a second, I told Mum I was slightly worried about the remoteness. Mum gave me a serious look.

"Do make sure you don't say you want to go just because you think that's what Rob wants, Rosal. You *have* to be honest with each other."

"Hmm."

"Is it very beautiful?" she wanted to know.

"It is. I mean, it's got nice mountains."

She looked at me, waiting. The unspoken 'but' was almost audible, I clearly wanted to say more.

"It's quite stark as well though, you know, bare. It hasn't got a sandy beach or anything."

Which if you're going all that way, to somewhere *so* remote, you'd really expect. Wouldn't you?

Day 50 — 9th February 2011

On the underground home after my meeting with Lorna, I was pleased. Pleased it had gone OK. After I spoke to Lorna I went round to say hi to everyone in each of the three departments. Everyone I saw was friendly and seemed happy to see me. Nobody looked at me as if to say, what's this lunatic doing here? Actually most people had curiosity in their eyes, as if they were trying to figure me out, work out why I'd been away so long.

Lorna had updated me on the forthcoming issue and told me that she hadn't told any of the staff anything about me being ill, because, as she put it, frankly it was none of their business. She'd just told them I'd decided to take January off. They'd have guessed something was up of course, you don't just take a whole month off work because you feel like it. But I was glad she hadn't told them anything specific.

She let me know about a couple of advertisers who had gone under and another one or two we were having problems dealing with. She also said that because she hadn't known how long I would be off, she'd put Michelle, my features writer, in charge of editorial for the time being. Fair enough, I thought.

The most shocking part of the meeting was nothing to do with me at all.

"There are a couple of things you need to know about what's been happening in the office while you've been away. One is that Shelley and Dom have split up," she said.

"Fuck!" I said, shocked. It only occurred to me later that this wasn't entirely appropriate language to use in the office.

"I can't believe that," I said.

Shelley was one of the salespeople and her and Dom had been together ages, about ten years I think. She was always going on about how in love they were. Shelley was very open about their relationship (too open, sometimes) and if you'd given me a hundred guesses, I'd never have thought this would be the big news from the office.

"As far as I understand it, Dom's been unfaithful and that's what's led to the break-up," Lorna said.

"Blimey, I didn't see that coming."

"Yes, well, you and me neither. I just thought you should know. And the other thing I'll warn you about is something I found when I came back from maternity leave. People don't think to tell you things about what's been happening in the business, which can get really annoying."

I couldn't really see myself getting overly annoyed with that sort of thing, but thanked her for the tip anyway.

When I got home Rob was totally stressed out. I knew he was preoccupied because he didn't ask how the meeting went. He was searching, slightly frantically, through boxes of admin documents, bills and official letters, that sort of thing. This was usually a bad sign.

"What's wrong?" I asked.

"Well, it looks like the sale's going to fall through, that's all," he said.

"Rob, tell me what's happened, please."

He quite often did that when he was worried; instead of just saying what happened in plain language, he'd not quite express it in an exaggerated style of mock-nonchalance. As if an attempt at dark humour would somehow take the sting out of it.

"Redpath Bruce have put the boot in, basically."

Redpath Bruce are our factors, the people who look after (I use the term very loosely) the communal areas of the building.

I thought back to a conversation I'd had with a neighbour of ours.

"I call them Red Mist Bruce," he'd said, "because that's what grips me every time I have to interact with them. Or even *think* about them."

I just laughed at first, unsure what he meant.

"Seriously, you know they rip us off all the time, don't you?" he'd said. "They play these 'divide and conquer' mind games; they prefer that to actually doing anything useful. But they do it so sneakily I can never quite catch them at it. Honestly Ros, my neck throbs every time I open their bills. We pay for services, for repairs we never asked for and they're so vaguely described on the bill that you can never work out if you agreed to it or not."

"Do you really think they're that bad?" I asked, more to stem the rant a bit than because a question was called for. I'd only just moved in and was shocked.

"Well, put it this way Ros, I'm pretty sure their contractors, their *cronies*, inflate their prices, do bugger all actual work and then give Redpath backhanders for the privilege of fleecing us."

I was stunned. Surely this couldn't be true? Or was I just naïve to think the world worked any other way?

"Of course, I can't *prove* any of this," he said with a humourless little laugh. "I mean, I hate to say it, but everyone who lives here is either too busy or too rich to care that much what the factors get up to. And even if we weren't, these people have decades of experience at, you know, being shady."

Well I certainly wasn't rich. But I was busy.

"So. What's going on?" I asked Rob, bringing myself back from the past.

"They've told Christina there's a meeting to discuss what's happening with the tower. Which is obviously going to fuck the sale up. Really bloody good of them to tell our *buyer* before we hear anything about it, isn't it?"

I hated seeing Rob like this. Hurt, kicked in the metaphoricals.

"Ah, bloody hell."

"I only found out when Elaine [a paralegal at our solicitors] told me," he said. There's always something to stress about.

"Rob, try not to worry. I'm sure it will work out OK."

I tried to sound reassuring, although I was pretty worried too.

"What if she pulls out? If she thinks there's a massive bill for tower repairs coming up, she'll change her mind and find somewhere else."

"What did Elaine say?"

"She said depending on what happens at the meeting, we could put the sale through with a retainer clause in the terms."

"What does that mean?"

"It means months from now, we could get a bill for thousands of pounds for our share of the repairs."

"Jeez... well, hopefully it won't come to that."

"What if she pulls out? I can't cope with putting it back on the market again. I hate this... being in limbo. With this tower thing hanging over us, we'll never sell the flat."

Rob sounded so despondent. I shared his concerns but, worrying as it was, I didn't see things as quite so black. At least not yet.

Neither of us wanted to mention the last time, the only other time, we'd sold a flat. We'd had a sale all lined up, but the buyer pulled out when the survey report came back saying the building had chronic subsidence. In the end we paid a bit extra for a more detailed report that showed it was actually 'historic settlement', not subsidence at all. It went smoothly with the second buyer. But I would never forget that feeling of helplessness, of thinking we'd be trapped in the same flat forever because nobody would want to buy it. We couldn't relax, couldn't believe it would really be OK, until the proceeds of the sale were physically in the bank. Surely we wouldn't have to go through all that stress again?

"Look, Christina loves the flat," I told Rob confidently. "Think about it from her point of view. She doesn't want to pull out. In her mind, she's already moved in. Think how much we loved this place when we first put an offer in. She'll do everything she can to make sure it happens. I'm sure it'll be OK."

I tried to convince myself as well as Rob.

Mum and Dad got the train back to Dumfries tonight. Rob's car is a sort of van type thing, with a big handy space at the back but only two seats at the front, none in the back. So to give them both a lift to the station he had to take my Dad first, then come back to the flat to pick up my Mum. I felt the familiar dull ache of guilt. I've never got round to learning to drive.

We waited in the atrium until we saw Rob's car/van pulling up for the second leg. We hugged cheerio and I stood behind the huge grand glass doors, waving goodbye. I was surprised to feel tears pop up into my eyes as a nasty unexpected thought occurred to me; this could be the last time I ever saw my Mum.

Day 51 — 10th February 2011

Rob was still very excited about moving to Scoraig, but I wasn't so sure. I wasn't *against* it as such, but it is very remote — and inaccessible — and I wasn't certain I could picture myself living there. I had doubts about our long-term plan working on Scoraig too. We wanted to start a holiday business renting out wigwams to tourists. But how many holidaymakers would be willing to make such a long journey for a little slice of wilderness?

Then again, I wasn't certain of very much at all just then. Was it just The Fear talking, holding me back? It's hard to make big decisions when you're still reeling from the mental ward. I had misgivings, but I didn't have any better ideas. We decided to spend the weekend on Scoraig to see how we liked it.

Rob contacted Chris, a lovely old guy whose brother owned the cottage we were thinking of buying, to see if it would be OK to stay in the house while we visited.

We were all set to go, until the night before we were due to leave. Chris phoned. I was amazed he owned a mobile; from what I'd heard he was very old school. He said there'd been some flooding at the house so it wasn't really habitable at the moment, but if we were still up for the trip we could stay at the bunkhouse, which was owned by some ladies called Aggie and Gill. Fine by us, Rob said.

We drove up to Nethy Bridge, a small town near Nairn, where our good friends Ronnie and Kaylie live. We spent Wednesday night with them, visited a few more highland properties on the Thursday, came back to Nethy Bridge that evening and headed off to Scoraig on the Friday morning, leaving our cat Jay with Ronnie and Kaylie. We would pick her up again on Sunday.

Day 52 — 11th February 2011

We drove to Badrallach on the north shore of Little Loch Broom, parked the car and started the five-mile walk to Scoraig itself. It was raining a bit when we started out and got progressively worse, so we were soaked by the time we arrived at the bunkhouse. Aggie, a hippyish-looking lady, possibly in her fifties, got there a couple of minutes after us. She had very long grey hair in plaits. She showed us the flower pot that the key was kept under. So people still do that? I don't suppose burglary is much of a problem round here.

Aggie was pretty friendly and showed us how to work the Rayburn so we could cook and keep warm. When she smiled I saw a set of crooked yellow teeth. I always notice teeth because mine aren't the best. They're not quite yellow but most people's are whiter and they're squint too. Aggie's were a lot worse than mine. I noticed she had really long curling nails, about the same shade as her teeth. Definitely a smoker.

"We usually ask people to pay £8 a night to stay here, but you can let us know if you think that's fair or not," she said.

We agreed of course. I could imagine how quickly the whole of Scoraig would find out if we'd suggested paying any less.

"Feel free to drop in to mine for a coffee once you've got settled in," she said.

She's very friendly, I thought.

"Oh, just one more thing. We're holding a cafe here on Sunday morning, to raise money for the local primary school. I hope you don't mind...? We'd love you to join us if you've got time."

"No, that's fine. We'd love to," I said. It was a lie, but I thought at least it was a chance to meet some locals.

"What time does it start?"

"Well we're expecting people from 10am but I suppose we'll need to start cooking about nine-ish."

Great! So much for a nice long lie-in on Sunday morning.

She left us to it and we made ourselves at home. The place was nice and warm once the Rayburn got going. There was a display to tell you how much electricity you were using.

Rob popped over to Chris's place in the afternoon but I stayed behind. I felt the usual pang of guilt from opting out of anything that threatened exercising my weak social muscles, but the weather was rubbish, giving me a fairly good excuse.

I was curled up on the sofa reading a book when Rob came back a while later with some eggs.

"Oh, have you been to the shop?" I said, a bit surprised. I wasn't even sure there was a shop.

"These aren't from the shop, Bosal," he said, grinning and looking especially pleased with himself. "These are freshly laid! I helped Chris get his neighbour's chickens in so he gave me these as a thank you."

"Wow, that's pretty cool. Nice of Chris too."

Chris phoned later and offered to take us out across the loch on his boat the next morning, assuming the weather had improved by then. Rob thanked him and we agreed to meet by the jetty at 10am.

There was no telly in the bunkhouse (a lifestyle choice or does a TV eat too much juice when you're off-grid?) so we played Scrabble that evening. Rob won.

Day 53 — 12th February 2011

It was unbelievably quiet at the bunkhouse and we'd slept well after our big walk. We got up, made some breakfast and headed down to the tiny wee harbour to meet Chris.

I was happy it wasn't raining. It was one of those lovely crisp sunny days that reminds you spring does actually exist. We helped Chris launch his little boat on to the water. I say we but, although I tried my best, I suspect Rob was more useful than me. Chris had some trouble starting the engine. Apparently this wasn't an unusual problem for him: "I was out on the water a few weeks back and I don't mind telling you that, although I don't particularly like these things," he gestured towards his mobile phone, "it probably saved my life."

It was taking so long I felt a bit embarrassed for Chris, not that he seemed bothered. After his little anecdote, I was wondering whether I even wanted to set foot on such an unreliable boat. But he finally managed to bring it to life. Soon we were cruising along the water. The trip didn't take long as the loch between Scoraig and Badluarach, on the south side of Little Loch Broom, is only about a mile wide. But with the sun and wind on our faces, it was a lovely experience. Chris kept talking but we just smiled and nodded because we couldn't hear a word over the engine. For the first time I could see how this wigwam idea might work here. Tourists would love this!

The reason Chris needed to go over the water was to move his car into its garage on the other side. When we reached the mainland there was an awkward moment as he tried his best to get the old banger up the little hill into its shed.

The tyres were spinning, mud flying everywhere. Rob and a few other blokes who happened to be around helped him push it up. He scraped the car along the side of the garage walls as he drove it in. Apart from that it went quite well.

Chris introduced a few people to us, including, which I was very happy about, a couple around our own age, maybe a bit younger. But then Laura told me she and her boyfriend, who both come from Scoraig, live in Edinburgh now and were only home for the weekend.

Chris's engine held out long enough to take us back over. We were planning to go for a wander after that but Chris offered to show us Hugh Piggott's house. Hugh is the main man on Scoraig, the guy who makes all the wind-powered turbines that enable Scoraig to exist off-grid.

"Hugh's away at the moment," Chris said, "but his wife Yette should be around."

We walked over to one of the best-looking houses on the peninsula. It had an amazing garden that struck just the right balance between swanky manicured features and pure wildness. The kind of place a child would have a brilliant time exploring. The house had big French windows and a large decking area. We met Yette, who had just a trace of a Scandinavian accent, and stood chatting with her for a little bit. Rob bought a copy of her husband Hugh's book, which is all about how to build your own wind turbine.

Yette was in her fifties. She was friendly enough but slightly aloof, and I wondered whether she'd been in the middle of something when we called. Rob asked her a technical question about turbines and she said it would be best to ask her son Jonah. So we all trooped off down into the cool garden to meet Jonah, who was busy tinkering with a tractor, rolled cigarette hanging from his mouth. He was about our age, with light blue eyes, shaggy blonde hair and a woolly jumper with a pattern borrowed from the eighties. What is it with the woolly jumpers round here? Is it some kind of uniform? Jonah said hello but was obviously a bit preoccupied with his tractor.

"When the weather's like this," Yette said, "we usually have drinks on the porch, if you'd like to join us later?"

"That would be great, thanks."

We arranged to come back at four.

Drinks on the porch. Now that sounds more like it!

Next stop was Chris's brother's cottage, the place we were hoping to buy. Only I wasn't very hopeful. We certainly weren't going to be bowled over by some quaint, immaculate little love nest. We were aware, even before we'd heard about the most recent leaks, that it needed some 'development'. Chris had been playing it down too, clearly trying to lower our expectations. Even so, I suppressed a sigh as we walked through the door. I tried to shake off the mental image of our bright beautiful Glasgow flat and concentrate on the cold leaky low-ceilinged cottage.

Bloody hell. It was bad. It was obvious nobody had lived there for quite some time. We ducked past the thickest cobwebs I'd ever seen, and I looked down as I heard a faint splash. The water damage was a bit depressing. The place was freezing. I knew the temperature wasn't relevant, but it certainly didn't help. It lacked a homely atmosphere.

Rob, of course, could see the *potential*. He actually looked excited. Whereas I just saw a hell of a lot of work. I knew it could be nice, eventually, but was it worth the effort? The living room had an open fire, something I'd always wanted. But the windows were tiny. Even on sunny days you'd hardly get any light.

Before we went back to the bunkhouse, we dropped in on Gill and Alan, the couple who co-owned the bunkhouse with Aggie. Gill looked friendly in a sort of mumsy way and Alan was a proper hippy, with baggy tie-dyed trousers and one of those daft-looking red waistcoats with lots of tiny little mirrors built into it. When we got there, Gill was unloading some food from her car for the cafe at the bunkhouse on Sunday, so we offered to take it over for her.

When we got inside she started quizzing us. Whereabouts on Scoraig are you thinking of moving to? Where do you live just now? Where do you work? How often do you have sex? OK, I might have made up the last one, but bloody hell!

"And of course the question people probably keep asking you, are you planning on having any children?"

I didn't really feel like explaining that we'd like to adopt eventually, but we're not ready yet and so on, so I dodged the question by throwing one back at her.

"Actually, nobody has asked that. Why, is that a big deal round here?"

She started explaining how they needed more young families on Scoraig if there was any chance of it surviving as a community. At the moment there was a decent number of children in the local primary, the problem was the lack of toddlers, younger kids due to start in a few years.

"We've been threatened with closure if we can't recruit more," she said, looking me right in the eye. Right. No pressure then.

I had a shower before we headed over to Yette's. Actually the shower was surprisingly decent, especially considering it's only heated by the Rayburn.

We took a box of red wine up and found Yette, Jonah and a couple of others sitting out on the porch. We were introduced to Jill, who's married to the postie Bill (Jill and Bill, did I really get that right?) and Joanie, a Glaswegian who moved to Scoraig a few years ago. Except for Jonah and us, everyone looked to be in their fifties. Everyone wore... yep, you guessed it, woolly jumpers! Except for Jill, the little rebel, who had the sheer audacity to wear a *fleece*.

Jonah brought out some cushions for us to sit on. I wouldn't say we were exactly bombarded with questions or anything, but they did all seem quite eager to suss out the potential new residents. I wondered how many of them came over just to check us out.

We asked them lots of questions about the place, what it was like living on Scoraig. Yette had a blanket on her legs when we arrived and kept commenting that it wasn't very warm. I kind of agreed but didn't want to sound like a big jessie from the city, so I kept quiet. Eventually we all trooped inside and Yette got out some old photographs to show us what Scoraig was like when it was even less developed.

I was very pleased to see that Yette had a lovely big flat screen on the wall. Aha! Tellies aren't banned altogether here then. Things were looking up.

After a little while Joanie and Jill headed home to make their dinner.

"Yeah, we should get going too, Rob," I said, keen not to outstay our welcome.

"I would ask you to stay for dinner but Jonah and I are going up to Cathy and Tom's tonight," Yette said.

But when she phoned Cathy to find out what time to come over, Cathy said Rob and I were very welcome to join them too.

"There's more than enough food," Yette said, still on the phone.

Rob and I looked at each other.

"What do you think, Ros?" I could tell from Rob's face he was dying to go.

A lot went through my mind in the few seconds before I answered. First, I can't really be bothered. Dinner with strangers was not on my agenda and could be awkward. I had been looking forward to snuggling up and relaxing on the bunkhouse sofa. Second, come on Ros, stop being so antisocial, it's lovely that this person has kindly invited you. Third, are they being kind or simply nosy? Do they just want to sneak a look at the potential newbies? Maybe a bit of both. Fourth, well, that works both ways; it's probably good for us to meet as many of them as possible too.

"Well, that's very kind. If Cathy's sure that's OK…? Oh, but we don't eat meat, will that be a problem?"

No, that's no problem at all, Cathy said down the line.

Before we left for dinner, Yette told us about another property for sale on Scoraig. It sounded fantastic.

"Is there any way we could go and see it before we leave on Sunday?" Rob asked.

"Yes, why not. I have to take a shower but Jonah could show you now if you like," she said.

It was only a five-minute walk and when we got there Jonah went straight to the flower pot near the front door where the owner had left the key. But before he picked it up, he said, "Oh, actually, they've probably left it open."

They had. Which just felt wrong to me and my city-living ways. I imagined me and Rob thirty years from now, grey-haired and wearing the standard issue woolly jumper, living on Scoraig but still checking we'd locked the doors and windows before leaving the house.

I couldn't believe it when we got inside. The place was beautiful, all wooden floors, with a massive open plan brand new fitted kitchen, tempting me in with its swanky chrome worktops. Wow. Maybe I could imagine myself living on Scoraig.

Off we went, the four of us. On Jonah's quad bike.

"Just make sure you hold on tight," he said with a mischievous grin as we got in. Or on. The ride was fast and bumpy and I kept wondering how much wine

Jonah had drunk. I suspected he'd smoked a few joints too, if his bloodshot eyes and perma-grin were anything to go by. But I tried to relax, he seemed to know what he was doing. His mother certainly seemed happy enough to trust him and she struck me as pretty sensible. She had a head scarf on, which made me think of the Queen.

The ride was great fun. The stars were out, and the wind zipping through my hair was refreshing after the wine. Nobody fell off and we got there in no time. Cathy ushered us all in and got us drinks.

Cathy had long thick black hair streaked with grey, giving her a slightly witchy look. I don't mean that as an insult. I couldn't work out how old she was, but with the regulation woolly jumper (hers was of the Arran variety, which I quite liked actually) she kind of pulled it off. Not literally.

Cathy's partner Tom, a stonemason, was quite good-looking, in a bookish, Louis Theroux sort of way. I pictured him doing manly stone-thrashing work. He was tall with glasses and the sort of unkempt brown curly hair that looked so soft I had an urge to ruffle it up. Luckily I wasn't that drunk. I immediately liked him. He was busy cooking and I offered to help but he waved me off into the living room with an easygoing smile, ordering me to sit down, relax. The cottage was lovely and cosy, with wooden beams and an open fire.

Dinner was informal; the idea was to help yourself to various dishes laid out on a big wooden table we were all sitting around.

"Whatever you do, please don't be polite," Cathy said.

It was all delicious and I told the hosts so.

"Everything here, except for the smoked salmon, was grown right here by us," Cathy said proudly.

"Wow, that's brilliant."

The conversation turned to Rob and me and what skills we could offer the place. I suddenly felt like this was a job interview and took a big gulp of wine.

"Well, Rob's very handy. He can build or fix most things," I said. They all nodded and looked approvingly at Rob, sizing him up.

"And what about you Ros?" Cathy asked.

"Well, if you want anything proofreading, I'm your man!" I said with an embarrassed laugh. I'd meant it as a joke really, but they all looked slightly confused. As if to say, why the hell would we want anything proofread? Rob started telling them what a brilliant writer I was, but Cathy interrupted to ask what sort of things I wrote.

"Is it poetry, or...?"

"Well, I'm working for a wedding magazine at the moment, so I mostly write about weddings."

Cathy looked horrified.

"But isn't that just… soul-destroying, working for a company like that?"

"No, not really," I said, trying not to sound as annoyed as I felt. "Actually I really enjoy it. It's great fun and our readers love the magazines we produce."

Cathy stared at me as if I'd just shat in her kettle, or admitted to paedophilia.

Then, even worse, she gave me a patronising 'you'll learn one day' look that infuriated me. I felt like punching her on the nose. How dare she automatically assume my job is worthless? She didn't know anything about it.

Tom deftly moved the conversation on to something more lighthearted and I forced myself to forget about it for now. I was a guest in her house, after all, so I bit my tongue. What I felt like saying was, "Oh, I'm sorry, what did you say you do again? Oh, you're an archaeologist. How very bloody *worthy* of you. Well you know what? You may not approve of my job, but digging around in the dirt sounds like absolute hell to me. So why don't you take your principles and your stupid jumper and feck right off!"

I'm not saying that's a reasonable, sound or particularly mature argument, but that's what I felt like saying.

I slowed down on the wine. The leaflet that came with my pills advised avoiding alcohol completely, of course. My GP told me it was "probably OK to have one or two drinks" while I was taking them, but I'd had considerably more than that over the course of the day and wanted to be careful.

Tom passed some kind of orange liqueur around after dinner. I was the only person who declined. When they started passing joints round I said no thanks to those too. I'm sure they all thought I was very boring or square (or whatever the non-square term for square is) but that was the last thing I needed.

Day 54 — 13th February 2011

In the car on the way home I tried to put my thoughts together. Had I enjoyed myself this weekend? Enough to move to that unusual, remote place? One of the things that bothered me was that we hadn't met anyone our own age who actually lived there. Another question mark was whether I could see myself fitting in there, making friends with all the woolly jumpers.

"Hey Rob, did you notice how all the women we met had a… similar look?"

"Not really."

I don't know what I was expecting him to say. He barely ever seemed to notice appearances, except in a very general way.

"Well, I mean, for a start, they all wore woolly jumpers."

"Of course. Wool's probably one of the best materials for keeping you warm, you know that."

"OK, OK, forget the jumpers. That was a bad example. What I'm trying to say is…"

What was I trying to say?

"I don't know, maybe it's just me looking at it through city eyes, but, well, it's not a crime to use hair dye and tweezers is it? Scoraig's like… like the opposite of 'The Stepford Wives' or something!"

Ah damn. I'd started the conversation determined not to sound mean, bitchy and judgemental. Rob was laughing at me.

"I don't think I saw any bearded ladies?" he said, pretending to look confused.

"Oh come on, you know what I mean."

Rob knew I wasn't one of those high maintenance women who spend thousands on the latest pointless lotions and potions. I might be a perfectionist, but only work-wise, not in the self-image department. Far from it. I was aware of my flaws. But I wasn't comfortable with the idea of letting myself go. Surely looking after yourself, taking *some* level of care over your appearance, is a good thing. Isn't it? Or at least not a bad thing. As long as you don't obsess. Or am I just a victim of social conditioning, a woman brainwashed into believing she should look a certain way? I was still thinking about how to express this without sounding nasty, snooty and shallow (isn't that an advertising agency?), when Rob broke into my thoughts.

"Maybe stuff like that… maybe it doesn't really matter as much when you live somewhere rural."

Possibly Rob was right. Annoyingly, he quite often was. Maybe it didn't matter. Maybe if I reach the age of 70 or 80, I won't give a toss about a few hairs on my chin, or having eyebrows that look like slugs. But I'm only 34. And at the moment I see no reason to leave the house without putting my face on. Certainly not if I've let that face develop a little moustache.

I promised myself right then that if we did end up moving to Scoraig, I would never get the uniform.

Day 55 — 14th February 2011

I went back to actual work today, my muscles still aching from our long walks on Scoraig. I felt a bit of a fraud. As if I was leading a double life, part of me settling back into my old role in the office, while the other half quietly planned my exit.

At the MMM (that's the Monday Morning Meeting) Lorna welcomed me back and told everyone that Michelle would remain in charge while we worked on the forthcoming issue. I suppose she had told me, or at least implied, this would be the case at our meeting, but I was still slightly surprised. I suppose it made sense. I hadn't had anything to do with this issue up to now, and I couldn't really act as editor for three days a week and then just bugger off and leave them to it the rest of the time. I managed to nod along with Lorna as if I had known this would be announced. Michelle, on the other hand, looked totally shocked that she was to stay in charge for now. When Lorna mentioned the words 'acting editor' Michelle turned towards me and mouthed the words 'Acting editor? Me?', with a disbelieving look on her face. I smiled back at her. It was quite sweet that she was taking her temporary promotion so modestly.

After work, I stopped in at Marks & Spencer on Byres Road to get one of those 'dine in for a tenner' deals. I don't buy this sort of thing very often, but seeing as it was Valentine's Day... And it was a bargain, because you got a bottle of wine thrown in too. Nice.

It was horribly busy in the shop and I tried not to get annoyed with all the middle class middle-aged ladies getting in my way. I failed. There's something about the typical M&S customer that really gets on my wick. I think it might be their sneeringly superior attitude. I resisted the urge to inflict a sharp elbow in the ribs of a particularly slow, overdressed lady who was (obviously) deliberately getting in my way.

I tried to remember where I was a few weeks ago. I tried to recall the happiness of wandering around Lidl that first day of my release. I tried to think of others less fortunate than myself. Those shopping in Iceland or Farmfoods, for example. (Joke. There are some great deals in Iceland.) Nope, it was no good. I could feel shop rage surging through me, waves of pointless irritation. They should hand everyone a glass of wine on the way in, I'm sure that would help.

I couldn't find the tenner deals for ages. Eventually I found what can only be described as the remnants of the deal. Of course, the whole of Glasgow's west end had had the same idea. There was bugger all left, especially if you don't eat meat. And... wait a minute! Oh, perfect. Even though only the dregs were left, the sign quite clearly explained that because it was Valentine's Day, they had a 'special' dine in deal. For *twenty* quid. Cheeky buggers! I took in the details as the physical signs of stress — heart racing, palms sweating — accelerated. Basically you were paying ten quid extra for a sorry-looking box of chocolates. There wasn't even any red wine included in the deal today, just some nasty cheap sparkling stuff that would probably taste awful and give us a headache. What a rip off.

Deep breath. Walk away. This kind of minor annoyance is just not worth the release of my stress hormones. Not exactly a 'fight or flight' scenario is it. OK, move on. It took ages to find an alternative, but I got a fish pie in the end. And some nice-looking asparagus on special offer because it had to be eaten today. Once I'd added a bottle of wine and some chocolate desserts, it all added up to nearly twenty quid anyway. But at least I had some things we might enjoy. Right, let's get out of here.

Over dinner we talked about Scoraig. I tried to be honest without totally pouring cold water on the idea.

"I suppose it's the remoteness that worries me the most. I know we both want to change our lifestyle, but... I'm wondering if anyone would come to visit us, and if I'd miss just being able to wander down to browse in some charity shops, that kind of thing."

I said it all quickly, before I chickened out.

"Well, we could still go into Inverness now and then, it's not that far. And I think people would love to come out for a holiday."

"I suppose..."

"Thing is Ros, I feel like I need to get out of the city. I feel like it's stifling me."

"I know, I know. So do I really..." I said, thinking back to my shop rage a couple of hours ago.

"It's just that Scoraig's *so* remote, you know."

"I don't know what else to do though, Ros."

Rob sounded upset now, and I felt one of my most familiar emotions. Guilt.

"And it's not like it has to be forever does it? Nothing's set in stone. If we don't like it, we just come back."

Rob laughed, but not in a happy or amused way. His voice was veering towards that 'this is all very simple, why can't you see it like I do?' tone. I went quiet and thought about it. I suppose he was right, it *wasn't* forever. What's the worst that could happen? I could at least give it a go, rather than letting The Fear stop me.

"OK, let's do it," I said, possibly emboldened by the wine.

I held my glass up towards Rob, who looked rather surprised, but clinked it to seal the deal.

Day 62 — 21st February 2011

The sale of our flat went through OK after all. We only had a few days of agonising before the meeting. As I walked downstairs towards the other owners I thought, hopefully, surely, this would be the last residents' meeting I'd ever have to attend. It was a very welcome thought. I used to dread these meetings for weeks beforehand. The whole thing was a stinking mass of cliques, cliques within cliques, backstabbing, false niceties, snide gossip about the people sensible enough not to go, and petty grievances. Oh, there were plenty of those. Important matters such as; "I'm sorry but I just *have* to say something about the food smells coming from the ground floor... sometimes it's like living in an Indian takeaway!" Or "Does everyone agree that any washing left in the communal laundry longer than 24 hours should be binned?" Or even worse; "Should we consider a selection committee for new residents?"

Jesus, get a *grip*. Have you ever actually listened to yourself? I didn't know it was possible to be bored and stressed at the same time until I'd been to one of these meetings. That nasty inner voice started haranguing me again as I thought about this; 'What did you expect, moving into a building like that?' I know, I know...

The outcome of my last ever meeting, the residents' consensus on the tower, was 'wait and see'. Everyone agreed, surprisingly easy, that it was just too early to tell whether the tower needed further repairs at this stage. So we were off the hook! We didn't actually celebrate then; the money wasn't in the bank yet, after all. But it looked like the sale would be all right.

We made a decision to put an offer in on the swanky newly built place, rather than the dilapidated old cottage. It was due to go to a closing date, but Rob got very excited after he'd talked to the owner on the phone. They agreed on a price and as far as Rob was concerned, that was it.

A couple of days later Rob was devastated when he talked to the owner again. He started swearing when he came off the phone.

"What's happened?"

"The guy's just being a cock," he said.

"Well, what did he say?"

"Apparently there's another 'interested party'."

"Oh. So what does that mean? He hasn't accepted our offer after all?"

"No, he hasn't bloody well accepted it. He's just a bullshitter. He told me he was happy to accept our offer. Now he's saying, oh these other people are offering ten grand more."

"OK. So... do you want to put in another offer?"

"I dunno. I just feel like... if I hadn't phoned him then, I'd be none the wiser you know? I'd be paying our solicitor to put in an offer he'd already decided wasn't enough. And the two-faced git didn't even bother phoning me!"

Rob was such a good bloke, such a kind, fair, nice person. I suppose, whatever you're like, you subconsciously assume that most people operate in a similar way. It hurt me whenever Rob was reminded that not everybody is as good-natured and honest as he is.

He got over it soon enough, but when he started talking about the clapped out cottage again, I discouraged him. All the houses for sale on Scoraig were cheap. Suspiciously cheap. I couldn't help wondering if that was because 99% of people, of potential buyers, would never even consider living somewhere like that. The more I thought about it, the more I was certain I didn't want to sink all our money into Scoraig. I imagined being stuck there for decades, unable to sell. I was surprised when Rob accepted my argument easily. Perhaps he was worried I'd go mental again if he pushed it.

So Scoraig was no sooner on the cards than we chucked the whole pack into the fire. I didn't realise how relieved I was until it was just another ex-idea. Another pipe dream snuffed out with a great big bucket of reality.

Day 65 — 24th February 2011

When we put our flat on the market before Christmas, the idea was to buy a place in the highlands, set up a wigwam site and make life a whole lot less stressful. Apart from the stresses of launching and running our own business for the first time. And moving to a completely different location. Oh and leaving all our friends and family behind, hundreds of miles away. Apart from all that, life would be entirely stress-free.

The problem was, quite apart from our little Project Scoraig diversion, we'd looked at dozens of properties since I'd got out of hospital and nothing seemed quite right. I just couldn't imagine myself living in any of those places, and decided I'd better tell Rob.

"Well, we don't need to buy somewhere immediately. In fact, the way property prices are going, it might be a good idea to hold off for a bit."

"But where would we go once we've sold? What would we do?"

"I don't know, but I feel like I need to get out of Glasgow."

"Me too. But if we're not going to the highlands what's the plan?"

I need a plan, always. Failing to plan is... well you know the rest.

"I don't know. I haven't got all the answers Ros."

Rob looked sad and I felt sad too. I need Rob to be in control at the moment, to know what we're doing and why. Otherwise what are we working towards? We're just floating along aimlessly. I need purpose. Goals. Routine. All that stuff.

I tried to think what I really wanted from life. I want a family, certainly. But not yet. What else do I want?

Eventually Rob broke the silence.

"I think Glasgow and the weather here... I don't know, I'm sick of it. It's just stifling me."

Another pause. Stifling is Rob's favourite new word for expressing how pissed off he is. I wish he would find a new one. It makes me picture someone's hands round his neck, literally stifling him. I shake the image away. We still need a plan, and I'm starting to feel angry that we don't have one any more.

More silence.

"Why don't we go travelling for a bit? I feel like I need some sunshine. We could buy a campervan, just bugger off round Europe for a while."

I can't believe we're changing the plan, again.

"But what would we do when we get back? How would we make enough money to live?"

He laughed. "Why are you worrying about what we'll do when we get back? We haven't even left yet!"

"I'm not worrying! I just like to know the plan, that's all."

"Well, we could do anything. Going away might give us some perspective on what we want to do. But with the proceeds from the flat sale in the bank, we wouldn't really have to worry about money too much, not for a while anyway."

That was true. We'll have a fair whack left after all the fees are paid.

Actually I quite liked the sound of this plan — no mortgage, no council tax or bills, no nosy neighbours, no tedious residents' meetings. Just me, Rob and the open road. I could get used to this idea.

We went out for dinner and started talking through our plans. I sent Sylv a text to ask whether she'd be up for fostering our cat for a bit while we went away. She said she'd talk to Mark about it. I wasn't sure that would work out though; Mark's allergic to cats.

Day 71 — 2nd March 2011

I asked Lorna for five minutes in the meeting room. I'd surreptitiously typed up a letter of resignation before the meeting, hovering around the printer so that nobody else had a chance to pick it up.

I had thought carefully about how to phrase it and in the end I told her I'd made the decision to "go freelance". Lorna was visibly shocked and while she took it in I emphasised that I wanted to continue working for the magazine, just not as editor.

"Well, OK. Wow. I'm sure you've thought about it long and hard before telling me, so... Of course it goes without saying that I'll be very sorry to see you go."

"Thanks Lorna."

"Who am I going to enjoy my hot cross buns with now?" she said. We were both big fans. I laughed and pushed the letter across to her side of the desk.

"In terms of dates, I said in the letter I'd give the usual month's notice, but if you need me for longer I'm happy to do another couple of weeks."

"Right, thanks. That'd be really helpful. Oh and Ros, if you wouldn't mind keeping this to yourself for now, just while I get my head round it."

"OK," I said, though I hadn't expected her to say that.

When we stood up Lorna did a strange thing. She hugged me. I don't think she'd ever hugged me in the six years I'd known her, so I was pretty shocked. Back at my desk, I took a deep breath, glad that was over.

Day 73 — 4th March 2011

It was Friday evening and I was about to leave the office when Michelle asked me about the budget weddings feature I was working on.

"Oh it's coming together all right. The only problem is the big budget wedding. I can't find anyone who spent over £25,000..."

She gave me a funny look.

"There must be loads of couples that spent more than that."

"Yeah, I found a few, but when I started asking them for a breakdown of how much they spent on each element, they all got cold feet, didn't want to publish."

"Well, we need a big budget wedding, the feature won't work without one."

This was weird, the most direct conversation we'd had with Michelle in charge instead of me. I didn't disagree with what she was saying, I just couldn't see how we were going to resolve it the way she wanted. I'd talked to a handful of big spenders and they'd all pulled out once I started asking for detailed information. My theory was that they had been happy to spend an obscene amount of money on their wedding days, but weren't willing to admit as much in print, in cold black and white, to the whole world. Perhaps they feared being perceived as vulgar, more money than sense, that kind of thing. Or they imagined readers looking at the photos and judging them harshly, saying things like,

"What? They paid over a grand for those poxy flowers? Idiots!"

"Well, I've got a couple who spent nineteen grand. I thought they could be our big spenders."

"Hmm. Leave it with me, I'll see if I can find someone else."

Good luck with that, I thought as I left for the weekend.

But she did. She tweeted our request and a couple who spent £28,000 came forward straight away. Damn, why hadn't I thought of Twitter? I checked my emails later on. I know, Friday night, what a saddo! But old habits and all that. And there was a very enthusiastic tweet. I emailed the bride straight away, before she could change her mind, copying Michelle in so she'd know I was on to it. I was very slightly vexed that Michelle had found the couple, rather than me, but for the sake of my feature I crossed my fingers that this bride wouldn't change her mind.

Day 74 — 5th March 2011

The big spender bride had emailed me back within a few hours. She was over the moon at the prospect of being featured in Real Life Weddings, had received my questions by email, made a start at answering them, promised to finish them over the weekend and send them to me first thing Monday morning. She'd even contacted her photographer on our behalf, copying me in so that I now had his email address. Which was perfect because more often than not photographers needed chasing up before they gave us the high-quality images we needed for print. I was impressed, this was my kind of bride!

I dropped Michelle a quick email to let her know it was all coming together nicely. Having been in her shoes, I knew she would appreciate having one less thing to worry about.

Rob and I decided to go for dinner in the Black Sparrow, a pub at Charing Cross that did nice scran. We'd got a 5pm deal so the food came with a free bottle of wine. Nice. I do love a freebie, especially one that makes you feel all warm and fuzzy inside. The pub wasn't full to bursting, but was busy enough to give it a lively atmosphere — and to offer abundant people-watching opportunities. Perfect.

I heard a text message arrive as we tucked into our mains. It was Michelle; Got your email, thanks for the update. Still in work... looking forward to you taking back the reins soon!

If you only knew, young Michelle. You'll soon be responsible for the reins, the horses and the unruly old stable boys. Mwahahaha!

Day 78 — 9th March 2011

Lorna called me into the meeting room today. When I got there, she shut the door, which usually signalled some serious or private business. Uh-oh, that was my first thought. Second was, hang on, you've already handed in your notice — what are you scared of exactly, getting sacked? But it was nothing major.

"I just wanted to ask you not to tell anyone about your decision until after we've gone to the printers."

"Oh. OK, if you like."

Bloody hell, that was ages away. I'd been looking forward to coming clean. I hate secrets and having to watch what I say to people.

"I don't want anything to interfere with production, or to stop deadline going smoothly."

I didn't really see how or why my news should have such a detrimental impact on those things, but outwardly I just agreed to keep schtum.

"And to be honest, I'm still getting my head round it and figuring out how everything's going to work..."

Ah, that made a bit more sense. I fleetingly wondered whether she wasn't too sure about making Michelle editor just yet. Lorna and Michelle were quite similar in some ways. Maybe Lorna thought they might clash if Michelle was promoted.

Oh well, none of this was my problem.

"And also, if you could put something down on paper for me, regarding how you think your freelancing could work, that would be great. You know, costs and that type of thing. I'm really glad you're still going to be a part of the magazine."

"OK, will do."

Day 84 — 15th March 2011

We're on deadline this week. Usually that means work is busy as hell, intense with mini highs and lows as one feature unexpectedly comes together and another falls apart while we're not looking. It means a promised image doesn't come through and we frantically look around for something else for the lead feature. It means an uphill battle as we painstakingly sift through the page layouts that need major redesigns.

It means the head of sales decides Photographers A and B have too many photos in this issue so we need to swap some out with the work of Photographers C, D and E. Everyone in editorial glares at our head of sales. The reason the designers chose so many pics from Photographers A and B in the first place is that their work is wonderful. C's, D's and E's on the other hand? Their stuff is blurred, out of focus, poorly composed, clichéd. Pish, in other words. But C, D and E pay for advertising space too, so we need to keep them happy. And so on.

It means getting home late, at least one large glass of wine, rocking back and forth like, well, like a nutter.

Being on deadline is just not the same now that I'm not the editor. As editor, deadline week completely consumed me, taking up all my energy, thoughts and time. Now that I'm not in charge, it amazes me how little it affects me. It barely registered, like rain off a Glaswegian's back. All this week I got home at a reasonable time and, OK, I wouldn't say I forgot about work completely, but I was certainly able to think about other things, other people.

It was weird during the day though. I'd see colleagues go up to Michelle with page layouts and questions. Querying stuff with her that they'd normally ask *me*. It didn't make me want to run off and hide in the toilets or anything, it just felt strange. Well, nobody's indispensable, I thought to myself. You knew that.

Of course, nobody knew Michelle had taken over permanently yet, not even Michelle herself. I was in the unusual position of watching someone else do my job before I'd even chucked it in. I shook off the feeling, whatever it was. I should have been happy nobody was bothering me. One of the most annoying things about being editor was not being able to get on with my own work because people were constantly badgering me with questions. I just hadn't realised that being needed like that made me feel good, important. I should really try to base my feelings of self-worth on something other than work. That would be healthy.

Day 94 — 25th March 2011

It was the day of the move and I felt emotional. Last night was strange enough, as I packed up all our mugs and plates and other bits and pieces. It didn't help having 'Junior Doctors' on in the background. Man, that programme is harrowing! So much has happened in this flat, hundreds of memories lodged here. I thought back to the little party we had here on the night of our wedding. I sat in my big red wedding dress on the sofa, surrounded by my favourite people. Someone had twirled fairy lights around my neck so everything glowed. Our friend Johnny had been to the excellent takeaway across the road, and enjoyed his first box of pakora so much he went back for seconds. He came back with dozens of boxes, having spent a hundred quid on pakora. It's funny the things you remember.

When everything was packed tightly into the van, with the help of our loveliest neighbour, Uncle Billy, I stood looking out the cathedral-style windows in the living room for the last time. I don't know why I was surprised to feel emotional, but there it was, water coming out of my eyes. Not enough to ruin my make-up or anything, but still. As soon as I started to feel sad about it, my inner critic piped up with a snidey comment; 'Oh boohoo! You had a nice flat and now you don't. Life's such a struggle isn't it? Dry yer eyes doll!'

The plan was to move in with Sylv and Mark in Edinburgh for a few weeks, while I was still working in Glasgow. I'd be commuting back and to each day, which was a bit annoying. (Again, 'Dry yer eyes! Ooh, has your hummus gone fizzy too? How do you bear the *horror*? You and your middle class troubles...' etc.) But it wasn't for long. There were people in Glasgow we could have stayed with, but Sylv and Mark had agreed to look after Jay while we went travelling, and we wanted to smooth the cat fostering process as much as possible by moving into her new home for a bit.

When we got to Sylv's and started taking the first set of boxes up the stairs, I had another emotional jolt. Our old place had the grandest, most opulent entrance you could imagine. Seriously, it looked more like a palace than a set of flats when you walked inside. It had an atrium big enough to host a ceilidh, huge pillars, plush red carpets, and the best bit, a fish pond surrounded by dozens of tall tropical plants. It was coolest at night when all the little floor lights made it look even more magical. I remembered the very first night we'd moved in, when I just couldn't believe that we lived somewhere so special. I nipped along the corridor from our flat, which was on the first floor, and looked down, marvelling at the sight.

The contrast between Trinity and Sylv's place stung me. Like most city centre stairwells, the one leading to my sister's place was OK, but to me it looked dark and drab.

Rob had been taking boxes of our stuff to various friends' places over the last few weeks, so getting everything else up a couple of flights of stairs wasn't too much of a pain. Thankfully people didn't seem to mind giving up some of their loft space for us, which would save us a load of cash compared to paying for official storage.

I felt a lot better once everything was inside and we were sitting down chatting to Sylv, eating homemade cookies and drinking tea. Sylv is good at baking (and chatting) and the cookies were delicious.

Day 98 — 29th March 2011

I dreamt we were back in the old flat last night. I was standing in the living room with Rob and we looked out the massive window and saw our life piled up outside, hundreds of boxes stacked far too high and just starting to topple over when I woke up.

Day 99 — 30th March 2011

I've always, as far as I can remember, been a glass half empty kind of person. I don't mean I'm a moany miserable git, but I'm always worrying about the worst thing that could happen. It doesn't occur to me to expect the best. A 'what if' sort of person.

I am also starting to notice what I think of as 'the waiting game' I play with my life. It's not much fun for a game. The main rule is I am always waiting for something to make me happy. I'm constantly bargaining with myself; if and when such and such happens, I will be happy afterwards. Oh I'll be so happy once these exams are finished, I think decisively. Then it's oh I'll be so happy once I find The One, the right man to fall in love with. Then I'll be so happy once we move out of this grotty flat, once we have enough money, once I've got a great job... but when you've got all that you've ever wished for and you're *still* waiting for happiness to kick in, where do you go from there? Maybe I should start trying to take more enjoyment from simple pleasures. Is that the way forward?

Perhaps that's why people have kids, because it gives you something other than yourself to think about. But I'm not quite unsatisfied enough to sacrifice my life for some ungrateful little bugger. Not yet anyway.

I was sitting on the underground on the way home from work tonight, when I found that watery stuff (water, I think it is) in my eyes again. How embarrassing. I'm lucky nobody makes eye contact on the underground. It had just sunk in that in only a couple of weeks, I was going to leave the best job I've ever had. I know there's a plus side; we're going on a huge adventure and it's clearly a good thing that I'm leaving the job that led to me being sectioned. But still, I feel some kind of sadness, some sense of loss. Will I ever have such a good job again?

I thought back to the first day I started my job. There was a company-wide MMM, or Monday Morning Meeting. The boss lady was introducing everyone to me in her own unique way; 'This is Stephen, whose job is... well, to make the pages look pretty.'

Stephen, a shortish guy with grey hair, cleared his throat and said, 'I'm Stephen, the creative director.'

Clearly not too happy to be demoted to the guy who makes the pages look pretty then, although that sounded quite important to me. There was another odd thing about the meeting. These people were all laughing and joking with each other. On a Monday? A Monday morning? I looked round for signs of drug-taking or madness or even just the forced jollity that people sometimes put on in front of the boss. But no, this seemed... genuine. These people were laughing and joking around as if it were a Friday night at the pub with their bestest pals. Rather than a Monday morning in the office with a random bunch of people you spend half your life tolerating so that you can pay the bills. Unbelievable. It was an office unlike any I'd worked in before.

Now I've opted out of this life where I'm needed, where my opinion counts for something, where people rely on me, where I'm valued, where I feel part of a team that's quite special. I know, logically, it's the right thing to do, it's time for a change and I've had enough of weddings. But I'm a married woman in my mid-thirties with no offspring — so what is there to define who I am, what makes me me, if I don't have My Fantastic Job?

Day 104 — 4th April 2011

Lorna sent an email round at work, offering everyone the chance to win a weekend at the Corsewall Lighthouse near Stranraer. The idea was to have a silent auction that would go to the highest bidder, the proceeds going to CHAS, the magazine's official charity. Nice idea, I thought and a good way to get rid of a contra deal in a fair way. There were plenty of contra deals at work, where hotels would offer us free stays in exchange for advertising space. I emailed Rob but he wasn't up for it seeing as he's not feeling very well and we have a lot to do this weekend. Ah well.

Day 106 — 6th April 2011

Got a nice surprise today, an email from Lorna offering me and Rob a weekend at the Corsewall Lighthouse on April 15th and 16th. The email said Craig and Lorna had been talking and they'd like to offer me the weekend, dinner, bed and breakfast, as a thank you for all the hard work and commitment I'd shown to the magazine. I was really pleased. What a lovely way to end my time at the company, especially as I'm due to finish up that weekend. They must have had a couple of contra deals from the lighthouse to give away; glad I didn't go for the silent auction now!

Day 107 — 7th April 2011

Michelle is off on holiday this week so I'm checking her emails every so often. When I had a look today I saw one that was headed April 15th / 16th. Right away I knew what it was. I felt like I'd been kicked in the stomach. By someone wearing steel toecaps. It was worded exactly the same as the one I'd received offering me and Rob a nice weekend at the Corsewall Lighthouse, right down to the phrase 'as a thank you for your hard work and commitment' and the 'Craig and I have been talking' line. Except Michelle's email was more specific, as it said '... your hard work on the April issue of Real Life Weddings'.

I looked at the date: Lorna had sent Michelle the email a couple of days before the one I got yesterday and Michelle had replied to say thanks for the offer but she couldn't make that weekend as she had tickets for the theatre. I suppose what Lorna had done was pragmatic, but it tainted what I had thought was a nice gesture.

I was still reeling when I scanned down and saw another email I wasn't supposed to see. I didn't read it properly but from what I could tell, Michelle had written some kind of editorial review and Lorna had gone back with comments. The first thing I noticed was the salary Lorna had offered Michelle to do my job. She was offering Michelle six grand more than me. And I've been doing the job three years! I couldn't believe it. I felt so hurt. Was I a complete mug for doing the job so cheaply? Did she value Michelle more than she valued me?

I should have just stopped reading then. But I spotted my name further down. Lorna was outlining her plans for how the department would run and was basically telling Michelle that not only can she take on a features writer, she can also hire another part-time regular to write for the magazine. She mentioned me working freelance five days a month, doing some proofing. In brackets after this, she had written, "if we want her to". So what does that mean, if Michelle didn't want me involved Lorna would be fine with that?

I felt wounded by everything I'd seen. My stomach was churning. Of course I couldn't say a thing to Lewis, the only person in the office I would even consider confiding in, because I shouldn't have been snooping.

Day 112 — 12th April 2011

Lorna has pissed me off again. When she met with Rob while I was in hospital, one of the options she offered was that I could go freelance but with a guaranteed level of work each month. But now, I've had an email from her suggesting that I would get a guaranteed five days' work for the first month only, and we would see how it was working out after that. So not really guaranteed at all then. The message was full of pish, with bollocks phrases explaining how she wanted to bring more editorial in-house and "restructure the department". An empty bullshit phrase if ever I'd heard one! Just say what you mean. Did she think she could pitch it to me so I wouldn't notice she'd gone back on her word?

Day 118 — 18th April 2011

We got to my parents' place in Dumfries, having spent a nice weekend up at the Corsewall Lighthouse in Stranraer, my last ever wedding mag freebie. Pretty much the first thing Mum said to me was, "Rosal, you've got an overhang!", pointing to my stomach. She was amused rather than horrified by my belly.

"Mum! We've just spent the weekend eating five-course dinners and massive breakfasts," I said, somewhat defensively.

Those damn pills.

Whenever I feel a bit fat I think of the Mr and Mrs Quiz I had to do on my hen night. I was to guess what Rob had answered to the question, "Which is Ros's best physical feature?" It was multiple choice; her sparkling blue eyes, her figure or her hair. I guessed eyes and got it wrong. We all laughed when my sister revealed the answer: "No, sorry Ros, it's your figure. Let's hope you don't pile on the pounds when you get married eh!"

Doesn't seem *quite* as funny now.

Day 119 — 19th April 2011

Didn't sleep well last night, just couldn't switch off. I feel like I'm in recovery, but from what? I'd feel more justified in feeling low if I had something concrete to go on. If I'd been through drug addiction or alcoholism, for example. Or if I'd been abused as a child or even attacked in the street by a violent mugger. But my psychotic episode was due to what, getting stressed over *job-related pressure?* So basically working a bit too hard? It sounds so pathetic.

Mum and Dad had gone to the hospital for my Dad's cancer check-up — he has to go every six months since he had bladder cancer a few years ago. Rob was on the phone sorting out insurance for our newly purchased motorhome, so I was left in charge of the dog. Lucky me.

For some reason, my 67-year-old parents thought it was a great idea to buy a completely mental English bull terrier puppy called Jacques, who thinks sinking his teeth into your flesh is the best game ever invented. The breed is not classed as a dangerous one, but he can be intimidating sometimes. He's all teeth and muscles. Oh and snout.

"Are you sure it wouldn't be better just to get a normal dog, you know, a collie or something? One that's a bit easier to handle at your age?" I'd said at the time.

"Oh no! Once you've had an English bull terrier, other dogs... well, they just don't compare."

You don't see dogs like Jacques very often (although you will if you watch 'Oliver' the musical; Bill Sykes' dog Bullseye is the same type), which makes taking him out quite good fun. People stare in amazement and often comment on his muscly physique. But he is so strong that I wouldn't feel comfortable taking him for a walk on my own. The one and only time I'd held the lead for my Dad for a second, Jacques had pulled and almost dislocated my shoulder. He's pulled my Dad over at least twice. He is fairly good-natured (the dog I mean, although Dad is too) but he's oblivious to his own power.

I was sitting enjoying a bit of sun in the conservatory when he started making whining noises from his cage in the dining room. Thinking he must need a wee, I gingerly let him out.

Big mistake. Instead of going outside, he just lay down and refused to budge. I tried to drag him out but of course I had no chance. Eventually he gave me a dirty look and headed out to the back garden of his own accord. Soon he started barking to come back in, so I opened the conservatory door for him, but instead of walking to his cage like a normal dog would, he dashed into the dining room and started running round and round the table like a maniac, smashing his head against a chair every now and then. He was like a demented beast. Every time I opened the conservatory door to come in and try to put him away again he went even more mental, jumping up all teeth and spittle, launching himself at me like an absolute loon. For God's sake, Jacques needs some antipsychotic meds or something.

I was basically trapped in the conservatory with the dog on one side of the glass door and me, now scratched and out of breath, on the other.

"Oh for Christ's sake," I muttered as Jacques gave me a look that said 'Ha ha, got you cornered now, loser!' I sat down feeling silly and sorry for myself until Rob finally came off the phone and easily guided the little git back to his cage.

"What did you let him out for?" he said testily.

"Because I thought he needed a piss!" I shouted back. "Look what he's done to me," I said, pointing to the scratches on my arm.

"Well you should have waited until I'd come off the phone," Rob said, as if I was a complete imbecile.

"Yeah well thanks a lot for the fucking sympathy," I snapped, storming off into the garden. I sat outside on a chair as I waited for that annoying emotional watery stuff to pop up in my eyes again. Bloody hell, I can't believe that little bastard got the better of me! Imagine being outwitted by a freaking dog. I was pissed off I'd let it upset me too, and that Rob had snapped at me.

After a bit Rob came outside.

"I'm sorry but I'm a bit distracted because I've got problems with the insurance."

"Whatever," I said, not ready to stop being annoyed yet. Bloody typical. Rob's the most laid-back guy in the world, except in two scenarios. One: something goes wrong with his computer. Complete disaster. Two: something goes wrong with his car. Never mind. At least Mum and Dad returned from the hospital with good news; he'd got the all-clear for another six months.

We were all sitting around chatting in the conservatory later on and before long the conversation turned to me and work and what happened at Christmas. I thought about Friday, my last day at work. I'd been on edge all day, knowing that my workmates would give me some kind of leaving present. I dread that kind of attention. I hate people seeing my reaction as I opened presents from them. It had been fun in the end though. They gave me lots of nice things, chocolates and wine, plus a £60 voucher for Amazon. I wasn't expecting anything like that.

Lewis, one of my favourite colleagues, had put on the 'Dirty Dancing' theme tune, 'I've Had The Time Of My Life' and tried to get me to dance with him in front of everyone. Of course, I refused, far too embarrassed. But he just acted the clown, dancing around the office by himself and coming over to look mock-wistfully at me every now and then. We all laughed and everyone had hugged me and said nice things about how much they'd miss me. We reminisced a bit about some of the most memorable nights out we'd had.

The only downside, although it was something of a relief in a way, was that Lorna hadn't bothered coming in to say goodbye. She didn't usually come in on a Friday anyway, but had told me the day before that she would be there. It was Craig, the sales director, who let me know she wouldn't be coming in. I understood that having a baby meant you couldn't always stick to your plans, but not bothering to phone me and say so herself seemed a bit crappy. However, I hadn't yet responded to her email about the freelance work, so at least she wouldn't have the chance to ask me about it in person.

Although I felt hurt by Lorna going back on her word, I also found it difficult to accept that she'd acted badly towards me. Apart from the way she'd changed her mind over the guaranteed freelance work, Rob was pissed off with her about my sick pay. My contract said that, at my manager's discretion, I could be off sick with full pay for up to three months. But Lorna had decided I only deserved a month's paid leave. That didn't really bother me as much as some of the other stuff, such as Michelle getting paid loads more.

When we started discussing it, Rob seemed almost annoyed with me that I wasn't more annoyed with her.

"Sounds like Stockholm Syndrome to me," he said, laughing in that obviously-not-amused way he does sometimes.

I thought about it for a second.

"I think that's a bit over the top. She's never kidnapped me or taken me hostage or anything. She just didn't keep her word."

Rob looked sceptical. I tried to explain how, even though my job made me very ill, I felt a bit lost without it.

"Oh yeah, you will do," Mum said. "You're experiencing a loss of status at the moment. I went through the same thing when I retired."

Mum and Dad and Rob are all wise in their different ways and I felt better after we talked.

While Dad and Rob were off somewhere, probably fiddling with radiators or something, Mum told me she's not sure I realise just how much Rob went through at Christmas.

"I felt so sorry for him when he told me about falling over and spilling the Chinese takeaway," she said with big sad wet eyes.

"About what?" I said, feeling my stomach tighten. The thought of anyone in my family falling over has always made me feel peculiarly, physically awful. It's such a nasty image to have in your mind. And this was even worse, because it was my fault.

"When did that happen?"

"Oh you didn't know about that? When he took a Chinese in to you on your anniversary, because it was all icy outside he slipped and fell and some of the food came out on to the ground."

I put my hands up to my face. Oh God, that's so *sad*. I hate feeling sorry for Rob.

"God, he never told me that. That makes me feel terrible."

I found Rob on the computer in the hall so I went over to him and put my arms around his neck.

"I'm so sorry baby," I said. "Mum just told me about you falling over on our anniversary."

He didn't say anything for a second. I hugged him tightly, yet again feeling horribly guilty for putting him through all that. I expected him to softly say, "It's OK, don't worry about it Bosal. Don't get upset."

But he didn't. He burst out laughing! Not just a little bit, he was absolutely pissing himself, as if I'd told a brilliant joke. I can't believe him sometimes.

"What are you laughing for? It's so *sad*!"

"That's not sad, that's funny!"

His reaction was so unexpected that I even laughed with him after a second.

Our friend Stuart, who laughs quite a bit himself, once said that Rob would laugh at a door closing, and it's true that he does laugh a hell of a lot. Weirdly, he never cries. I wonder if those two traits are connected, that he needs to recalibrate his emotional gauges or something. I've seen his bottom lip tremble a few times but I've definitely never seen him cry in the seventeen years I've known him.

When I tackled him about his inability to cry, he said he had cried once since we were married.

"When was that?" I was intrigued and, strange though it sounds, glad in a way. Glad he wasn't completely emotionally stunted.

"It was when we got that massive bill in for the car last year, do you remember?"

Then it was my turn to laugh. His wife goes mental and he retains a stiff upper lip, but the thought of shelling out a big wad of cash, *that* pushes him over the edge.

We went out for dinner to celebrate Dad's news. I still felt pissed off with Lorna, lost without my editor status and guilty about what I'd put my family through. But it's almost impossible to stay angry while you're eating banoffee ice cream.

Day 120 — 20th April 2011

Got a check-up appointment with the head doctor later today. So they can check I'm not about to go mental again. It's with a new psych doctor, Dr MacReadie, and to be honest I'm relieved it's not with Dr Ali. Not because he's rubbish or anything, but every time I see him I'm slightly embarrassed. Not just because he's young and male and good-looking (happily married though I am, I'd still rather act like a loony in front of an ugly old female doc) but because every time I see him, I get a flashback to the first night I was in the hospital. When I was so deranged that I addressed him as Scarface, due to the rather large scar across his cheek.

I don't think I did it in an aggressive manner... having said that, I'm not sure it's possible to do such a thing in any other way. My little messed up brain must have been looking for something, anything, it could relate to. Unfortunately Al Pacino's gangster character popped into my head, at a time when my inner monologue wasn't working.

Ever since then, when I saw him I not only cringed as the memory came back, I also tried so hard not to stare at the scar that I probably overcompensated by staring at anywhere else on his face. I wondered whether, while concentrating on not staring, I'd accidentally fixed him with such an intense look that he still thinks I'm a weirdo.

So we're back at Shawpark, the mental health facility in Glasgow's Maryhill area. During the meeting I was surprised to find out that the doctors didn't actually diagnose me with depression, something I always assumed I'd been labelled with. Dr MacReadie told me that technically what I experienced was "a psychotic episode". I'm not sure if that's more or less scary than depression. Just different I suppose.

The doc seemed happy with my progress and the answers I gave. As usual I found it difficult to answer the one about how my mood had been since my last visit. I didn't want to say, 'Well I was pretty merry in the pub the other night'. I think I managed to come across as normal enough.

While we were in Glasgow I took the opportunity to go for a massage. Nicola, my masseuse (sorry, holistic therapist), said my decision to leave work definitely agreed with me.

"You had much less tension in your neck and shoulders this time," she told me.

On the way home I mentioned to Rob that the doctor was happy to reduce my dose of mirtazapine now.

"She said it's up to me, though. I suppose there'd be no harm in keeping it at 30mg for a while."

But Rob was adamant I needed to start reducing it straight away.

"I want *you* back Ros," he said, surprisingly strongly.

"But... how do you mean? I'm back to normal aren't I?"

"Don't be offended when I say this, but you're still not quite right. I only notice it because I know you so well."

I felt slightly stung by what sounded like criticism.

"Well, how do you mean exactly? Can you give me an example?"

"It's very subtle, and you're only about 1% different, but there are little practical things that you just don't think to do."

"What kind of practical things? I'm not really that practical at the best of times, am I?"

"Look, I can't think of anything at the moment..."

"Well next time I do or don't do something, you let me know."

"OK."

Day 121 — 21st April 2011

The adventure becomes a little more real today — we're off to pick up the motorhome we bought a couple of weeks ago. Once I see it I'll be able to imagine our big trip a little better. It's all very exciting but I'm also vaguely nervous about seeing what will be our home for the next six months.

We got up ridiculously early (6.30am) to go down to Birmingham and pick up the dream machine, the tin can of fun, the mega piece of machinery for our magical mystery tour, helping us shake off the shackles of thirtyness. Or something like that.

Rob's parents drove from their home in Somerset to meet us there, so that they could take our car back down with them and we could bring the Hymer back to Dumfries. If I could drive, they wouldn't have had to bother, so I felt slightly guilty about the arrangements. But they have plenty of friends in the Midlands — that's where Rob's family is from — so they claimed not to mind making the journey.

The Hymer was massive, much bigger than I'd realised from looking at the photos. A nice older guy called Pete, a Brummie with a moustache and shaky hands, talked us through all the features and showed us how everything works.

"I'm a caravan man myself, but this is a lovely piece of kit, lovely."

He said that a bit wistfully, as if he couldn't quite believe we'd be taking this lovely bit of kit away and out of his life forever. He took absolutely ages showing us all the bits on the outside. I couldn't wait to get a look inside.

"What do you think?" Rob said slightly nervously, once we were in. "Do you like it?"

I told him I thought it was pretty cool. It really has got just about everything you need inside, from a largish fridge-freezer and wardrobe to a shower, flushing toilet, hob and gas oven. (The oven even had a rotisserie, not that — as veggies — we'd have much use for it.)

Because it's a German motorhome it comes with a 19-inch boot horn as standard. I didn't realise that's what the long grey plastic thing was when I pulled it out of the wardrobe.

"What the...?" I said, showing Rob what I'd found while Pete was outside dealing with another customer.

"Ah, I ordered this specially. That's for me to keep you under control with if you get out of hand," Rob said, taking it off me and slapping it up and down in his palm trying to look menacing.

"Very funny."

I whipped it back and tried to whack him on the bum with it. He was fast though, so I had trouble making contact.

"Stop it! Pete'll see you. Don't! Stop being a daftie," he said, laughing and jerking his rear end out of the way.

Bonus: the motorhome has a built-in TV that Rob didn't notice when he first looked round! And you can watch it from bed. Or from *one* of the beds, I should say. There's a double at the front and another at the back. How good is that? Almost as impressive as the electric step. I loved this; you press a button by the side door and two steps miraculously emerge from the underside of the van, to aid your exit or entrance. Cool! Pete guided us through a whole host of clever little features, but the electric step was my favourite. He pointed out all the hidden storage spaces. Almost everywhere you looked contained some kind of cupboard or shelf. For example, large comfy fixed seats were set around the dining table, but when you lift their cushions they revealed empty spaces waiting to be filled with shoes and clothes. Or camping equipment, if Rob gets his way.

There was even storage space inside the steps that lead to the back bed. So well-designed.

Pete was talking about "catering quality water".

"Does that mean we can have a big party in here?" I said with a grin, but the blokes didn't seem to find this as funny as I did.

When Pete started talking us through the toilet cassette system and how to empty them, I said, "Oh there's no point me listening to this bit, Rob."

I'd said it more to wind Rob up than out of any serious intention never to help with the smelly stuff.

"Unbelievable, isn't it?" Rob said to Pete, shaking his head.

"The women always say that," Pete told him wearily. They shared a 'women, eh?' look.

After a very quick catch up and vehicle handover with Rob's parents, we headed back up north just after lunchtime. The first song that came on the radio when we set off was 'Street Life' by Randy Crawford, one of my all-time favourite tunes.

"I think that's a good omen," I smiled at Rob.

We got stuck in loads of traffic in Birmingham and Manchester. But it wasn't too gruelling because it was fun cruising around in such an unusual vehicle. People peered up at us from their cars and I noticed how high we were positioned; we were level with massive trucks and lorries rather than normal cars and vans. Our Hymer was a left hand drive, which is perfect for Europe, but in the UK it meant every now and then Rob needed me to check there was nothing coming up from the right hand side, before he pulled out.

"OK," I shouted, to make sure he could hear me all right.

Rob hadn't stopped smiling since we picked up the Hymer. He loved the automatic gears and — best of all — its cruise control function.

"This is brilliant," he said, laughing. "Literally all I have to do is move the steering wheel. You know, I have an amazing feeling of freedom now that we've got this. You realise we can go literally anywhere we want? Well, as long as we get the right visas."

When we got back to Dumfries my Mum and Dad were standing waiting for us in the driveway, eager for a look at the new machine. The other day we'd been chatting about motorhomes and someone mentioned that you sometimes spot women in the passenger seat with their feet up on the dash. Mum had screwed her face up in disgust and said vehemently, "Oh it looks so common when women do that. You might as well tattoo 'slag' on your forehead!"

A bit harsh, I'd thought. I thought it would be hilarious to stick my feet on the dash now to annoy my Mum, as Rob reversed in. She pretended not to notice.

Day 122 — 22nd April 2011

I've started using my Mum and Dad's Wii Fit thingy. It's great fun. I've done everything from rhythm boxing to juggling and even snowball fighting. Burning off a few hundred calories a day is the only way I can hope to compensate for my parents being shameless feeders. Every night we have a lovely big dinner, then dessert, usually ice cream or cakes or BOTH or maybe my Dad's homemade roly-poly. Whenever he made one of those I hoped I wasn't starting to ape the human Roly Polys, the group of fat older dancing ladies who used to perform with Les Dawson.

About an hour after tea, my Mum will get the chocolate biscuits or the Pringles out and we'll munch through them too. It's crazy. Whenever we get close to the end of a packet of anything, my Mum will cheerily announce, "Oh don't worry, we've got three more packets of those in the cupboard!"

If it wasn't for the Wii Fit I'd probably be morbidly obese by now. As it is I'm only just hanging on to my chubbier-than-ever status, rather than losing weight, which is what I need to do. I have a naturally slim frame but since Christmas I've started to develop an alarming beer belly. Or chocolate belly, since I don't drink beer.

Every time I complete an activity on the Wii Fit, it gives me a ranking, such as 'roaring fire' if I've done pretty well. When I do badly, it tells me I'm 'unbalanced'. You have no idea, I think to myself.

Day 153 — 23rd May 2011

We're down in Somerset for a while, giving Rob a chance to work on his Mum and Dad's loft; he's put a hatch in and has been insulating and flooring it too.

We're also getting ready to go on our big European adventure! There's a lot to do before we head off. We need to get inoculations and sort out our finances a bit, plus a hundred other little jobs.

The equally big news is that I now officially have a therapist. Not sure how I feel about that. It sounds so American. But I want to understand myself better and to understand what happened to me and make sure it never happens again, so I think it's a good idea. I have spoken to him on the phone and explained a bit about why I'm coming to see him. He sounded nice enough. He talked about "re-framing" what has happened to me; he believes thinking of it as a nervous or mental breakdown isn't helpful.

Today is Monday and I'm seeing him for the first time on Wednesday. He's asked me to compile a list of significant events in my life, from being born up to now. So here goes;

1976 — Born in Seaford, a small town near Brighton on the south coast. Mum, Dad and big brother Clive are around.

1979 — Sister Sylvia born.

1980 — Brother Adam born.

1986 — Family moves to Dumfries. I don't remember the move itself being traumatic but we move into temporary accommodation while we look for a permanent place. This means all four children living in one not-huge bedroom. There's lots of fighting between the siblings. I get the nickname 'donkey' because I kick a lot. My big brother regularly calls me ugly; I've got short hair, look like a boy and believe him.

September, 1986 — I start secondary school in our new location. Some kids make fun of my southern accent but I make friends OK.

1987 — We move house and I get my own room.

1993/4 — A friendship with a boy at school, let's call him Fred, goes wrong. He gets obsessed and when I try to break off communication with him, starts stalking me (I feel bad that I may have led him on), following me home etc. He pours a pint over me in the pub one night. The police are called and come round to the house to interview me, but I don't press charges.

September, 1994 — I move to Glasgow to go to uni, make some brilliant lifelong friends and have the time of my life.

September, 1995 — I find out that my school stalker lives in the next street to me in Glasgow, but he never contacts me. Just in case, my Mum gives me a pick axe handle to protect myself with. Me and my friends call it a Fred-basher. I never have to use it.

May, 1998 — Right before my final exams, I split up with Tinning, my boyfriend for the last three years. He doesn't take our break up very well. Dealing with the aftermath is stressful.

Summer, 1998 — I graduate with a 2:1 and start seeing a work colleague (he's a bouncer at a nightclub) who then cheats on me. It was never very serious (clearly not to him) but I am very upset about it. Then I start going out with Ewan, a good friend and housemate. This turns out to be a poor decision. We were much better as friends.

November, 1998 — Having split up with Ewan, I start seeing Rob, but we keep it quiet at first in case Ewan is upset. This doesn't make it more exciting, it feels horrible being deceitful.

New Year's Day, 1999 — Rob tells Ewan we are a couple. This causes massive problems within our close group of friends. Ewan and his sister Kirsty stop speaking to us for a while — this is devastating and has a massive impact on me and Rob. It's around now that I start smoking dope. Soon I'm smoking every night.

2001/2 — Unhappy with my career path (I can only get sales and marketing jobs, which I find unsatisfying) I go back to uni to study journalism.

January, 2005 — I get made redundant from my job writing and editing for a music magazine. This is a sacking disguised as a redundancy after I unwisely get a bit snappy with the boss one day. I was irritable at the time because I was trying to give up smoking cigarettes. He won't speak to me for three days then makes an example by firing me. I am upset and give up on giving up the fags.

July, 2005 — I start working for the Scottish Wedding Directory as a features writer. This is a good move for me.

June, 2007 — I'm promoted to editor.

Oct/Nov, 2007 — Dad gets bladder cancer, has an op and gets the all-clear. My sister is also unwell, though not for long. Our cat is diagnosed with terminal cancer. Not a happy or easy time then.

December, 2007 — I get married to Rob.

January, 2008 — Our cat dies, just before our honeymoon.

New Year, 2009 — I stop smoking cigarettes.

May, 2009 — Rob gets made redundant.

July, 2009 — I get really stressed out about a meeting at work and don't sleep much for about a week. This culminates in my boss coming to my flat for the meeting and basically (in a nice way) telling me to get a grip. A week later I get antihistamines from the doctor to help me sleep. I realise I'm a workaholic. All this is not helped by having a friend of ours, Malky, move in with us for a while. I feel I can't relax properly at home.

August, 2009 — I decide I need to leave my job so Rob and I come up with a plan to escape the rat race: we're going to buy some land in the north of Scotland and open a wigwam-style campsite. I stay on as editor but we work towards realising this plan.

January, 2010 — Rob decides to abandon the LED business/project he's been working on in favour of becoming a professional photographer.

August, 2010 — Rob launches his photography business. This means extra work for me helping out when I come home from my actual job.

November, 2010 — We put the flat on the market.

December, 2010 — I don't sleep properly for over a week due to work stress and eventually I'm sectioned and checked into a psychiatric ward, where I stay for three weeks. Once I'm allowed to go home I keep taking mirtazapine, an antidepressant to help me sleep.

February, 2011 — We don't find a property up north that's suitable for our wigwam project and decide to sell the flat, buy a motorhome and go travelling instead. In the meantime I go back to work.

March, 2011 — We firm up our plans and I hand my notice in.

Day 156 — 26th May 2011

Went for my first therapy/counselling session yesterday. Not really sure what to make of it. The therapist, Mike, is pretty old, maybe early sixties, with sticky out ears. He's bald apart from little bits of hair at the sides. I got a bit impatient at the start because he kept going on about 'sleep hygiene'; things like winding down, regulating waking and sleep times, exercising, not having too much caffeine or alcohol. The sort of stuff I've read about millions of times over the years.

He did make some interesting suggestions though. He recommended writing down my worries before trying to sleep, rather than waiting until I couldn't sleep and then making notes. He talked a lot about synchronising the mind with the body, so that you're always in the moment. He talked me through a few new techniques to help with that, and gave me a CD of guided meditation. He also recommended having worry space, so you set aside a time every day to write down worries, then leave it for 24 hours. At that point you start to write the way to deal with them, which makes it about problem solving rather than aimless worrying.

"What do you think would happen if you didn't worry so much?"

I thought about it for a minute.

"I don't know. I think it's to do with a fear of failure, of not doing things properly."

"OK. Well you should know that everyone has an element of them that is a 'hurt child', made up of bad experiences that they carry around with them. Most people have an identity and sense of purpose that overrides this hurt child, but I think your purpose and identity have been taken away by leaving your job."

"So what I'm left with is this hurt child version of me?"

"Exactly. And people in this position then tend to self-sooth. We do this in many ways, whether it's gambling, alcohol, drugs or food or a combination of these. Friends and family fall into the self-soothing category too."

He reckons it would pay to arm myself with some 'mindfulness' techniques.

"Going travelling could be the experience of a lifetime but when you look back in five years' time you might think, what did I do? If you don't learn how to appreciate where you are and what you're doing at that moment, you'll look back and wonder why you didn't appreciate the richness of the experience, because you were too busy worrying about what would happen next."

Interesting.

He asked how much anxiety I'm carrying around with me. I started to explain that at the moment things were a bit chaotic because of staying with my in-laws, who have two foster daughters...

"Yes," he said, cutting me off. "Our circumstances are not always ideal."

"Well, no."

I suppose that was his way of saying, life's not perfect and it's never going to be — get over it.

Later on, I sat in the study at Rob's parents' computer thinking about what Mike The Psych had said. I could hear Rob drilling or sawing stuff up at the loft hatch. I imagined a set of 'Shallow Grave' holes coming through the ceiling. Now, what was I going to Google again? Oh yeah, mental health stuff. I did what I usually did when something really interested me, researched the hell out of it. I loved immersing myself, knowing all I could about a subject. I found lots of stats. 3% of the population get sectioned at some point in their lives, one in four people has some sort of mental health problem in any given year. According to one study, around 300 people out of every 1,000 experience mental health problems every year. Of those 300, six will become inpatients in a psychiatric hospital. I prefer words to numbers, but that sort of statistic does interest me.

I discovered women are more likely to have mental health problems when they're premenstrual, which, with all those hormones flying around, makes perfect sense. I discovered that left-handers are more likely to go mental and are more likely to be insomniacs too. One study found that while 10% of the general population are left-handed, 20% of those with psychosis are. A later study put the second figure even higher. In that context, they meant psychosis as in conditions such as schizophrenia, rather than the state of being psychotic, which was more relevant to me. Anyway, this explains a lot doesn't it; a left-handed premenstrual female insomniac with perfectionist tendencies?? Surely it was only a matter of time before I succumbed to my natural disordered state. Joke.

After getting side-tracked for half an hour by all the things left-handers were more likely to do and be, I made the mistake of clicking on a link to a Guardian article by the irritating psychologist Oliver James, the guy who used to explain why all the 'Big Brother' contestants did the crazy stuff they did. The phrase from the piece that stuck in my mind was 'a weak sense of self'. Basically he was saying that anyone could go mental, but people who weren't strong-minded were more likely to be fruit loops. I got annoyed before remembering the idea of the supposedly subtle difference between genius and insanity. I just stumbled over the line, that's all. Way over the line. Got so far from the line I couldn't even see the line. The line went a bit wiggly. Etc.

Day 162 — 1st June 2011

Went for my second counselling session today. It was sunny outside so as we sat down I said, "It's a nice day isn't it?"

"Yes it seems that way doesn't it?" Mike answered.

No it doesn't *seem* that way, it's just a freaking nice day — fact! For Christ's sake.

This session was harder than the first one. Mike said we were going through it at about ninety miles an hour because he knows I don't have much time before I go travelling. I wish I'd written more notes but I was so busy thinking I didn't write much at all.

At first we talked about 're-framing' the hospitalisation. He doesn't like the word breakdown much, so I started using the term psychotic episode instead. He wasn't overly keen on that either.

"The thing about labels is they can be sticky and once you stick a label on yourself it can affect what you perceive as your ability to deal with stressful situations in the future. Psychotic episode is OK as a medical term but it's generic and what we need to do is personalise it."

"Well, how should I think of it then?"

"Perhaps something along the lines of, the situation exceeded my ability to cope. Think of it like a container, and all the stress gets added to the container and it goes down a bit and up a bit depending on what's going on and when you had the breakdown, the container overflowed. What led to it happening?"

"Basically I had one really bad week of not sleeping."

"It's not possible for something like that to happen in a week. It would have been building up for weeks or months. The thing about being stressed is you get so used to feeling like that that you don't even notice after a while. It often creeps up on you, it's insidious."

We spoke about how I feel having left my job and my negative thoughts about my relationship with Lorna.

"From what you've told me, I'd say you're grieving for your job."

I started laughing.

"I'm sorry but that just sounds ridiculous. How can you grieve for a job?"

"Well, what you've described is feelings of sadness, anger, loss... what does that sound like to you?"

I laughed again.

"OK, you're right, that sounds a lot like grief."

"You can grieve for all sorts of things, you know, not just people."

We talked about the things Lorna had done that pissed me off.

"It sounds like Lorna has been quite manipulative," he said.

"I don't know..."

However much she's annoyed me, I find it difficult to accept this. I still think of her as basically a good person, a nice, kind person. It's hard to accept that she didn't have my best interests at heart.

"It's interesting because workplaces are familial, as in we tend to revert to type there. We can think of it like a family and you would be naturally inclined to act as the big sister, because that's your role in your own family."

That makes a lot of sense.

"So who would be the mum and dad in your work family?"

"That would be Lorna and Craig. This is interesting because when I felt I'd been treated badly by Lorna, it felt like I'd been let down by my Mum or something. I wish I didn't care about her opinion so much but there you go, I do." Mike gave me a look that said 'that's your hurt child self talking, not your rational intelligent adult self'.

"But it's understandable you feel like that, because there were all those things Lorna could have done to ease the burden on you, which she didn't do. If we get back to this idea of the hurt child self and the adult self, think of it as the hurt child being in the executive chair when you're in a stressful situation. What you need to do is put the adult back in charge and say to the child, 'I acknowledge your presence but you're not in charge here. So you can stay but you have to sit on my lap.'"

Mike said from what I'd told him he felt I had a tendency to worry about other people too much and ignore my own needs, that that was part of what led to the hospitalisation.

"It's true that when I couldn't sleep, I was often thinking about other people."

"So what would you do differently if you could go back to before the hospitalisation?"

I found that quite hard to answer.

"Maybe I would have confronted Lorna about her not being on the ball. I suppose I should have externalised my feelings more. I definitely should have talked to Rob more as part of the problem was the uncertainty of where we would live after selling the flat."

Next we talked about guilt. I told him I felt guilty about what had happened to me, that it felt like such a *stupid* thing to have allowed to happen. My homework is to complete 'a pie chart of guilt' where I attribute slices to all the factors in my downfall. Mike says I'm driven by guilt and there's got to be another way.

***

Oh man! I've just been trying to get my repeat Mirtazapine prescription and it's a total nightmare. Why are doctors' receptionists so bitchy and unhelpful? Well, mine are at least. Maybe they're not all like that. They were supposed to have posted out my prescription last Friday. It's Wednesday now and it still hasn't turned up. I've only got two pills left. I phoned Shawpark to see if they could fax down a prescription and they said they couldn't do that as they're only advising the GP. Which meant I had to phone the Glasgow GP again and leave all the details with a nurse. Then some cow called Kirsteen phoned back and said they couldn't possibly fax the prescription.

"We're not allowed," she said.

"What do you mean you're not allowed, as in it's against the rules of the surgery?"

"Yes because we don't know where it's going, it might not be a secure line. All we can suggest is that you register with a doctor down there temporarily and ask for an emergency appointment."

I considered mentioning that they'd been willing to post my prescription, so obviously thought Royal Mail was *entirely* secure, but didn't think it would help. Instead, I went with, "Well, can I speak to a doctor please?"

"There isn't anyone here at the moment."

"What, you're telling me there are no doctors in the whole surgery today?"

I knew that my tone was becoming irate and that this wouldn't help the situation, but I couldn't stop myself. Her attitude was pissing me right off.

"There are no doctors available, they're all in a very important meeting together."

"Well I'd like to leave a message then."

"You can leave a message but it won't make any difference because we're not allowed to fax prescriptions."

What a cow! So now I've got to phone the local surgery at 8.30am to see if there are any appointments tomorrow morning. At the doctors round the corner they only have a surgery in the morning and it's very busy, but the receptionist (this one was actually quite nice, I must say) reckons the earlier I call, the better the chances of getting an appointment.

I can't believe how difficult it is just to get some bloody pills!

Day 163 — 2nd June 2011

I phoned the local docs first thing as advised, and they gave me an appointment for 11:45 this morning. Excellent. That was a lot easier than it had ever been getting seen at my Glasgow doctors. Now I just need to explain the situation to my new doctor and hope he agrees to prescribe some more pills. I sat in the surgery admiring their high-tech system; there's a big LED display that tells you when the doctor is ready for you and which room to find him or her in. And they have an automatic check-in machine. Very cool. While I was waiting I heard my phone ring. It was Rob.

"Hello. Guess what came in the post this morning?"

"Not my prescription?"

"Yep."

"No way! Right, I'll be back soon then."

I went over to the receptionist and explained why I no longer needed to see the doctor. When I got back to the house I looked at the envelope. No wonder it took so long to arrive — the postcode was marked 'PA14' instead of 'TA14' and rather than Stoke Sub Hamdon, they'd spelt it Stoke Sub Hampden, as in Hampden Park. Sheer incompetence! I'd spelt the whole thing out to them. Never mind, at least it's turned up now. I took it down the road to the pharmacy that's right next door to the doctors. Now I just have to sort out another prescription for enough pills to keep me going while we swan off travelling for six months.

Day 164 — 3rd June 2011

I was thinking back to that amazing feeling of freedom I had when I first got released from hospital. I was so happy just to be in the car, or browsing the food aisles of the supermarket. Everything felt new and amazing. I soon lost that appreciation of just being alive. I wish I could learn to enjoy simple things the same way again.

Day 170 — 9th June 2011

My medical notes have finally arrived! I've been trying to get my hands on them for ages. They even waived the £10 admin fee it usually costs, because it took so long.

It's weird to read comments about yourself written by medical people. Some of it made me quite sad, other parts made me laugh. I was pleased to see myself described as a "slim-looking woman".

I'd forgotten one of my consultants was called Dr Sowerbutts. I mean, come on! Surely you would change a name like that, wouldn't you? The bits when I kept asking for 'Nurse Rab' were quite amusing too. One thread that consistently runs through the file is how much Rob means to me. I'm either asking why he's not there, asking other patients if they are Rob, or worrying that he's going to leave me. I come across as obsessed!

I laughed when I saw the phrase, "Does not know where hospital is in relation to own home." That's completely normal for me!

Day 181 — 20th June 2011

We were on our way back down to Somerset after going to a wedding in Glasgow. I smiled as I thought about the way our friend Ally had greeted me when we arrived at the evening do.

"Ros! I haven't seen you since you were sectioned under the mental health act."

I laughed.

"Ally, it's so refreshing for someone to come out and actually say that. Most of the time I get an awkward look and they say, 'How *are* you?' or 'How are *you*?' I can almost see the italics, you know?"

My phone went as we hurtled down the motorway. It was Dr Scott from the Somerset surgery.

"Mrs Nash, I've received a fax from your doctor in Glasgow, a Dr MacReadie," he said.

That would be the fax requesting the Somerset surgery write me a prescription for a six-month supply of mirtazapine to see me through our travels.

"Right, OK."

"The thing is, your doctor didn't quite think it through. It's really not possible to give you the six-month prescription, certainly without having ever met you."

"OK."

"I think the best thing you can do is phone Dr MacReadie and she can explain the situation properly to you. If, after that, you want to discuss anything with me, by all means please do phone for an appointment."

"All right, I'll do that. Thank you," I said.

Bugger.

When I got through to Dr MacReadie she told me there were a couple of problems with asking Dr Scott to give me the prescription. Firstly, because I was still officially registered in Glasgow, he didn't have my medical notes to refer to. Also, official NHS guidelines state that a doctor shouldn't give a patient more than a three-month supply of any medication. She said some doctors were willing to make an exception to this rule, others weren't. Dr Scott sounded like the kind of person who fell into the latter category. Furthermore, as he'd said on the phone, part of the problem was that he'd never met me and therefore wasn't comfortable handing over hundreds of pills. All of this made sense, but was a pain in the bum for me. As I responded on the phone, I tried not to sound irritated or neurotic in a way that could make Dr MacReadie think I was going mad again.

Day 182 — 21st June 2011

Just back from my third and final therapy session with Mike. We talked about my propensity to worry, and recognising that.

"It's important not to overlook your innate perfectionism, which is typical of the experience you've had. What you need to do is notice when you have that tendency. To consciously learn that good enough is OK. Remember that striving for excellence motivates you, but striving for perfection demoralises."

Wise words, Mike, wise words.

"OK, but aren't high standards a good thing?"

"Yes, they can be. But it's important to learn to switch them on and off. Have no fear of perfection, because you can never achieve it. Think of having sentries on guard, looking out for perfectionism."

He started going on about being honest about "the beast in the cellar".

I think I'm right to assume this is a metaphorical beast, a part of me.

"What we do, what we all do, is we check the windows and the locks in this cellar by keeping ourselves clean, by paying attention to the details. Now we should be familiar with that part of ourselves and acknowledge that we feel this way for genuine reasons. Once we've acknowledged that part we can gently make peace with ourselves. Then we can open the windows and doors and say, 'This is who I am.' Once we've done that we can let some light in the cellar."

A bit wacky but I think I get his point.

I phoned Dr MacReadie's office again to see if there was any progress with my prescription problem. Her secretary told me she was still working on it. Damn, I would have liked this sorted out before we go to Glastonbury.

Day 188 — 27th June 2011

The Monday after Glastonbury was always a weird day. Back to reality... That phrase might imply I spent the whole festival stuffing my face with mind-altering drugs, whereas strawberry cider was about as wild as I got in the psychoactive stakes. The most addictive substance to pass my lips was a very moreish Mint Aero milkshake.

I stood in the shower at Rob's parents' house for a long time, thinking about the festival and luxuriating in the endless supply of lovely hot water. Luxuriating is really the right word, though it sounds like you should only ever read that on the side of a bottle of bubble bath. Showers were available at Glastonbury, though not readily. This year our little group of Glasto chums had gone for a bit of (relative) luxury. We'd paid a couple of hundred pounds extra each to camp in the tipi field, which not only boasted not-completely-minging composting toilets, but solar showers too. Queuing for twenty minutes or so was a very small price to pay for starting the day nice and fresh and squeaky clean. I wouldn't say everyone in our group was as bothered about the personal hygiene benefits of the tipi field, but for me those solar showers made the whole experience a great deal more pleasant.

Almost as amazing was the tipi itself. Normally at Glastonbury this is the order of events: 1) start out very early in the AM battling the immense traffic to get to the mammoth site itself, 2) queue for a couple of hours to get inside the gates, 3) walk several miles (I'm not exaggerating) from the Glastonbury gates to your chosen camping field, 4) collapse on the grass, fatigued having carried your stupidly heavy bags and tent and booze and wellies, 5) groan when you have to get up and move everything again because your friends decided to pitch their tents at the opposite end of the chosen field, 6) groan again when you remember that after all this, you haven't even begun pitching your tent yet, and because by then it's raining and your face is red from exertion and you're hungry and above all else you really just want a comfy chair and a cup of tea, not the beers people keep offering you, and you've just remembered you forgot to pack your comfy camping chairs too. It does get substantially better. But that's how I always think of the first part of Glastonbury.

However, for tipi dwellers, it's not like that at all at the beginning. At the tipi field you get a wristband. (Top tip; when readying yourself to offer a wrist, consider which hand you normally wipe with and *be sure to give the steward the wrist attached to the other one.*) Your smiley helpful volunteer gives you a map pointing out where to find your – this is the best bit – already-built, ready-to-collapse-in and complete-with-ground-sheet tipi. When you get to it, you just dump your bags inside and marvel at the huge canvas structure that is your home for the next five days. No pitching necessary, blooming marvellous! It's big enough to comfortably sleep six people, making it possible to slob around and socialise simultaneously (bonus), tall enough for even a very tall person to stand up in and – unlike most tents – protects you from whatever elements Mother Nature fancies blasting down on you. In warm weather, in a tent, you're forced to get up early, horribly dehydrated, because your tent has become an oven. Sun, wind, rain? They're nae bother when you're cosied up in your lovely big wigwam.

I don't think I could go back to pitching a tent at Glastonbury, after the wonderful tipi experience. It had felt slightly like cheating, living across two tipis with our little 'Glastonbury family'. There was a whiff of guilt, as I'd imagine you'd feel living in a gated community. But it was so comfortable, despite having five people in close proximity each night, with all the snoring and sleep talking and grunting that entails.

I'd been slightly worried about how I'd cope with the festival this year. There are lots of things I like about Glastonbury – the food, the heady atmosphere, the costumes, the lying around in the sun only half watching all the silly strange sights floating by. Oh and the performances, some of those are good fun too. Not just bands, musicians and DJs but comedians, acrobats, activists... and countless others. But Glastonbury can be overwhelming too. Could a bad festival experience trigger a relapse? I didn't think so; workplace worries had been my weak point and at the festival I would be among friends. But I wondered about the assault on the senses that Glastonbury feels like sometimes, whether that could push me over the edge again. That was my general worry. Specifically the worst thing that could happen to me was getting stuck in human traffic, in a big crowd I couldn't escape from. That could make me panic at the best of times, that hemmed in claustrophobic feeling. But I didn't really consider not going. My strategy was to keep Rob as close as possible without being irritatingly clingy. He could calm me down if I started to get anxious.

From experience – me and Rob had been six or seven times – I knew that I would sleep well; even with music going on all night, it was easy to drift off, probably because of all the walking (and daytime drinking) we did.

I'd mostly avoided the biggest crowds (and stayed calm when we did get caught up in them) and all in all had quite a lovely time. Sylv and Mark were there this year and the Robinsons (Charlotte and Mikey) had come along for the first time ever, all of which made it loads more fun for me. On the second or third day I didn't see Charlotte for a few hours. When we met up again she was completely Glastonbury-fied, with a massive henna tattoo down her arm and bright red dreadlock extensions in her hair. Charlotte is nearly always up for a good laugh, but it still made me smile to see her getting 100% in the spirit of things. She would never go for that hippy look in the normal world. We called her Rasta Robinson for the rest of the week.

Musically it hadn't been a bad year either. I saw Pulp, one of my all-time favourite bands, doing a special surprise gig at the Park Stage. Well, 'saw' isn't quite the right word. The position on the hill where Rob, Mikey and I ended up meant I couldn't actually see Jarvis at all, except on the big screens. But I definitely heard them. I looked around enviously at the skinny young girls getting a great view by balancing on their boyfriends' shoulders, but didn't think I'd feel safe up so high. Anyway, Rob had some strength, but the sad truth was I wasn't sure he could comfortably take my newly increased bulk. I might have broken his neck.

During the first few days of the festival, the collective crowd was split. Half the revellers were wetting their figurative pants at the thought of seeing headliners U2. The other half thought Bono was a bit of a wally (that wasn't always the exact word used) and would rather have gone to see Cliff Richard doing a turn in the hip hop karaoke tent. Actually that sounds unmissable.

Anyway, when the huge news broke that Bono had hurt his back and U2 couldn't therefore play, there was a lot of feverish speculation about who would replace them. Madonna? Kylie?? CHAS & DAVE??? On the day, Damon Albarn's Gorillaz stepped in, which made me very happy.

But the Glastonbury memories that lodge themselves properly in a little corner of my brain aren't necessarily musical. Sometimes they're comical little encounters with strangers, daft conversations with friends, seeing a policeman, in uniform, doing a backflip. I smiled thinking back to Sylv's outrage when Rob woke up, very early one morning, and immediately started talking, pretty much non-stop and to no one in particular. I can still picture her face as she swiped off her eye mask and looked at him, disgusted.

"Rob, it's half *seven*! It's far too early to start chatting for God's sake."
I think he was quite quickly forgiven, especially when he made the most of his early bird status, heading down the hill with Mikey to bring coffees and breakfast rolls back to the tipi. Breakfast in bed negates nearly all sins. Sylv's reaction had made me laugh because I suddenly realised I was so used to Rob's rambling early morning chats. It would never occur to me to be annoyed by them, despite my weak relationship with good sleep.

Now that I was back at Rob's folks' place, I felt the usual relief that I'd survived, not to mention quite enjoyed, another year at Glastonbury. I hadn't got trampled to death by the Beyoncé crowd. Or slipped over in the mud and broken an ankle. Or got food poisoning. Or mistaken hash cakes for normal ones, eaten three of them and come up smiling on Tuesday. Or tripped over a guy rope in the dark and knocked myself out. Or had any Portaloo experiences bad enough to scar me for life.

Day 189 — 28th June 2011

I checked my post-Glastonbury post and found a letter from Dr MacReadie, explaining that my new local doctors aren't able (willing, more like) to give me the six-month prescription, but that my Glasgow doctors are. However, it states that I will need to pick the prescription up in person. Well, that's clearly not going to happen. I'm not making Rob drive all the way up to Glasgow just to pick up a bloody prescription! I tried to think how else I could do it. Maybe I could ask someone to pick it up for me. I phoned the Glasgow surgery and must have caught the receptionist in some freaky kind of good mood, because she said, "I don't think that should be a problem."

Brilliant. I sent a text to my good reliable mate Jo, who replied to say she would be happy to go and pick it up for me. I felt bad asking her as she's pregnant, but needs must. Right, almost sorted then.

Day 191 — 30th June 2011

Bugger. Jo just messaged me to ask for the address of the doctors as she'd accidentally deleted it. Baby brain... I was kind of hoping she'd already have posted the damn thing, but she had to wait in for a parcel yesterday so couldn't go then. I tried not to sound demanding as I replied saying I really need it ASAP. She is doing me a favour, after all.

Later she messaged back to say it's done now and she's sent it next day delivery, so it should get here just before I run out of tablets. Phew.

Day 192 — 1st July 2011

I went to check the post as soon as I got up and was very relieved to see that my prescription had turned up. Good old Jo! I can't quite believe that I have the thing in my hands after all the trouble it's been. I should say 'things', because for some reason they sent two prescriptions, one from Dr Chapman, a doctor I haven't seen for a while, and another from Dr Ali, who I have seen recently.

As relief washed over me, I looked more closely. That's when I noticed it said 'six month supply, to be dispensed monthly'. What!? Monthly!? Are they having a laugh? The whole point is that I need six months' worth of pills to take *with* me, not to bloody well pick up once a month! I couldn't believe it and grabbed the phone to call the surgery. But as I was dialling I looked at the other prescription, which didn't say anything about being dispensed monthly. I hung up before anyone answered. Oh. So that's OK then. Thank flip for that.

I took it straight to the pharmacy down the road and handed it over to the friendly lady behind the counter. I paid and waited for the tablets, ready to be happy when they were safely in my possession.

I saw the lady who served me give the piece of paper to the beardy guy I remember from the last time I came in. I suppose he must be the pharmacist. He furrowed his eyebrows and said something to the lady. Oh blimey, what now? They talked for a minute before the woman came over to me with the prescription in her hand. Why has she not got a nice big bag of pills in that hand? And why is she frowning?

"I'm sorry, we're not allowed to take Scottish prescriptions."

Eh?

"But... but," I stuttered, looking over at the guy, "I got my prescription here last time, just a few weeks ago, and it was no problem then."

He came out from the back.

"Yes I know you did, but we had something in our bulletin not long after that, saying we couldn't take them."

I was completely stunned and asked him why they couldn't take them. I couldn't believe this.

"I don't know why," he said, in a kind-but-definitely-not-budging sort of way.

"I just know we're not supposed to take them any more. I think you could be a victim of NHS politics."

The woman at the till obviously felt sorry for me and while I was getting my money back, she asked whether I was registered with a doctor down here.

"Maybe they could help..."

"I'm registered next door," I said wearily, eyes close to bulging over with water now, as I tried to succinctly explain why I couldn't get a prescription there.

"Why don't you come with me and let's see what they say?" she said, leading me next door. The nice pharmacy lady explained what was going on to the receptionist, who said Dr Scott was free just now. Scot-free? Ha-ha. She phoned him and then led me down a long corridor. Dr Scott, a short thin wiry guy, came out of his office and met us in the hallway.

"Actually I'm just in the middle of something rather important," he said, talking to the receptionist instead of to me. Whereas me and my problem are rather trivial, I suppose.

"Can you add her to my list please?"

Why the hell didn't he just say that when she phoned him a minute ago?

Back down the corridor we went. I waited in reception.

"I'm sorry about that," the receptionist said.

"That's OK," I told her, although I thought Dr Scott was a bit rude not to acknowledge me.

I couldn't quite believe that five minutes ago I was about to get my tablets and now I'm here, without them. I didn't have long to wait before Dr Scott generously found a window for me. My name flashed up on the LED screen and I went down to his room and knocked before going in.

"Hi Rosalind, sit down please. Sorry to have had to keep you waiting there. Now, what can I help you with?"

I felt he already knew the answer to this but patiently explained what was happening as best I could.

"Right. Well first of all I'm sorry about this. I'm not sure about why the pharmacy next door couldn't process a Scottish prescription, you may want to double-check that with the local HCA."

He carried on talking while I wondered what the hell an HCA was.

"I'll just give you a little background into your situation from my perspective, and of course you don't have to agree with me. We received a fax from your doctor... sorry, I can't remember the name, a female doctor?"

"Dr MacReadie," I reminded him.

"But I telephoned Dr MacReadie and the thing is, what she was asking me to do was prescribe a medicine to a patient I'd never met. Now there were two problems there. First of all, she was asking me to prescribe to a patient whose history I had no prior knowledge of and whom I'd never met. Now don't get me wrong, it's great that I've met you now, but-"

I could see where he was going with this. It struck me that he should have my records, because I'd officially registered as a new patient here a couple of weeks ago. There hadn't seemed much point staying on at the Glasgow surgery when I didn't live there.

So I butted in to say, "Surely as my new doctor, you've got access to all my health records now?"

"No," he said. "At the moment I don't have access to any of your health records, not the records from your GP nor any of your mental health records. We wouldn't normally get these from your last doctor for at least six weeks after you'd registered."

I felt worse when he said this. Before that I was embarrassed because I thought he knew my 'mental health history'. Now I know that he doesn't; all he knows is that I've accessed mental health services. At least if he had my records he'd know I've only gone mental once!

I wanted to justify myself, to say, 'Look, you should understand that usually I'm quite sane. It's just I'd been working too hard and not sleeping properly...'

Of course I might as well have said, 'I'm not bonkers, honestly!' But you don't usually find sane people explaining that they aren't mad, do you?

He carried on talking, but I already knew he was leading up to saying he couldn't help, one way or another.

"There's also what's known as an oath of responsibility, which the prescribing doctor has to all their patients. That means if anything were to happen to you as a consequence of what I'd prescribed, I would be held responsible. What's also important here is that the medicine your doctor asked me to prescribe is an antidepressant, which potentially could kill you."

He paused for effect, let the phrase sink in. Great, so basically he won't give me the tablets in case I top myself. He used the same phrase two or three times in the course of the conversation, as if to underline that he's only refusing to give me a prescription for my own good. This struck me as a somewhat bizarre argument. I mean, if I wanted to kill myself I could easily just take a load of Paracetamol I'd bought from a shop. I thought I'd better not say that, in case he thought I was actively considering this.

"The second problem is that NHS rules state doctors are not allowed to prescribe more than three months' worth of any medicine. Some doctors choose to ignore this rule, but those are the rules."

"So I take it you wouldn't even consider giving me a prescription for one month then?"

"No," he said firmly.

I can grudgingly take his point about not knowing me or my history, but really can't see much logic in his arguments, apart from covering his own bony arse. I tried to emit a radiance of calm, rational, logical thinking, but what I really felt was anger that he wouldn't help me and embarrassment that he seemed to believe I could be a suicidal nut job.

"So where does that leave me, bearing in mind that I only have a couple of days' worth of tablets left?"

"Well, there are two courses of action open to you. You could try other pharmacies, or the only other thing I can suggest is that you post your prescription back up to Scotland, where someone can then go to a pharmacy there and post your medicine back down to you."

The thought of posting the damn thing back up to Scotland, when I've had such a palaver getting it here in the first place, and then relying on bloody Royal Mail to deliver the actual pills after that, just seems ridiculous.

I got up to leave and said, "Well, thanks for your time."

What I really wanted to say was, thanks for nothing you pompous little shit!

I shut the door to his office slightly too loudly, though I don't think you could call it a slam. Which I immediately regretted, because now he's bound to think, well, I did the right thing there didn't I? She's obviously unhinged. A bit like his door would have been, if I'd slammed it as hard as I wanted to.

As I wandered back to the house, dejected, I couldn't help wondering about the other side of his 'oath of responsibility' towards me. OK, it's natural he wants to cover himself, to not have a potential whack job ODing on his watch. But his sole focus appeared to be making sure I didn't neck all the pills at once. Surely he also has a responsibility to make sure I don't run out of the tablets that help keep me right, that supposedly help prevent me being a whack job in the first place?

I also think he's conflating two issues. He doesn't like the idea of breaking the rules by prescribing so much of a drug that could kill me, but I'm sure even a one-month supply could do that.

When I told Rob and his parents about the latest developments, they suggested phoning Rob's sister Catherine, who's a technician in a pharmacy. I was just going to use up some of my free mobile minutes to call her, but Rob's Dad dialled the number for her branch on their landline for me.

"Just ask for Catherine," he said as he passed the phone.

"Yeah, thanks for that Barry," I said, fairly irritated but trying not to sound sarcastic. Does everyone around here think I'm completely incapable? Who did he think I was going to ask for, the Easter Bunny? I felt bad for being short with him though, I knew he was just trying to be helpful.

I told Catherine the problem and she went off to check with someone whether her own pharmacy, Lloyds, accepts Scottish prescriptions.

"Sorry Ros, we're not allowed to take them either. Something to do with not being able to process them."

I couldn't believe this. I know it's an extremely minor difficulty compared to some people's problems, but that logic doesn't always make you feel much better. I suppose I could post the prescription to my parents in Dumfries. And I do have a few pills left over from my stash of the higher 30mg dosage that I was originally on, which I could halve for now to keep me going.

It's all just such a pain in the arse.

"What you could do is try the big Boots in Yeovil," Catherine said. "They might dispense it, because they've got a kind of drop in centre that's meant for travellers... I mean, people who, you know, aren't really registered anywhere."

"OK, thanks Catherine. I'll give that a shot."

I was pretty sure I would get the same answer from Boots. But amazingly, when I phoned them, the answer was yes, they'd process my Scottish prescription no problem. I felt lots better but didn't quite let myself stop worrying until Rob had driven me to Yeovil and I had the damn tablets in my hand. True to their word, they took my non-English prescription without raising so much as an eyebrow. Good old Boots!

Now that it was sorted out, I felt a bit silly for getting upset about it. I thought back to Barry advising me to ask for Catherine on the phone. He has a tendency to state the obvious and, looking back, that was all he was doing. This trait is legendary within the family. It had made for some great comedy moments over the years. I remembered a discussion between Rob and his Mum about how long it normally took to drive from Somerset to Wolverhampton. Barry had been silent throughout. Until he said, "Well, it depends how fast you drive." The rest of us looked at him for a second and then burst out laughing.

Day 197 — 6th July 2011

I dreamt last night that we went travelling, but we weren't in the campervan, we were in a horrible hostel where we had to sleep in the kitchen. Sylv was there too and she was asking questions about the next place we were going to stay at, which was in Tampere. Finland must have been in my mind because my brother Adam lived there for a while. Sylv asked 'Is it a proper flat?' and the crusty-type lady who ran the place said, 'Well, no. Actually it's just a wooden shed.' When she heard that, Sylv started getting a bit upset. When we went to sleep I realised I felt really odd and woke Rob up in a slight panic. That's when I noticed he had blood coming out of his ears and his belly button. Although I told him I felt strange, he didn't seem too worried, until we realised the carpet was wet because the crusty lady had spilt her LSD-tainted water all over it. As you do. The drug had seeped into our stuff and poisoned us in our sleep. An everyday story of country folk, as my Dad would say.

Day 208 — 17th July 2011

Finally, we're off! We've been planning this trip for so long I can't quite believe we're on the road at last. We spent our last night in the UK on the car park of the Golden Galleon, a pub restaurant in Seaford, the small town on the south coast where I grew up. I went inside, feeling a bit shy, to ask if it was OK for us to park overnight on the car park. The manager said that was fine, as long as we bought food there in the evening. Which suited us well enough.

This afternoon a group of Iraqi holidaymakers spotted the motorhome and came over, hugely curious about the vehicle.

"Did you rent it?" one of them asked, craning his neck around the door to get a better look inside. I wondered if it was impolite not to ask them in.

"No, we moved out of our flat and bought this," Rob told them.

"How much does this cost?" another guy asked. A tad nosy, I thought, until I remembered it's only the British who get uptight talking about money.

Rob, being British, avoided the question.

"Well, we sold our home and bought this instead."

"They were nice, weren't they?" I said when they left a few minutes later.

"Yeah, they were. I think this vehicle might attract quite a lot of attention," Rob said, looking pleased.

We drank wine over dinner, and talked about which countries we might go to over the next few months. My sister's Danish friend Sara had invited us to her wedding in Copenhagen in September, but apart from that we had no deadlines.

Day 209 — 18th July 2011
E15 Motorway, France

The adventure began in earnest today. Well, tonight actually, as the cheapest Channel Tunnel crossing turned out to be at 1.30am. We drove from Seaford down to Folkestone and waited in the car park until we could board. It was lashing down with rain and very windy.

Eventually we went through passport control. There was a very friendly policeman at the kiosk. He was easy on the eye too, with big chocolatey brown eyes and a good manly square jaw. I tried not to smile too much at him and let Rob do the talking. What is it about men and uniforms? Something to do with power I suppose.

Although we arrived at the check-in area well before all the other vehicles, we were the very last to be let on. It felt like we had to wait forever, probably because I was impatient to get our journey started. But when Rob finally got the nod and went to drive on to the train, he sat still looking at the barriers on either side.

"I'm not sure we can get through there, Ros," he said, looking worried. The assistant noticed our hesitation and came over. Rob opened his window and told her with a nervous laugh that he reckoned it looked a bit tight.

"Well that's actually the width of the train, so if you can't get through there..."

"Oh right. Well, it should be OK," Rob said.

It was. A minute later we were on board and the train was moving.

I was surprised by the size of the carriage, which was only just bigger than the motorhome itself. It felt more like a shipping container than any train I'd been on before.

"Isn't it amazing to think that we'll be travelling underneath the sea in a second?"

"Yeah. I reckon I'd rather not think about that too much," I told Rob.

For a split second I started to get The Fear, or maybe even just fear of The Fear, wondering if I was going to get claustrophobic. I realised I needed distracting, so we started playing cards and I forgot all about it.

It only took about half an hour to get across the Channel. By which time Rob had beaten me at Shithead, our favourite card game, four times. Damn!

We had our passports ready to show the French dudes as we drove on to foreign soil for the first time, but there was no one to show them to. We just saw a few signs reminding us to drive on the right. Nobody stopped us and within a couple of minutes we were on an actual French road. It all seemed a bit, well, unofficial.

Once we were on our way I felt a rush of overwhelming nervousness. I looked over to Rob but he appeared perfectly calm as usual.

We drove towards Paris for a few hours and, gradually, cruising along French motorways started to feel less nerve-racking and more normal. When we got tired around 3am we stopped at an aire. Europe has a network of aires, overnight parking spots designed for motorhomers. By sleeping at an aire in a motorway service station, we were breaking one of the golden rules of travelling by motorhome. When we researched the trip we read a hundred times how dangerous it was to do this, how you'd be gassed while you slept by gangs of criminals who would rob you of all your belongings while you were incapacitated.

We figured this place couldn't be too bad, since there were plenty of lorry drivers happy enough to stop for the night here. Anyway, all our valuables were in the safe and we had a gas alarm on the go too. Plus, we were pretty knackered. We were a little jumpy and hyper-aware of any strange noises outside. But eventually we fell asleep for a few hours.

Day 210 — 19th July 2011
Paris, France

We have just arrived at Paris De Camping, managing to avoid the city centre roundabout that everyone reckons is completely mental. Phew. This is a proper campsite, rather than an aire. Which means we are now 112 Euros poorer! And that was only for two nights. Gulp. That's what you get for camping in a capital city, I suppose.

Rob went to buy some food over an hour ago. I was starting to get slightly worried. I didn't want to phone him unless I really had to as it would cost us loads.

Eventually he came back, loaded up with quintessentially French shopping; baguettes, various cheeses and red wine. I was a bit disappointed he didn't have a stripy jumper, a beret and a string of onions round his neck.

"What a nightmare I had!" he said, laughing. Turns out in France you don't get your veg weighed by the person at the till, you weigh and price it yourself after you bag it. But Rob didn't know that until he got to the till.

"The woman at the counter just picked up the bag of tomatoes and shrugged, like 'what the hell do I do with this?'"

Luckily a nice Parisian lady took pity on Rob and nipped out of the queue to go and weigh his stuff.

We got stuck into the food and Rob took great delight in making me guess exactly how cheap each bottle of red wine was. I got it wrong every time, completely underestimating just how little a decent bottle can cost over here.

"But... that makes it cheaper than *milk*!" I said, thinking he must have got mixed up on the exchange rates.

"I know, it's brilliant isn't it?" he said, a massive grin on his face.

Everything — the wine, the cheese, the bread — tasted amazing. I could get used to this.

Day 211 — 20th July 2011
Paris, France

The aim of today was to have a nice time doing Parisian touristy things. We decided to walk from the campsite to the city. We told each other this was so that we could get a better 'feel for the place', and see more of it. But really it's more to do with our reluctance to fork out for an expensive taxi or figure out how the public transport systems work.

It was a long way into town.

We tried not to stare at the prostitutes peppered along the streets on our way in. Which was hard because I was so curious. I wanted to see how young they were, how downtrodden they looked, what kind of clothes they wore, whether I could spot any signs of substance abuse. There were so many of them! I wished I'd worn my glasses. Many of them jumped into vans, presumably to do the deed. They were completely blatant about it. Which makes sense considering it's not a crime here. I couldn't help feeling sorry for them, especially as it wasn't exactly warm and they were wearing next to nothing. Maybe getting cold is the least of their worries though. They looked pretty desperate to me.

We took photos of the Eiffel Tower and checked out the Champs Elysees. Both were impressive, but the aggressive begging at the big tourist draws was unbelievable, worse than I could have imagined, despite having been warned about it.

The kids were the worst, the hardest to sidestep. One little girl — she couldn't have been older than eight or nine — had a clipboard that she doggedly pointed at, using a pen and her eyes. She looked as determined and frustrated as she was desperate. She must be mute, I realised. I quickly scanned the form on the clipboard and understood that she wanted me to sponsor her in some way. I said no thank you and stepped to one side, but she mirrored my move and looked even more frantically from me to the clipboard. She was in front of me, blocking my path. She might have been determined, but physically trying to stop me leaving irritated me, taking the edge off my sympathy. As we pushed our way through the crowd I wondered whether, if I'd given in, one of her friends would have pickpocketed me as I filled the form in.

Not long after that we were conned into giving an African guy ten Euros. We had probably let our guard down a bit because we'd wandered into a less busy area, despite still being pretty close to the tower. As soon as he stopped us and asked Rob to put his arm out I realised this was a scam I'd read about. I told Rob not to do it but it was too late. The guy was quickly weaving a few different coloured threads together, throwing questions at us to keep us talking, obviously trying his best to distract us. Where are you from? What are your names?

"It doesn't matter what our names are," I said, pissed off and at least wanting him to know his falsely bright banter wasn't fooling me. Wanting him to at least know I wasn't stupid enough not to know we'd been had. When we mentioned Scotland, he was over the moon.

"Ah! Scotland! So do you like Glasgow Rangers?"

Bloody hell. Despite my mood I was amazed that this African Parisian guy had heard of the team.

I still couldn't believe this was happening. Now he was speaking some shite about how tonight we'd be making love and we'd see a flash and the Eiffel Tower and the bracelet would give us the best night of our lives. For God's sake, now he was trying to embarrass us into acquiescing. The whole process only took a few minutes and when the bracelet was plaited and tied on Rob's wrist he asked for ten Euros "for coffee". Rob tried to give him five, but he was well practised at being fairly insistent. While it's clearly a con, it was hard to argue with him, especially as — on the face of it — he'd sold us a bracelet. Bollocks.

Rob was incredibly pissed off but I just wanted to forget it now that it was over. I certainly didn't want it to ruin our day.

"Never mind, it's a lesson learnt I suppose," I said, once we were out of his clutches.

"Nightmare. I did hear you telling me not to put my wrist out by the way, but I kept thinking about all the money I was carrying… and there was no one around at all except a couple of his mates across the street."

"Yeah, I know. He could easily have robbed us instead. Or worse. The whole thing was pretty intimidating really."

On the plus side, I had the best hot chocolate ever today.

Day 213 — 22nd July 2011
Hamoir, Belgium

We arrived quite late at the aire. It was pretty dark but eventually we found the place where motorhomes were allowed to park.

"This is strange Ros," Rob said once he'd parked us in a good spot.

"What is?"

"Well, from what I've read it's pretty unusual to see caravans at an aire. They're usually just for motorhomes."

"Looks nice though doesn't it, from what you can tell in the dark. I'll put the kettle on shall I?"

A couple of minutes later, once my eyes had adjusted, I noticed an area nearby with a few tents pitched. I pointed it out to Rob.

"That's even stranger for an aire. Funny how we seem to be the only motorhome here as well," he said.

"Mm. I suppose they must have different ways of doing things in different countries."

I started getting set up for the evening. I was considering what I fancied for dinner when Rob came back inside with a big smile on his face.

"What have you found?"

"This place is brilliant! You get free electricity!"

He started fiddling with the knobs at the back, swapping the central heating and fridge from our own LPG supply to 230V, now that we had a free source of power.

"Look, it works fine," he said, pointing to the electronic display where the little plug symbol was showing.

"Blimey, that's well good isn't it. I didn't realise you'd get free lecky at these aire things. How can they afford that?"

"Dunno. I suppose it's a way of attracting tourists to the area," he said.

"Yeah but still... I mean, we're in a recession and everything."

In the morning Rob did a scout about outside, exploring now that we could see properly. I was making our first cup of tea of the day when he came back in, a funny look on his face.

"We need to move," he said, barging past me to start packing things away.

"Eh?"

I was still half asleep and none too pleased at the thought of moving, especially pre-caffeine.

"Why?"

"We're in the wrong place. I've just found the aire!"

I was too confused to question him so I just helped tidy things away, although Rob's mode of packing was much faster and slightly frantic.

When we started driving off I was about to enquire as to when I could realistically hope for a cup of tea, when I noticed we were slowing down again at the entrance to the aire. There were about ten motorhomes parked just outside the main gates.

"Oh! *This* is the aire then, not the bit inside?" I said, as the penny started dropping.

"Yeah, when I walked round I saw those signs," Rob said, pointing up. The signs were written in English and several other languages. They made it perfectly clear that the holding pen-style area outwith the gates, where all the motorhomes were parked, well, *that* was the aire. We'd inadvertently parked overnight in a municipal campsite, which you were supposed to pay for of course. Hence the 'free' electricity.

"Whoops," I started laughing. "Well, it did seem a bit too good to be true didn't it?"

Rob was laughing as well but he did look a tiny bit concerned.

"Do you think we should try to go and pay for last night?" he said, looking around as if he thought an angry Belgian campsite manager might be about to confront us.

"Nah! It was an innocent mistake. And anyway, it's really nice in there so it could be dead expensive. We're in the right place now, that's the main thing."

Day 214 — 23rd July 2011
Hamoir, Belgium

We've met some very nice Belgian people. We've also met some who seem a bit unusual. Take this morning, for example. We got woken up at 7.10am. By the sound of engines being revved right outside.

"Is that like… a lorry or something?" I moaned, groggy and bad-tempered.

Rob got out of bed to have a look.

"Oh. It's the other motorhomes, they must be about to go."

"They're taking their bloody time aren't they."

Why do old people get up so early? They didn't go though. They just sat there, revving their stupid engines!

"Why are they *doing* that?"

I put the kettle on, resentfully giving up on sleep.

"I dunno. I thought maybe they were just waiting till the condensation on their windscreens went or something. But they don't seem to be going anywhere."

"For God's sake…"

About twenty minutes later, the place was quiet. All the Belgian motorhomers had switched their engines off again. Some were making coffee, others were reading books or newspapers. They clearly weren't planning on going anywhere any time soon. So why waste the petrol?

"Oh I get it," Rob said a little later, when my morning grumpiness had worn off. "They were running their engines to charge their batteries."

I thought about it. He was talking about their leisure batteries, rather than their engine batteries. The leisure batteries power the motorhome's lights and taps. The inverter also feeds off the leisure batteries, converting the batteries' 12V into 230V, meaning you can, for example, charge up a laptop or a phone. You're totally reliant on leisure batteries when you don't have hook up or for devices that don't work off gas. And they cleverly charge themselves back up when you start driving again.

"I suppose that *kind* of makes sense," I said. "Although it seems a bit wrong to just sit here wasting petrol doesn't it? They could at least drive into town and buy some bread… or go for a day trip or something."

"Yeah it is a bit weird. Especially when they could just drive down there and get free electricity."

I got a shiver down my spine when the Kindle's free 3G finally kicked in and I read that Amy Winehouse had died of a suspected heroin overdose. What a sad cliché. She was 27 as well. Just like Jimi Hendrix and all the other creative self-destructive people who have gone over the edge. I felt even sadder when I read some of the nasty things people had written about her on Facebook. 'Good riddance to that junkie'. Jesus. Whatever happened to compassion?

I thought about my Mum's often-repeated warnings that there was a history of depression in our family. Surely you could say that about most families? I wondered if there was a history of insomnia too. Insomnia makes you feel incredibly lonely, as if the whole world is asleep except for you. Obviously this would never happen, because of time zones and when it gets dark, but that's how it feels. I suppose what I need to remind myself in the middle of the night, when problems always seem blacker, is that if I was to start getting anxious about not sleeping again, I wouldn't be alone. I'm not the only person who's ever felt like that. It's quite a comforting thought. I thought about the people in my life and the problems they've had over the years. I could think of a friend my age who had post-natal depression. (Not that we ever acknowledged it of course, we are British after all!) I could think of several older people who had suffered nervous breakdowns. I could think of a friend who suffered from SAD (Seasonal Affective Disorder) every year. I could think of lots of friends who were taking antidepressants for various reasons. I could think of people who had contemplated suicide, a few who had actually tried it and even a couple who succeeded. There were undoubtedly a lot more that I didn't know about.

I really wasn't alone. Even if most people experienced their problems on a less dramatic scale.

I liked the analogy that Rob used once, likening the human brain to a computer. My mind overheated, crashed and needed rebooting. A software update? I don't think I need a new hard drive. I thought of the TV programme 'The IT Crowd', when Moss gets knocked out and comes to again, to the sound of the Microsoft jingle. It feels less painful, less embarrassing to think of it like this, more a technical fault than a weakness of the mind, or a character flaw.

Day 215 — 24th July 2011
Damme, Germany

We're in a nice little aire with plenty of room for each motorhome. We're surrounded by Germans, funnily enough. They are all very friendly. There are washing machines here so we cleaned our clothes and hung them on a makeshift washing line (a bit of rope tied between two trees), hoping none of our neighbours minded us ever so slightly lowering the tone. Rob asked one of our German neighbours whether they minded our washing line.

"No of course," he said heartily. "You need to wash? You need to wash," he shrugged matter-of-factly.

Once we were settled in and had had our tea, I turned to Rob and said, "Right, what's next then? Another game of Scrabble?"

I was quite up for this as we'd had numerous games and I was in the lead, ha! Which is only right of course; my prowess in the word department is dominant in this partnership. Not that it's easy. Rob is very good at reading the board.

"Weeeellll, I could try and have a go at setting up the satellite dish, get a bit of telly going?"

"Ooh, go on then."

An hour later we were still struggling to get anything except a plain blue screen. I was about to suggest giving up when suddenly loads of channels popped up.

"Yay! We have TV," I told Rob, whose body was currently halfway out the back skylight.

"Nice one," he said, squeezing himself back in.

But that was the highlight of the telly watching. When we started flicking through the channels we found nothing at all we'd even consider watching. We dodged past one God channel after another — not really our thing — and loads of porn channels. Also not our thing. I'm using porn in the loosest possible sense of the word. Really it was just big-boobed women lying around in their underwear waggling mobile phones and other things at us, breathlessly encouraging us to call. No, thanks all the same.

"Ah, this is rubbish!"

I looked round at Rob but he was pretending to be hypnotised by the provocatively dressed lady filling the screen.

"Can you pass my phone please?" he said, with a wild lusty look in his eyes.

I punched him on the arm.

"Very funny. Come on Rob, flick!"

Eventually we came to some film channels.

"Brilliant, we haven't watched a film in ages," I said.

But most of them were on channels like Movies For Men, which should have been called Movies For Men Who Have Very Poor Taste In Movies. Or they'd play films in Arabic and no subtitles. Worse still, you'd spot a great film but about two milliseconds in realise something was very, very wrong. Al Pacino/Robert De Niro/Your Favourite Actor had been brutally dubbed into German.

We wasted another half hour searching for something we could bear to watch, and were about to give up when hey presto, what looked like a pretty good old World War 2 film lit up the screen. War films aren't exactly my favourites, but still. I could definitely watch this. It amused me that we couldn't bear anything dubbed, but we'll now happily forget how silly it is to hear German soldiers speaking to each other in English.

"Crank it up a bit, would you Rob."

It was one of those films that was so old the audio wasn't great. All the incidental background sounds were quite loud, but you could barely hear the dialogue.

It was when they started goose-stepping that it hit me.

"Rob," I said slowly, darting a quick look outside.

"Mmm," he answered, in that way I could tell he wasn't really listening.

"Rob," I repeated, in the insistent tone that makes him tune in.

"I'm not sure we should be watching this... you know, *here*," I gestured around us where plenty of nice old German couples were still milling around outside their motorhomes.

"Oh yeah," he said, looking from the Nazi uniforms and Swastika-adorned German army base on our telly to the real life people outside. The soldiers were really going for it now, hundreds of them marching along, only stopping to do the Hitler salute.

"Ah, I see what you mean. Maybe it does seem a tad inappropriate."

"Scrabble?"

Day 217 — 26th July 2011
Buxtehude, Germany

This is a great wee aire (or stellplatz, as they're called here), surprisingly close to the actual town. And it's totally free to stay here; the only cost is one Euro a night for electricity, so we really can't complain.

I was a bit freaked out that the friendly Germans kept saying 'hello' to us as we walked or cycled by. Shouldn't they say 'guten tag' or something? Had the word hello become international or did we just look incredibly British? A few days later we worked it out. It wasn't just us; Germans say hello (really it's more like 'hallo') as often as Brits.

Day 218 — 27th July 2011
Buxtehude, Germany
We made a huge mistake today; attempting to drive our three-metre high, seven-metre long motorhome into the centre of Hamburg. Cue raised blood pressure, going the wrong way down a narrow cobbled street, several near misses with hapless pedestrians and other hazards, and wasting lots of diesel while we failed to find a big enough parking space. We eventually gave up and drove back to our stellplatz, dejected. Thankfully Neil, Caroline and their young daughters Marin and Katie — who are on holiday here and were set to meet us in the city — didn't mind coming out to see us here in Buxtehude instead. It was nice to see them, and we all went out for a meal together. It felt surprisingly normal to see them in Germany, hundreds of miles from Glasgow.

Day 219 — 28th July 2011
Buxtehude, Germany
Rob has repaired the kitchen tap that broke yesterday. I'm lucky he's one of those handy-to-have-around men. He somehow knows how to fix just about anything. I do know a few other men (and women) who are skilled in this practical sort of way (they're not as brilliant as Rob, of course), but I feel a wee bit sorry for women married to the kind of bloke who would just 'get a man in' and *pay* someone else to install things and do repairs.

While I was pottering around in the motorhome today (it is possible to potter in it, though not as easily as in a larger space), I found the bon voyage basket our friend Linsay gave us when we said our goodbyes last month. It was filled with Scottish goods to remind us of home; oatcakes, Scottish tea bags, shortbread, there was even a Scottish beer. Such a sweet, thoughtful thing to do.

Day 220 — 29th July 2011
Flensburg, Germany
We are parked in a town right by the Danish border, at the harbour, a lovely setting.

I started thinking about being on deadline at the magazine, about how I just wanted it to be over when I was in the midst of it but missed the buzz when it was over. I wrote a poem about it while we drove through Germany.

Missing Deadline
It's that time again

hours vanishing
under your pen
And the only thing faster
than the tickety-boo clock
is the twitching your heart makes
like a jangly old lock

Between pangs of panic
you are having such fun
but how will you ever
get this thing done?
People ask how you are;
what they really mean
is tell me the end
can nearly be seen

Time plays cruel games
with its cryptic tricks
Mac/PC won't talk,
makes your patience itch
Now your senses are beaten
so restless and wired
No one mentioned all-nighters
when you were first hired

Instead of dreams
either sour or sweet
your brain hits replay
it's stuck on repeat
Your psyche's swept up
in a deadline loop
How many apt words
will colleagues dispute?

Now you're still awake
cos you care too much
But those typos, just one

is a kick in the guts
Perfection's your issue
a ridiculous aim
But you're always wondering
why don't they feel the same?

9am gatecrashes
in Groundhog Day vein
just work, sleep (no play)
keep going, and again
You can't wait till it's done
till this damn mag is away
yet when it's finally over
you don't feel so yay

There's just emptiness left
the end's so abrupt
When the pages are printed
your soul's not clear cut
What was that feeling...
fear, joy or some sickness?
Either way it's gone now
and you'd only just glimpsed it

Day 221 — 30th July 2011
Ringsted, Denmark

We've just left the strangest aire yet. This one was basically just a nice Danish couple's driveway. Which would have been odder, more awkward, except that they were very warm and welcoming. And the drive was quite big. They didn't want any money for us staying the night and even offered to hook us up with electricity. How nice is that? They're in their fifties and I think they run some kind of farm and bed and breakfast business. The guy's English wasn't brilliant (still a hell of a lot better than my Danish) but we got by as his wife's was damn good. Even though he wasn't fluent, when we said we were from Scotland, his eyes lit up and he started talking about whisky. Unfortunately we didn't have any whisky with us, so when we said goodbye he had to make do with a bottle of French plonk from Lidl and a couple of Innis & Gunn beers as a thank you. At least the beer was Scottish.

I've found that cruising along in the motorhome gives me the perfect opportunity to think clearly. Because we use a satnav I don't have to bother map-reading or looking out for road signs; on a normal day the most I do is key in a postcode or consult the aires book to find the next motorhome stopover. Random thoughts are free to wander up and down any avenue or back alley. And there's just enough happening on the road to keep me 'in the moment' (what an irritating phrase that's become!), which means I don't have too long to stew over unpleasant feelings. As we drove along the quiet roads towards Copenhagen, I started thinking about my stay in the hospital, specifically what led to it. Jane Austen said to think only of the past as its remembrance gives you pleasure. But I think she meant that in a slightly tongue in cheek way. My hospital stay had often popped back into my head, but I didn't push it away this time. How do you learn from your mistakes unless you look back?

I think the only way to describe my behaviour then — when I was delirious with sleep deprivation — is regression. My brain stopped working properly, broke down, operating on an increasingly simple wavelength that made less and less sense to normal people.

I'd been working really hard in the run up to Christmas and looking forward to almost two whole weeks off work. Nothing unusual there; it's always a busy time of year for me because the magazine deadline falls right before the holidays.

But it was worse than usual. I'd done fifty hours of overtime in the three weeks before it all kicked off. There were extra stresses too. We were launching a new online bridal forum in January and while it wasn't really anything to do with me, my Features Writer, Michelle, was spending lots of time on it, so she had less time to write articles for me.

My boss, Lorna, the owner of the company, wasn't really her usual self either, and hadn't been on the ball since she'd come back from maternity leave earlier in the year.

Even the weather made things more difficult. We'd had an absolutely ridiculous amount of snow and ice, it had been around for weeks. So I was constantly worried about whether my team, especially the graphic designers, whose workloads were particularly heavy in the last few days before deadline, were going to make it into work each day or not.

But all that still doesn't quite explain how I turned from a normal functional being into a mentalist.

I thought back to the few days before I went into hospital. What's surprising is how quickly I went downhill. I remember the week before Christmas being pretty tough. But again, that was normal. I remember not sleeping much in the last few days of the week before I went into hospital, taking antihistamines to try and get me through the week. Lots of people take antihistamines to help their minds relax enough to sleep. The downside is that you wake up with a very foggy head, and, of course, the more you take them the less effective they are.

Usually I am able to relax at the Product Design Christmas lunch (an annual get-together of Rob's old uni course mates and partners), which always falls on the Saturday before Christmas. This time I couldn't. I was so sleep-deprived I couldn't feel my teeth, and I was worried about the pages we had to complete on Monday. So het up that I wasn't able to function properly at the lunch. I felt paranoid, self-conscious and too edgy to concentrate on a proper conversation. I felt incredibly uncomfortable in my own skin. I was premenstrual and bloated and none of the clothes I tried on had felt right. I have a tendency to be indecisive but I literally couldn't make a decision about anything that day. I couldn't even decide whether to go to the damn lunch or not.

I was a wee bit hungover that day too. I'd worked late on the Friday. All day I'd felt like crying because I was so tired that everything seemed a huge effort. Part of the effort was putting a brave face on it, when I felt anything but brave. Because I was the editor, my theory was that people took their lead from me; so if I was outwardly stressed and tired and struggling, the rest of the team would be too. That's why I tried so hard to hide my fears. I'm not sure if I was kidding anyone, but that was my strategy.

Bizarrely, Lorna had decided to base herself at my desk that day, which made work a little more awkward for me. I kept wondering why she was doing that. Was she implying I couldn't do my job and she had to take over my role? The low point of the day was when I went over to grab a printout from my desk and spotted Lorna on my work email account. What the hell was she doing, checking up on me?

I went to the toilets and sat down in one of the cubicles, breathing deeply to try to keep calm. I was angry that she'd done that when I was working my arse off as usual, but more worried really. Why did she feel the need to do it?

Another niggling worry was the forty or so pages still left to do after the weekend. Usually by that point on the Friday we'd have nearly everything done. So when I got home I drank lots of wine, but clearly not enough to send me off into a lovely deep sleep. I woke up early feeling anxious and unable to switch off from work mode. What I should have done was talk to Rob about my day, express my feelings and all that. But I didn't. Maybe I didn't want to bore him with it all. Or maybe I was trying to put on a brave face again.

I had all but decided not to go to the Product Design lunch, but as usual my FOMO (fear of missing out) kicked in so I forced myself to get ready, even though it was the last thing I felt like doing.

I went home at 7.30pm because I just couldn't pretend I felt normal any more. I couldn't function well enough to socialise properly. I felt better once I got in the taxi home, like I'd just escaped from a fate worse than death. The taxi went past George Square and I noticed how pretty all the Christmas lights looked. I was breathing hard, so relieved I no longer had to pretend to be merry. But once I got home I realised there was no point going to bed because Charlotte and Mikey were staying over; they would come back with Rob and wake me up in a few hours anyway. I hoped they wouldn't bring anyone else back with them.

So instead of trying to sleep I watched TV for a bit, but everything on telly freaked me out. I watched some of 'Catch Me If You Can' with Leonardo Di Caprio, a film I thought might be comforting because I'd seen and enjoyed it before. It's about this total fraud guy who blags his way into different cool jobs; he has no training as an airline pilot, surgeon, whatever else, but talks the talk and gets away with each job for a while. I started to think the story mirrored my life, that I was a fraud and a liar, just like Leo's character. I flipped through the channels and settled on 'Blackadder', one of my favourite comedy programmes. But I started to think Baldrick was the only character I could relate to; I felt like I was really thick and everyone I thought was my friend was actually laughing at me and taking the piss. Or was I nasty and two-faced like Blackadder himself? Instead of laughing at the jokes Rowan Atkinson was making, I was a bit scared of him. He seemed so sinister, not at all funny. Was I like that?

A few days later, when I was further down that dark path, Rob and I watched a Christmas-themed episode of 'Miranda'. Every time she looked straight at the camera, I was convinced she was looking at me, that she was trying to give me some kind of message. When I think back to this now, it is clearly completely ridiculous, inexplicable. But that's how I felt.

Obviously by that stage on the Saturday night, the telly wasn't helping me.
I went to bed but found myself restless. I couldn't switch off from work and when I wasn't thinking about work I was busy worrying about other stuff. I started to worry that Charlotte, who likes a drink, would get too drunk, wander off from the crowd and something terrible would happen to her. Then I was worried that

everybody who was out that night would come back to our flat for a post-pub party, which sometimes happened after the Christmas lunch.

I should have known that Rob would never do that when I was not feeling good, but I didn't. I felt lonely and wished Rob was there so I could talk to him.

Eventually I phoned him, around 1am I think, trying to hide the fact that I'd got the heebie-jeebies, The Fear. I instantly felt better when I spoke to Rob but when I came off the phone I started to worry again. Was I a controlling person? He'd said they were coming home soon, but was that only because I'd phoned? Had I ruined their night?

I started to liken myself to horrible characters from TV programmes. I was almost completely convinced that I was just like Tony Soprano's mother. Which again is utterly ridiculous when I look back on it now — she tried to have her son whacked! I don't have a son but I'm pretty sure if I did, I wouldn't do that.

I felt very bad about myself at that point. I felt guilty that I'd taken a couple of antihistamines on Thursday night to help me sleep. I wondered whether I was experiencing some kind of comedown or payback rather than a hangover from last night's alcohol. All sorts of weird thoughts started going through my mind as I struggled to understand why I felt so bad. I wondered what I'd done wrong to be punished like that. I even thought there must be some big secret to life that everybody else knew about and I didn't, that I was being taught a cruel lesson.

My thoughts took such a weird turn that at one point I was convinced there was a God. This might not sound so outlandish, but since the age of about ten I've firmly believed that organised religion is a load of old mumbo jumbo, codswallop that people fool themselves into believing because they can't handle the idea of death.

This is around the time that I started to get stuck in a loop. Like a broken computer that doesn't know whether it's starting itself up or going into shutdown. I was trapped in a senseless circle. The old Mars Bar adverts kept popping into my mind, but was it time to work, rest or play? My body clock's instincts were out of whack so I didn't have a clue whether to eat, sleep or get up and work. Instead I spent time going round in circles, trying to do one after the other and not succeeding in accomplishing anything properly.

Not long after I spoke to Rob I heard them come in. I couldn't decide whether to go downstairs or not. I could hear them making cheese on toast and watching cartoons. They didn't sound particularly drunk. Had I *made* them come home? Had they been out having a good time then had to cut it short because I phoned?

Did they roll their eyes when Rob said they'd have to come home and look after me?

I sat on the stairs, undecided about what to do. I got a horrible feeling of déjà vu, the briefest of flashbacks... but to what? Had I been here before? Charlotte walked through the hall and spotted me on the stairs. She looked very glamorous and beautiful, with eye make-up showing off her thick eyelashes and hair all curly for the night out. Her eyes went wide with concern.

"Are you all right, Ros? You look like you've just had a really bad dream."

"I feel like I have, but I haven't been to sleep."

"Oh dear. Do you want a cup of tea or something?"

"Er, no but can you just ask Rob to come up and give me a big hug please?"

"OK."

I went back upstairs and heard her pass on my request. It felt like ages before Rob came upstairs but it was probably only a few minutes.

As soon as he put his arms around me I started to feel better, almost human again. Rob always had a calming effect on me. He pulled away and said he was just going downstairs to make some more cheese on toast for Charlotte and Mikey. I made him promise to come back upstairs as soon as he could. He was a bit drunk so didn't notice there was anything wrong with me. After a little while he still wasn't back but I couldn't stand being alone with my thoughts so I went downstairs.

"Are you OK Ros? You look really freaked out," Charlotte said. She might have been a bit drunk but I couldn't hide much from her.

"I don't know, I think I've got The Fear. I'm sorry, I don't know what's wrong with me... Do I always do this? Honestly, I'm not negative attention-seeking."
This last phrase is something I've picked up from 'The Sopranos'. Basically it's to do with displaying fake negative emotions in order to make yourself the centre of attention, acting as if you're going through terrible experiences so that people are forced to stop what they're doing and sympathise with you.

I'm not sure why I thought I would be guilty of this, I don't like being the centre of attention at the best of times. Charlotte, Mikey and Rob started being silly to cheer me up, repeating some of our favourite daft sayings in regional accents. They even managed to make me laugh for a second and I relaxed a bit. What was I so scared of? These people were on my side.

But then it was bedtime, and The Fear came back because I knew I wouldn't be able to sleep. In bed Rob's big open-ended hug made me feel better while it lasted. But eventually he fell asleep and I was left alone with my brain again. I couldn't believe it was Sunday already and I was still knackered and stressed out. The idea on Friday was we all took the weekend off and came in fresh on Monday morning. I was running out of time.

I managed to get a couple of hours' sleep but at 7am I was wide awake again. I would have been better getting drunk last night, I thought bitterly. At least that would have knocked me out for a while. I went down to the kitchen and Charlotte was at the sink, bleary-eyed, filling the kettle. She was such an early bird I wasn't surprised to see her.

"Have you slept?" she said with sleepy eyes.

"Not much. I think I might go for a run, get rid of some of this nervous energy."

She looked a bit surprised, probably due to the early hour and horrific weather, but only said, "Good decision."

But I couldn't face going for a run, especially with the ground so icy. I'd probably slip over and break my ankle or something.

"I so need to find another job," I said to Charlotte as she made tea.

"You've really got it bad this time, haven't you?" she said sympathetically.

She'd seen me stressed out before, but never in this much of a mess.

"I know. I'm sorry, I'm a rubbish host aren't I?"

"Don't be silly, you've got nothing to apologise for."

A little while later Charlotte and Mikey went home, but even when it was just me and Rob I couldn't relax. I had the feeling they only left so quickly because I was in a sorry state. That made me feel bad. What must they think of me? Then I realised we didn't even cook our best mates any breakfast before they went, and that made me feel even worse. What a rubbish friend I am! So self-obsessed.

I was also worried that I hadn't slept properly, that I wouldn't be fit for work tomorrow because of it. I felt miserable. Rob looked miserable too. I bet he wished he could leave too. I took a hot water bottle to bed, to see if the warmth would help me drift off. It didn't.

I came downstairs to see whether I could fall asleep to an old film on telly. 'Cleopatra' with Elizabeth Taylor was on. I thought a change of scene would help. It didn't. Nothing worked. Every time I got close to sleepiness I realised what was happening and got so excited by the idea of being asleep soon that I woke myself up before getting there. It felt like chasing a plastic bag down a windy street. Every time I got near, a new gust propelled it in the opposite direction.

I thought about the difference between tiredness and sleepiness. Most people can sleep if they're tired. For me, the two didn't always work in tandem. I read somewhere that sleep is like a cat. It only comes to you if you ignore it. My problem was I was doing the opposite; obsessing, desperately coveting that sweet restorer.

By Monday morning I'd only managed a couple of hours' sleep and Rob phoned in sick for me. But the idea that I didn't have to worry about going to work that day didn't help me relax. In fact it was even worse, because I kept thinking about what was happening without me. How was it going with the cover? Had they managed to get those last forty pages done? How many typos would go unnoticed because I wasn't there? Would they miss my help or resent my absence? Why did I care so much anyway?

I was still stuck in a loop, couldn't think clearly. I was semi-aware that I'd started talking in riddles. Rather than proper fully rounded thoughts, little phrases or sayings went repeatedly through my mind. I kept clutching a heart-shaped cushion, for example, saying, 'Home is where the heart is.' I was so sick of trying to sleep. Why couldn't I just sleep easily, like a normal person?

By Monday afternoon I was getting cabin fever. Rob decided a little walk might do us good; we'd get some fresh air and it would hopefully tire me out.

It was cold out and I felt a little shaky, unsteady on my feet. Everything was going in slow motion. Rob had his camera with him. I felt like a naughty little kid because Rob kept having to say, "Come on Ros, you can't just stop there, we've got to keep going. It's well below freezing out here."

I had the sensation that we were being watched. What if someone from work saw me? I was supposed to be off sick. I also thought Rob was trying to give me some kind of coded message, conveyed through the various places we stopped at along the journey.

When we got to the tunnel under Kelvinbridge, there was a really long icicle hanging from the roof. I was captivated by it.

"Look at that Rob, it's beautiful!"

I stood right underneath it and opened my mouth to catch any drips. I'm not sure why but it seemed a great idea. Rob looked annoyed. I couldn't understand why he wasn't fascinated by it too. Just then someone walked through the tunnel – I can't remember now whether it was a man or a woman, let alone anything else about them – and I tracked them with my eyes, even turning my body as I followed their path. They noticed me noticing them and said hello. I didn't react, except to continue following their progress with my eyes as they walked off. About a hundred yards out of the tunnel the person turned and looked back, saw that I was still looking. This didn't deter me. I carried on looking until Rob tugged my arm.

"Ros, please stop this, it's rude to stare. Come on, we've got to keep going." What was this obsession with 'keeping going'? The freezing temperature didn't bother me. I enjoyed being cold. It made me feel more awake, more alive.

The tunnel made me think of one of Rob's best photos, Don't Walk Away, which was taken from one end of the tunnel. The photo was of me from behind. I was wearing a red jacket, walking through the tunnel wrapped in a halo of sunlight. I thought Rob had deliberately taken me there, again to give me some kind of message. But what message? It wasn't as if I had been thinking of walking away. Or was he trying to tell me *he* was about to walk away?

Walking along the river, I saw a bench and it reminded me of Rob's parents, who got engaged on a park bench in winter. I wanted to stop and sit there for a minute but Rob thought that was crazy.

"It's freezing Ros, the bench is covered in snow. I'm not going to sit here in this weather."

I thought it would be romantic so I was unusually insistent, but Rob got even more annoyed.

"Ros, please listen to me. You promised you'd never stop listening to me."

Blimey. His face and voice were really serious. I stopped going on about it but didn't get why he was so bloody moody.

When we passed The Big Blue, the pub/restaurant we had been to loads of times, it made me think of my brother Adam and his ex-fiancée Catriona. That's where we'd taken them out to dinner when we first met her. I felt sad that it hadn't worked out between them, and wondered if somehow that could have been my fault. Maybe if I'd been nicer to her when they visited, she would still want to be with him.

Back at the flat after our long walk, the exercise hadn't done its job in making me sleepy. I was too far gone. The main theme going through my mind was worry, not just about work, but about why Rob seemed so annoyed with me. Of course, it didn't occur to me that he was not so much annoyed as concerned about me and my strange behaviour.

A weird phrase kept running through my tired mind; 'All I want for Christmas is a cup of tea and a nice sit down'. I kept thinking of my Mum.

Rob had to visit his printers in Partick that day, to pick up a couple of huge abstract photographic prints for a customer in Edinburgh. He'd promised her a pre-Christmas delivery. I was acting so strangely by then that Rob didn't think it wise to leave me alone in the flat. So we got in the car. We had Radio 4 on; there was a programme about professionals binge drinking. I was convinced that the presenters were talking for my benefit and nobody else's; not just that the item was relevant to me but that it was literally being played as a personal message. I thought Rob had set up the broadcast; it was his way of telling me I had a drink problem.

When we got to the printers I was supposed to wait in the car while Rob went in. But a few minutes felt like hours in my spaced out head. While I sat in the car I convinced myself there was a big secret that I wasn't in on. Rob and the printer were (obviously) part of this secret/trick/big joke/conspiracy. I felt compelled to find out what was going on. I don't remember locking the car but eventually, breathing hard, I chapped the door.

Rob looked surprised to see me but introduced me to the printer guy, who gave me a friendly smile. I started looking round the place, picking up random things. Rob kept telling me to leave the printer's stuff alone.

The next incident, of all the embarrassing things I did, is the most painful and difficult to look back on. I can still hardly bear to think of it. I'd got it into my warped head that Rob and the printer guy thought I was a skiver; they were working hard and here I was, not at work but off sick. I thought Rob had engineered this meeting to teach me a lesson. To teach me that lots of other people were working hard, that I wasn't the only one with a demanding job. This preposterous train of thought, the idea that they were judging me, led me to suddenly shout, "OK, OK, I get it! We're all in the same boat!"

I can still see the look on his face now, as the pleasant smile slipped, fading away to complete shock and dismay at this very weird outburst.

I wish I'd stayed in the car.

I shuddered as I brought myself back into the present. In some ways it's even worse to think of those times, of falling into the abyss, than of my three weeks actually in the hospital. I remember it more clearly, since I wasn't on a trolley-load of drugs then.

So how do I stop it happening again? I need to learn not to worry so much. To relax more, stop bottling things up, talk openly about my worries. Often when I'm awake in the middle of the night the thoughts go round in a loop. It's not a helpful loop, it's unproductive. I need to look for solutions during the day, rather than stressing about problems at night.

I looked across to Rob's placid face. I like it when he's driving because I can sneak a good long look without him noticing. I'm so grateful to him for pulling me through those three weeks. I'm annoyed with myself though, because as I got ill, I lost my focus, forgot to focus on him. I forgot for a while that as long as he's with me, there's no need for fear; I can cope with anything. God I'm so cheesy sometimes.

Day 222 — 31st July 2011
Copenhagen, Denmark

Blimey, Scandinavia is expensive. I am in shock. We have just shelled out what works out as about £50 — fifty! — for one night in a campsite six kilometres from Copenhagen. Again, city prices suck. This grates even more than Paris because we're still 6km from the actual bright lights and excitement of Copenhagen. But we really needed to use a laundry so we went for it.

I'm feeling vaguely annoyed with Rob, but I'm not sure why.

Rob, the sociable little imp, has befriended the nice young German couple in the camper next door. They're called Sven and Jess, and Rob's just informed me that they're coming over "for a beer" soon.

Jess was pretty and blonde with rosy cheeks and Sven had brown eyes and wore a baseball cap. I thought he was in his mid-thirties, like us, until he took his cap off. His baldy head made him look older. Their English was very good, so it was easy to chat. As usual, I was embarrassed that I couldn't return the favour and talk in their language. I can't even count to ten in German.

Their campervan was pretty clapped out looking, and they told us all about the problems they'd had with it so far. They broke down and got rescued by a Swiss family in the wilderness of Denmark, eventually getting towed to a hotel where they had to wait a week for the right parts to arrive.

It struck me how nice it was to talk to someone other than Rob for a change. That must be why I felt irritated by him earlier, sheer overexposure.

It turned out Sven and Jess were doing a very similar trip to ours. They'd both given up jobs to go travelling for a while. We all agreed it must be good for the psyche to see different places.

"You are so lucky to travel for six months," Jess said. "We are going for two. But when you are just working, working, working you can feel like you are on..." she paused, looking around as she searched for the right phrase, "a hamster wheel," she finally said, with a satisfied smile.

"That's definitely true," I said. "But I find it funny, some of our friends' reactions to our trip. So many people are jealous, saying, 'Oh I wish I could do that', but I keep telling them, you could do this if you wanted to!"

Jess and Sven were nodding.

"It's strange how people think we're brave for doing this," Rob said. "It's not really brave at all," he said with a laugh. "It's not like we're camping, or doing the trip on foot or something."

"Yeah, that *would* be brave," I said.

"But many people think it is strange to leave a good job and a good life," Jess said, "because they are scared of losing things. But you can go back to that conventional life. You can always get back on the hamster wheel later."

That's very true, I thought to myself, you can opt back in. It's fantastic to have the chance to try living in a different way, but it doesn't have to be forever.

We sat outside, between the two vans, drinking and chatting until it got dark. I was vaguely aware of mosquitoes and made a half-hearted effort to put some repellent on, but I'd drunk enough wine to not really care.

The next morning I wasn't quite as blasé about it. I counted eighteen bites on my legs, arms and face. Insects love me so I always get about twice as many attacks as anyone else. I also had a nasty fuzzy red wine head. Ugh. Rob claimed to feel not bad but I had the feeling Jess and Sven felt at least as rough as I did.

Day 223 — 1st August 2011
Kristianstad, Sweden

We've found an amazing spot in a car park just a couple of minutes away from a beautiful sandy beach. We were surprised not to find any other motorhomes parked up.

After dinner, we went for a walk and then settled down to a game of Scrabble. But when it got dark we started hearing strange noises; it sounded like someone dropping bits of scaffolding. Although we couldn't see where the weird noises were coming from, we noticed some strange behaviour in the car park. Cars kept pulling in, waiting about twenty seconds and then speedily driving off again. What were they up to? It didn't make any sense.

"Rob, I don't like this."

"What do you want to do? Find somewhere else?"

"I don't know, I just have a bad feeling."

We waited for a while, peeking out the tiniest of gaps in the blinds at the back and the side of the vehicle. No cars turned up for a bit but we could still hear the scaffolding noises every now and then. It all seemed very odd but we had been drinking last night. I wondered whether we just had the heebie-jeebies.

Were we making something out of nothing? That's when I saw a guy walking right past the motorhome, wearing what I'm pretty sure was a holster. It was very dark, but I'm certain he was carrying a shotgun. That was enough for me.

"Rob, can we find somewhere else? There's no way I'm gonna be able to sleep here."

We took a look at the aires book and found a place that was only a ten-minute drive away. Which was good, because it was nearly midnight by then. But when we got there we spotted the dreaded sign; a motorhome with a red circle round it and a diagonal line going through the middle. Damn, no motorhomes! We looked at the book again, and found that the closest aire was about an hour from there. We drove to a place called Sandviken, where the aire was basically just a big car park. It was easy to park, because there was loads of space and only a few other motorhomes.

"What do you think was going on at that other place?" Rob said when we'd settled in.

"I don't know, but I'm really glad we're not there any more."

I fell asleep almost as soon as my head hit the pillow.

Day 224 — 2nd August 2011
Eksjo, Sweden

I woke up to the sounds of people laughing, chatting and slamming car doors. I pulled the blind down a notch and looked out the window by the bed.

"Bloody hell Rob, it's totally mobbed!"

What had been a very quiet car park when we turned up in the middle of the night was completely packed out with cars full of beachgoers this morning.

We got out of there pretty fast, Rob adeptly manoeuvring his way through the car park without hitting anything or anyone. We drove to Stallplats Lyckarp in Eksjo, Sweden. It's pretty with lots of big old trees everywhere and, best of all, it's nice and quiet. It costs seven Krona a night plus three for electricity. All of which you put in an honesty box. How quaint.

Talking over our sharp exit the night before, Rob remembered that he had spotted a huge factory quite close to the beach, which could have accounted for the strange clanging noises.

"What about the guy with the shotgun though? That was well dodgy in the middle of the night."

Rob agreed at the time. But later in the trip we got more used to seeing people out with guns; we soon learnt that it was quite an everyday activity all over Europe.

The weather was lovely and warm today so I sat outside writing my diary.

We met a lovely old man who is either the gardener or the owner. It was impossible to tell as he didn't speak a word of English, which at least made me a bit less embarrassed not to know any Swedish. He looked a really sweet old guy with twinkly eyes and a constant smile. But he started doing that thing British people do, thinking, oh surely they must speak a *bit* of my language? Perhaps if I say it again, slightly louder this time, they'll understand me. So we kept saying stuff that he didn't understand and he did the same. This went on for some time — one party speaking, the other concentrating, thinking it through, then shaking our heads and looking blank — before we all started laughing about it and resorting to sign language.

Then clever old Rob had a brainwave. He got a map of Scotland out and pointed to Glasgow to show him where we'd come from. Turned out the old guy had been to Orkney on holiday and he took great delight in tracing out his route for us on the map. It feels like whoever you meet, there's always some connection with Scotland.

As I sat enjoying the sun this afternoon, my mind wandered back to the hospital. I remember thinking I was on trial for something, that I was in prison, then trying to find answers to a non-existent puzzle. I remember worrying that I'd done my memory some serious permanent damage. And I kept getting stuck in the same loops, physical and mental ones. I felt so sorry for the other patients, and then I'd realise with horror that I was one of them. Other people must have pitied me in the same way.

What's that Shakespeare quote again? Something about doubts? I looked it up on the Kindle: 'Our doubts are traitors and make us lose the good we might oft win by fearing to attempt.' I think when I was ill, the traitors took over.

Day 225 — 3rd August 2011
Eksjo, Sweden

Certain things you take for granted at home need a little more planning when you're living in a motorhome. Having a shower, for example, is only possible when we know we have a source of water nearby. You have to wait about half an hour for the water to heat up. Rob isn't too bothered about showering, but I can only go a maximum of about four days between showers without feeling really grotty.

Washing clothes can be a challenge. Hand washing is OK, but it's quite labour-intensive and takes ages. It's difficult to rinse properly so that all the soap comes out and because you're not machine spinning, unless the weather conditions are perfect clothes can take days to completely dry. Plus, there are only certain places you can do it because some aires don't allow washing lines. And of course it's not as effective as a machine wash.

Using a launderette brings its own set of problems. They're difficult to find when you don't have the internet, they're expensive, and they're usually located slap bang in the middle of a town or city, which makes it difficult to get the motorhome anywhere near them. And once you're in, you have to figure out how to work the machines using instructions in a foreign language.

On the plus side, because these mundane chores are a bit more of a hassle, we definitely appreciate the results more once mission's accomplished. It's as if you take a couple of steps down Maslow's hierarchy of needs; you become satisfied just by achieving the really basic, simple things. The other stuff doesn't really apply. For example, having a whole set of clean, dry clothes is brilliant and the lovely clean feeling you normally get after a shower is multiplied tenfold when it's your first for four or five days.

For some reason food tastes better on the road too. And there's also a lovely feeling when everything is right within the motorhome. When we're stocked up with food and LPG — the gas that powers the heating, oven, cooker and fridge — the waste has been emptied and the water tank is full, it's almost as if we're invincible; nothing can stop us now!

We both love riding round new places on our bikes. It's a quick, free and environmentally-friendly way to explore. I do have a rather bad case of 'biker's bum' though, which, I would like to point out, is nothing like 'builder's bum'.

While we were out on our bikes today, we met a guy from Durham. I thought he was a Geordie at first, but not quite. He introduced himself as 'Mr Simmons'. A very formal way to say hello! He was parking up his Hymer when we met him, so Rob and Mr Simmons had a nice blokey chat about chassis and engines and all that stuff that sparks my auto-tune-out button. Now, Rob likes to chat, there's no denying that, but Mr Simmons gave at least as good as he got on the word count score. The man wouldn't stop! I wondered whether he was always as talkative, or whether it was a consequence of travelling alone, grabbing conversations whenever he got the chance.

By the time he'd reached his seventh or eighth fairly detailed anecdote, I was feeling quite an urgent need to go to the toilet. Too much tea. I was too polite to try escaping just yet though; I'll wait till the end of this story, then that's it, I bargained with myself.

"I met this guy who was sellin' Es," he was saying.

Oh, well this sounds a bit more promising than the stories he'd shared so far. But he got to the end of his tale with no mention whatsoever of drug dealing. Or anything even half as exciting. I was confused.

"What about the ecstasy?"

He looked blank, as did Rob.

"How d'ya mean?" Mr Simmons asked.

"Well, didn't you say this guy was selling Es?"

They were both looking at me as if I'd said something incomprehensible.

Everyone was quiet for a minute, unsure where to go from there. Then Mr Simmons started laughing, a big rocking laugh so genuine I suddenly found him quite endearing.

"I never said he was selling Es, woman, I said he was Ceylonese! He was from Ceylon."

"Ohhhh, I see! Sorry. From Sri Lanka you mean?"

"Ah, they're always changing the names of these places aren't they."

We laughed a bit more, and I managed to cut off his tenth story at the pass, before I wet myself all down my bike.

Day 226 — 4th August 2011
Riksettan, Sweden

We're in a lay-by (I must start calling them picnic stops, it sounds ever so much nicer) with no facilities, but it's nice enough with plenty of trees and greenery. We've just been out on our bikes, which allowed Rob to invent a new game, called How To Annoy Your Wife On A Bike Ride. The rules are easy to learn. First, make sure you're naturally fitter than her even though she looks after herself a lot better. Second, simply pepper the conversation with any or all of the following 'helpful' phrases during the bike ride, preferably when it's 25°C;

"If you used your gears properly, this would be easier than walking, you know."

"What do you mean you're tired? We've only done fifteen kilometres so far!"

"Well, I hate to say it, but you'd be finding this a lot easier if you'd practised using your gears on the flat yesterday, like I told you to."

"Did I bring water? For a piddly little 20km cycle?? Don't be silly!"

"WRONG GEAR! You'll know when you're using them properly because you should be able to maintain the same number of revolutions per minute, whether you're going uphill or not, like I'm doing – see, it's easy!"

"Come on, work a bit harder or we won't get rid of our beer bellies."

Just before a massive hill: "I seem to remember this is a really flat road coming up..."

On seeing a 70kph speed limit sign, gesticulate sarcastically towards it as you say, "Now try not to break the law won't you."

At the end: "Blimey, you're not out of breath are you? That's really funny, I haven't even broken a sweat!"

The game ends with The Wife hurling a volley of expletives in your direction, getting off her bike and walking home with an angry look on her big red face. No one wins, except possibly the divorce lawyers.

Day 227 — 5th August 2011
Stockholm, Sweden

I take it all back about driving into city centres. We are currently parked right on the harbour and getting here was a doddle. What a brilliant location. And best of all, it's free!

We took a wander round the city and got caught up in some changing of the guards ceremony. Once it started the police refused to let anyone leave the area until it was over. It went on for ages with hundreds of tourists trapped in a little square together. I was getting hot and thirsty and it was all a bit tedious, until some dude in a tatty old Volvo found himself in the middle of it all. Instead of reversing out, he started doing a three point turn that escalated into a thirty point turn. He took ages doing this, but what made it really funny was that you could tell from his face he wasn't the slightest bit embarrassed or flustered. Meanwhile the police and army guys were increasingly aggravated by the lengthy hold up and gesticulated more and more wildly at him, frantically blowing whistles until he finally left. As he drove away, still looking completely unfazed, the crowd started clapping and gave him a great big cheer. What a cool guy!

Back at the motorhome I burnt my hand. The way it happened was silly. I went to put an oven glove on so I could move a hot tray. But before I got there Rob touched the tray and said, "That's not hot, feel it." Like a fool, I did.

"Jesus fuck!" I shouted, dropping the tray and knocking over two full glasses of red wine. I'd stupidly forgotten about Rob and his asbestos hands. I swear he must have some kind of freakish incapacity to feel pain. I mean, the boy actually enjoys getting an injection at the dentist. The skin on three of my fingers immediately started blistering and throbbed painfully. I glared at him.

"For fuck's sake, Rob."

"Sorry, but it didn't feel hot to me," he said, shrugging sheepishly. A couple of hours and an ice pack later, I'd just about recovered.

There's a Gay Pride Festival on in the city this weekend. It is also free. So we wandered around looking at the random stalls and admiring the costumes. There was some live music but it was pretty cheesy in a Europop (ie not good) sort of way. We bought a couple of glasses of red wine. They cost more than a three-course meal back home. Ouch.

Day 231 — 9th August 2011
Nikkaluokta, Sweden

We are in a car park next to the start of the walk up to Sweden's highest mountain, Kebnekaise. Rob completed the walk in record time. Most people do the walk in (the part that gets you to the base of the hill) on the first day, camp overnight, walk the mountain itself the next day and then camp out again that night, walking out on the third day. Rob decided it was daft to waste three days on one little mountain. Even though it's over 2000 metres high, starting almost from sea level. So he did the whole thing in a mammoth twenty-hour stint. Which is pretty mental. Especially because it's a year since he's climbed a munro. To be fair, he felt under pressure to get it done quickly because we had less than a month to reach Copenhagen for the wedding.

I was quite relieved when he got back to the motorhome safe and sound. However, he was absolutely buggered and walked like an eighty-year-old for about three days afterwards.

Things have gone crazy at home. There were riots in London and the violence spread across England. Apparently a black guy called Mark Duggan was shot and killed by the police, and that sparked off all the trouble. The chaos in the UK triggered thoughts of my own personal chaos just a few months ago. I was surprised I hadn't felt more scared of going mental again since we'd been travelling. You might imagine I'd be full of anxiety. Waiting for The Fear. Worried the worries would take over again. Or nice and calm on the surface, with a seething mass of neuroses bubbling just under the surface, invisibly but inevitably spiralling out of control off camera. Like a pot on a hob, happily simmering away but essentially volatile, ready to boil over if someone cranked up the gas.

Especially because I'm a natural born worrier, and travelling around in the middle of nowhere, hundreds of miles from home, could feel like a frightening scenario if you stopped to think about it. And I certainly had plenty of time to think. I had flashbacks every now and then, but they didn't cause much anguish. The worst ones made me feel uncomfortable for a minute, but very often that was followed by a feeling of relief that I wasn't in hospital any more.

In general though, I didn't feel bad at all. Maybe there was an element of levelling out, an emotional recalibration where little things affected me disproportionately. But on the whole I was pretty relaxed. I was pretty sure that insomnia and work stress had been my main problems, rather than some deep-rooted underlying psychological susceptibility. Even as that thought popped out, I wondered whether this was self-preservation. Whether it was just easier, more convenient, to blame the madness on a combination of sleep deprivation and work stress. Instead of believing it was a core part of me. It's impossible to be 100% sure.

It was odd that I had such an unbending (surely unjustified) faith in the pills I was taking. I kept thinking there's no way I'll have a relapse while I'm on these anti-depressants. As if they were magic beans. I did feel nervous if I had two or three consecutive bad nights' sleep, a slight knot of fluttery anxiety in the stomach, but I was learning not to bottle up my fears. Of course, insomnia is much less frightening when you have bugger all you have to do the next day. And I was confident that if I started going loopy again, I'd spot the signs and shout for help before it went too far. Fairly confident.

Day 233 — 11th August 2011
100km south of the Finnish border, Sweden

We're in a lay-by/picnic-style stopover with no facilities but quite a few other motorhomers, all silver-haired as usual.

We stocked up on red wine today, because although Sweden is expensive, it's not nearly as expensive as Norway. Much later in our trip, we found out that we had so much wine squirreled away in the back of the vehicle, we were unwittingly carrying far more alcohol across the border than you're legally allowed to bring into Norway. Whoops.

I phoned Mum today, as it was her birthday.

"So you're OK then, you two?"

"Yeah, we're fine Mum."

"You sure?"

"Yeah, of course–"

"You would tell me if you weren't, wouldn't you?"

I laughed.

"Mum! I just said so! What makes you think we're not?"

"Well… it's just… to be honest, Rosalind…"

Oh God, my full name. That always meant trouble.

"Go on Mum, spit it out will you?" I said, trying not to sound impatient.

"Well, you know when you went round to see your friends before you left?"

We'd dropped in on a couple of mates on our way south, so I knew what she meant.

"Yeah," I said, wondering where she was going with this. I hated the thought of worrying Mum and worried was exactly how she sounded.

"That wasn't you… saying goodbye was it?"

"Eh? Well, sort of. We probably said, 'Cheerio, we'll see you when we get back', that sort of thing. But–"

"I thought you were… you know, p'raps permanently saying bye."

"What? You mean you thought we were gonna… like… Jesus Mum!"

"So you're not then?" she said in a quiet voice.

"No!" I let out a kind of half-laugh, half-cough, more shocked than anything else.

"How could you think we'd do that?"

"Well we were telling our friends about what happened to you and they said they understood exactly how we felt because their daughter had tried to kill herself. I had no idea…"

"Mum, there's no need to worry about that, OK? I promise. Just because your friend's daughter… bloody hell. So, anyway, what did you get for your birthday?"

We had a fairly normal conversation after that. I got off the phone and told Rob he wouldn't believe what Mum had just said. He looked shocked, vaguely annoyed.

"Seriously?"

"Mental eh."

"I can't believe she'd think that, of either of us."

"I know."

This was a classic example of something that had been bothering me on and off since I was sectioned; other people's newly formed perception of me in the light of my Mental Health Problem. I've always been a worrier, but while I feel that being sectioned is something that happened in the past, I also now find myself worrying about other people worrying about me! What I should be concentrating on is not worrying so much at all.

***

At 2am, we were rudely awoken. Rob heard someone trying the side door, and then there was a knock. Some guy was talking to us in Swedish. Rob walked over to the door where the voice was coming from.

"In English please?" he said, croaky with sleep.

"Oh, sorry," the guy replied, switching effortlessly.

"Do you have a dog?" he wanted to know.

"Er, no, we don't."

"OK. Do you know if anyone else here has one? We find him wandering along the road by himself."

"Er, sorry, no I don't know."

"Well, sorry to disturb you. Goodnight."

And then he was gone. I was slightly concerned that he had tried to open the door before knocking – was he attempting to rob us? – but as Rob said, he might have knocked first, while we were still asleep. Rob peeked through a gap in the blinds and saw the guy going over to the motorhome parked about a hundred metres away from us.

"Ah, the dog's gone in. Must be theirs then."

"Right, good. Back to sleep."

Day 235 — 13th August 2011
Alta, Norway

What a beautiful spot. We passed some unbelievably stunning scenery to get here and even spotted a reindeer on the road. Amazing. I can see why everyone raves about the fjords. Now we're parked by a lake, right by the water's edge, with mountains in the background. It's completely gorgeous, like the highlands on steroids.

Day 236 — 14th August 2011
Alta, Norway

Rob wasn't feeling too well today, so I went for a long walk on the beach by myself. We're still in Alta, but at a different place now. We're right by the water again, but closer to the road now. It's lovely and sunny.

Good news: we managed to tune in to BBC World Service on the radio tonight. It was lovely to hear English and Scottish voices.

Very very bad news: the iPod broke today. So when we can't get a decent radio signal (most of the time) we are music-less. Our quality of life on the bumpy Norwegian roads has plummeted to a new taciturn low.

Day 237 — 15th August 2011
Near Hammerfest, Norway

It's amazingly warm considering how far north we are. We're above the Arctic Circle and the land of the midnight sun. Actually we're a couple of weeks too late to see the real midnight sun, but the lack of darkness is strange nonetheless. Even now it never gets properly dark. Generally you see a big orange sun dip under the horizon, producing a tangerine sunset. A couple of hours later the sun pops back up. It's quite something. And it has the weird effect of not triggering the usual feelings of tiredness, even late at night. I'm glad we have blackout blinds.

Hammerfest is a beautiful coastal town, with each house painted a different bright colour.

Rob met some Norwegians who told him to avoid Nordkapp, the most northerly point in Europe. We had planned on going there, but apparently it's very commercial, touristy and expensive. They reckon Nordkinn, the most northerly point on the mainland, is much nicer, so we're going to head there instead.

I'm getting a bit tired of Scrabble, even though I'm winning 8-6.

Day 238 — 16th August 2011
Near Gamvik, Nordkinn, Norway

The landscape on the way here was so weird. It's unbelievably remote and barren, making me think of the surface of the moon. The roads are strange too. I was wondering why a country as rich as Norway couldn't afford to tarmac a few more of their roads, but Rob told me tarmac wouldn't work this far north.

"Tarmac would be completely destroyed by the freezing conditions here. That's why they use these dirt tracks instead. And even then, every year in the spring they have to re-lay them, because they get washed away when the snow and ice melt."

"What a pain in the bum."

We parked up, had some scran and decided to go out to watch the sun setting. But we were running a bit late by the time we'd had dinner and washed up and ended up running down the road to get to a nice spot in time. The sun disappeared much faster than we'd reckoned on so, we pretty much missed it. I thought it was quite funny, but Rob was really upset.

"Bloody hell."

"It's OK. We can always see it tomorrow can't we?"

"We need to get going tomorrow. We don't have time to stay here another night."

"Oh. Well, OK. But I don't get why it matters so much," I said softly.

"I just thought it would be romantic, that's all, watching the sun go down together."

He said this in such a small, sad voice that a huge wave of sympathy washed over me.

"Why do I always mess things up? I can't seem to get anything right at the moment."

"Don't be silly, you haven't messed anything up. You're brilliant Rob."

He is usually such a happy person that it shocks me when he gets melancholy like this. Back at the van we had some wine and Rob said he might stay up to see the sunrise instead. I thought about it for a second.

"Well, why don't we both go? We could stay up and watch the sunrise together. That would be nice wouldn't it?"

He looked at me. "But wouldn't you want to go to sleep before then?"

"That's OK, I'm sure I can handle one night without much sleep."

So we packed some snacks, red wine and a couple of hot water bottles in a rucksack and made sure we were well wrapped up.

At 1.20am we walked a little way until we found a great spot at the top of a cliff. All we could see was the ocean. We drank red wine and stuck the hot water bottles underneath our jumpers to keep warm. Although the sun had dipped down under the horizon it wasn't really dark and it started getting lighter again around 2.30am. I couldn't believe how fast it happened. It was beautiful and we had such a good laugh, talking and taking silly photos of ourselves. All of which looked really really bad, which made us laugh even more. We'd had enough wine that even though every single one looked terrible, it didn't put us off trying again. After each shot, one of us would say, "OK, one more try. Now try and look normal this time."

I started snorting with laughter, very ladylike.

"Rob!" I punched him on the arm to get his attention, even though I already had it. "Rob, look at this one. You look really fat!"

When we'd both stopped laughing Rob said, "Thanks for cheering me up, Bosal."

"Oh that's OK."

"You always manage to do that," he said softly, putting an arm round my shoulder.

"Hey, look at that!" I pointed towards the most beautiful fox. He had snuck up and was sitting just a few feet away looking up at us.

"Wow," Rob whispered, trying to get his camera out without startling him. But he didn't look the least bit frightened. He looked curious, if anything.

"You know, he's probably never seen a human being before."

How does Rob *know* these things?

"You realise what it is, don't you?" Rob said. Does he think I've gone gaga again or something?

"Er, yes Rob. It's a fox," I answered, leaving the 'well, duh!' unspoken.

"Yeah, but it's an *Arctic* fox."

"Oh, I see what you mean. But... wait a minute, if that's right shouldn't he be snow-coloured?"

"Noooo," he said, barely containing a snigger. "They only develop white fur in the winter, don't they."

Of course. How silly of me. Why would their fur be the same colour all year? That would just be mental. He disappeared for a second (the fox, not Rob) then popped up even closer.

"Look Ros, he's sniffing the air."

"I told you you should have had a shower. Or maybe he wants some red wine," I said, laughing at my own stupid jokes.

"Throw him some chocolate, quick."

I gently chucked a few pieces of dark chocolate in his direction, hoping it didn't look like an attack. He looked a bit unsure, sniffed it for a while and then snuffled it up.

"Cool, look, he likes it," I said. I threw him a wee bit more but then remembered something that stopped me.

"Hey, you aren't supposed to give chocolate to dogs are you. Doesn't it give them a headache or something? What if it's the same with foxes?"

"Ah it'll be all right," Rob said, throwing him another piece. "He's obviously enjoying it, look."

"Yeah but it could be like diabetics and sugar. You know, they love the taste but it'll kill them if..."

"Oh stop worrying, Ros. It's very unlikely to kill him."

When he scampered off we checked out the pictures on Rob's viewfinder. There was one really excellent shot; the image was totally sharp and the angle and expression of the fox were perfect.

"Oh Rob, that's brilliant."

"Yeah, it's not bad is it."

"You'll have to call it Fantastic Mr Fox."

We sat admiring the image for a minute.

"See," I said, whacking him on the arm again. I really must stop doing that. "If we'd made it to the sunset we'd never have met him, would we?"

"That's true," he said, smiling.

Day 239 — 17th August 2011
Landersfjord, Norway

After our late night with the fox we woke up at 2.23pm. We drove back into town and although there wasn't a whole lot going on, there was a cool wee shop attached to a place called the Red Tree Hotel. It had loads of quirky things for sale, including some unusual, pretty glass-blown ornaments.

We ended up chatting to a South African guy called Ruan, who runs and owns the shop as well as an expedition company, with his Swiss wife Tina. Ruan had a part-time job in a fish factory as well, which he was planning to keep until they'd built the business up. He told us a bit about an amazing trip they'd taken together, walking all the way from Norway to Romania, in aid of a medical condition called CHARGE Syndrome. I'd never heard of it before and made a mental note to look it up later.

I was amazed to hear that when he got back, his feet were one and a half sizes bigger than before he went. That's mental.

"All the walking must have got really tough towards the end?" I asked, wondering if that was a completely stupid, obvious question.

"To be honest, it wasn't so much the walking that was tough. By the end we were so fit we were literally running up mountains. What was difficult, though, was the media constantly following us around. At one point, I couldn't even go for a pee without someone watching me."

Blimey. Now I felt even more ignorant for not having heard of the condition.

"What about walking in Russia?" I wanted to know. "Isn't it quite difficult to get a visa?"

"Yeah, well we originally asked for a permit to stay in Russia for a month, but they only gave us permission to stay seventeen days, so we just had to do it, had to walk it much faster than we'd have liked."

"Wow," I said, thinking what a huge country it is.

"It must have been a big test for your relationship," Rob said.

"Well, a lot of people wouldn't have put up with what Tina did. I mean, we just slept under bushes on the street some nights. The amazing thing is that we didn't have one fight in all the time we were away. We know each other so well we don't even have to speak sometimes to know what the other one is thinking." Very admirable. Although I couldn't help *slightly* thinking, oh shut it you smug git.

We took a look through his photo books of the trip. When I say photo books, I don't mean photo albums with little prints stuck inside under pages of cellophane. He'd gone to the trouble of having a proper hardback book produced, filled with stunning, colourful full-page images and minimal text. As we looked through, he explained that they'd had to curtail the trip they'd originally planned because Tina became seriously ill and had to be flown back to Switzerland for emergency medical treatment.

"Oh no. Is she OK now?" I asked, really hoping there wasn't a tragic reason why we hadn't met her.

"Yes, thank goodness, the doctors were amazing," he said, putting his hand on his heart. "She isn't 100% recovered yet, but I think she will be soon."

He had some amazingly beautiful photographs, and we told him so.

"Thanks, we're still working on the written version."

A written version too? Blimey, talk about overachievers.

Since moving to Norway Ruan had been lucky enough to see the northern lights several times.

"Oh wow, that must be amazing. What's the proper name for that again, aurora...?" I could never remember the second word.

"Borealis," Ruan reminded me. "Yeah it is pretty spectacular."

"How do you find it here when it's dark for months and months?" Rob asked.

"Well, although there's no sun, what you do have is a big open sky, plus all the snow. And the moonlight reflects off the snow, so it's actually not as dark as you'd imagine. The other thing is you often get pretty good weather here in August. It's warm, maybe 20 degrees or so. So that's a nice little bonus before the snow comes in."

We bought one of Ruan's glass-blown plates as a present for Sara and Anders, the couple whose wedding we are going to in September. Made by a local artist, it was blue and white and quite pretty, decorated with a little reindeer design. I hope they like it. Especially as we are in Norway, so of course it cost about the equivalent of a couple of months' mortgage payments back home. On a *mansion*. In Mayfair... I exaggerate, of course. It was only one month's worth.

Having reached the most northerly point, there was only one direction possible. But before we headed due south, we did a four-hour walk to a cliff and peninsula where the Sami people used to offer sacrifices to the sea. The route had been recommended by Ruan.

I did pretty well on the walk. There were some steep parts but I never got very out of breath. We got back to the van at 10.20pm and then drove till 1am, stopping at Landersfjord. This all felt perfectly normal, because it was still light.

Because there's less traffic, driving at night can be easier. But not on this occasion. There were loads of little rodent-type animals who kept running out into the middle of the road. They looked like hamsters or guinea pigs and there were hundreds of them along a particular stretch of road. Rob kept having to swerve to avoid them but it was tricky because there were so many of them.

"Oh watch out Rob, there's another one! Oh no, I think we got that one."

Every now and then we definitely failed to miss one and I cringed to think of its little squished body lying in the road. "Oh God, this is awful! I think I heard a little squeal then. Surely that's not possible, is it? Above the engine noise? Surely?"

"I don't know," Rob said. "Why do they wait till we're going past to run out into the road?"

I felt terrible. But it was almost like they were deliberately running into us, a mass rodent suicide. It reminded me of the film 'Withnail And I', when the two main characters are on the road in some godforsaken place. Withnail, who's very drunk, sees an 'Accident black spot' road sign and scoffs, "Accidents? These aren't accidents, they're throwing themselves into the road! Throwing themselves into the road gladly to escape all this hideousness."

I was horrified to think how many creatures we'd murdered. When we finally stopped the massacre and parked up for the night, Rob sent a text to Ruairidh, a friend of ours who knows loads about animals.

"Oh of course," Rob said, talking to himself more than to me, when Ruairidh replied.

"What did he say?"

"Those little creatures were probably Norwegian lemmings. They're attracted by the headlights; that's why they kept running towards us."

I was hugely shocked by this.

"Lemmings? But… they're not real are they? Are you joking?"

Rob was looking at me, amused, as if I was still mad. He started laughing and didn't answer the question.

"Lemmings, as in… the computer game? The ones that chuck themselves off cliffs?"

I felt quite tired and couldn't work out if I was an ignoramus or if Rob was just pulling my leg.

"Yes, lemmings are real," Rob said, making an obvious effort not to laugh now I was getting weary.

"No way."

Day 240 — 18th August 2011
Alta, Norway

We've given in and bought a new iPod. The lack of music over the last few days was completely unacceptable. Although I'm relieved the musical blackout is over, I'm also cursing our bad luck in having to make a major purchase in one of the world's most expensive countries. Damn you, Apple! I'm sure they programme their products to self-destruct. (Only kidding, if any Apple lawyers are reading.)

We're back in Alta, heading south, but this time we have a guest with us, a young Polish student called Przemek, who's hitchhiking his way around Scandinavia this summer.

We saw him sitting at the side of the road, with a little sign that read 'Alta'.

"Should we stop?" Rob asked. I was in two minds.

"Quick," he said. "Make a decision."

I took a second glance. He looked so forlorn, as if he didn't expect anyone to stop for him ever again, that I told Rob to go for it. He put his sign down on the ground when he saw us coming and looked extremely surprised when we pulled up beside him. He pointed towards himself as if to check that we'd stopped to pick him up. We nodded and smiled and he looked incredibly happy as he grabbed his bag and came over.

"Campervans never stop," he said with a surprised laugh, as Rob sorted out his seatbelt. Later he mentioned that Audis and BMWs never stop either.

"I'm sorry it's so messy in here," I said, wishing I'd brushed out the mats this morning.

"No, no, it's amazing here," he said, grinning. He's got blonde hair, bluey-green eyes and a great tan. He looks young, maybe nineteen or twenty.

It turned out that Przemek didn't really have a plan as to where he was going to stay once he got to Alta, so Rob suggested he pitched his tent next to our motorhome, at the amazing wild camping spot we'd stayed at here before.

"Wow, it's beautiful here," he said with a huge smile.

He had clearly prepared well for his trip, with a good quality tent and sleeping bag and a little stove to cook on.

Not long after we got there a helicopter appeared overhead, hovering and eventually landing just a few hundred metres down the fjord from us. As ever, the sight of a helicopter immediately made me think of Ray Liotta in 'Goodfellas'. We were all quite curious, but Przemek was so intrigued or excited that he ran over to find out what was going on. Rob and I looked at each other and smiled. Ah, the enthusiasm of youth. Quite endearing really. He ran back a few minutes later, informing us that it must be some kind of training exercise.

I made us all some dinner — I was pretty sure it was Przemek's first Quorn sausage experience — while the blokes built a campfire. Very gender appropriate. Afterwards we sat round the fire drinking red wine while Przemek told us about his trip.

"Do you usually stay on campsites?" Rob asked.

"No, most nights I try to camp out in the wild, maybe in a national park or something like that," he said.

"Don't you ever feel scared?" I asked.

"No, because I have something to protect me," he said, disappearing into his tent. Rob and I gave each other a quizzical look. He came out brandishing some kind of black plastic police baton about six inches long and two inches wide. It looked fairly non-threatening until he shook it and it flipped open to double the length. He waggled it about and the end bent from side to side.

"Well I wasn't expecting that," Rob said, and we all laughed at his unusual weapon.

"It looks like something James Bond would have!" I told him.

He nodded, quite proud.

"When I tell my parents I am going to Russia they said I must get a weapon."

"Wow, you hitchhiked in Russia?"

I was impressed and eager to hear more; it's somewhere I've always wanted to go.

"Yes, but I did have some problems getting there because there is a rule that you cannot walk across the border into Russia. You need to go in a car. So I asked a policeman to help me. I said, 'What can I do? This rule is a problem for me.' So the next car he catches driving too fast is a Porsche Cayenne and the policeman says to the guy, 'You can either pay the fine or give this guy a ride to St Petersburg.'"

"So they gave you a lift?"

"Yes, but you should see this guy; he is definitely a gangster. He has a bodyguard and he told me everything about St Petersburg corruption, prostitution and drugs. Corruption is everywhere in Russia, and the people are very poor," he said sadly.

"What an adventure though," I said.

"Yes, but it is very difficult in Russia because nobody speaks English, even in the big cities. All the road signs and menus, everything is in Russian."

At some point in the evening I realised we'd got through four bottles of wine between us, plus quite a bit out of one of the four-litre boxes. I told Rob and Przemek.

"Yes, I think this is the first time I have been a little drunk on wine," Przemek said. He explained that in Poland, wine isn't something you'd drink to get drunk; that's what straight vodka is for.

We got on to the subject of ages and Przemek was surprised when we told him Rob was 35 and I was 34.

"No! I thought you were maybe 27 or something," he said.

I was really pleased until I remembered that when you're *very* young, older people just seem older; it's difficult to tell just how much older. And now that I'm getting a bit older myself, I find it difficult to tell the age of younger people. Sometimes I'll do a double take when we're in the motorhome; I spot someone behind the wheel and think, surely that wee baby-face can't be old enough to drive? Then I remind myself that a new driver could be just half my age. And that makes me feel really old. Still, at least Przemek didn't think we were 47.

Przemek's phone went and he started yapping away in Polish. I love how it sounds, like Russian but softer. I could listen to that all day.

It was getting cold but I kept close to the fire for warmth, pointing my feet towards the flames. I must have got a bit too close though, because Przemek shouted, "Ros! Your shoes, they have smoke on them!"

I looked down and right enough there was a stream of smoke coming from the underside of my boots.

"Shit."

I whipped them off and had a look. There was a big hole on the bottom of each one where the rubber had started melting. Whoops.

Day 241 — 19th August 2011
Halti, Enontekiö, Finland

When I stepped out of the van, Przemek was already up and eating his breakfast.

"Did you sleep OK?" I asked, worried he might have been a bit cold.

"Totally," he said. "I don't know whether you say this in Scotland, but in Poland when we sleep very well, we say we slept like a dead one."

"Er, no, can't say we do," I laughed. "But I might start using that."

When we dropped Przemek off later that day he said he was very grateful for everything and had never been given such a long lift by anyone before. He gave us a really sweet little thank you note and hugged us both.

"If you ever go to Gdansk, I will show you a great time," he said.

We said our goodbyes and left him by the side of the road with a new sign. This time it said 'Narvik'. I imagined him sitting for hours waiting for a lift.

"Do you think he'll be all right?" I said to Rob as we drove away and he got smaller and smaller.

"Yeah, I'm sure he'll be fine."

***

We are currently 800 metres above sea level at the start of Rob's walk up Halti, Finland's highest mountain. Although the mountain itself is in Finland, the best approach to the walk actually starts in Norway. The drive here was a white knuckle ride for me, with loads of steep windy turns and narrow roads. I was pretty relieved to get here safely.

Rob cycled the seven kilometres to the start of the walk, then left his bike in the car park. I started my own (much less intense) walk up the road towards the car park, thinking that I didn't need to do the whole fourteen kilometres if it got too much for me. I was slightly scared of getting lost but Rob reckoned there were no turn-offs, so as long as I stuck to the track it should be pretty much impossible to go wrong.

I felt really good for some fresh air, even though it was cold and blustery. I had the iPod on and the tunes kept me going. I made it to the car park and saw Rob's bike chained to a tourist information sign. I looked up to the hills and wondered which one he was climbing. I hoped he was OK in this weather. It looked pretty cloudy up there.

As I was walking back down, pleased with myself for not getting lost, Rob suddenly appeared by my side.

"Oh hello, how did you get on?"

"Bloody hell, didn't you hear me shouting? I've been calling you for ages!"

"No, sorry. I had some tunes on."

"I saw you in the car park but I couldn't get your attention. I suppose it was pretty windy."

"Oh well. Aren't you impressed how far I've walked though?"

"Yes, you've done very well Bosal."

We took it in turns to ride the bike back.

We left that evening, even though Rob was knackered, because we still had plenty of driving to do to get to the wedding on time. We also really need to do some washing soon.

I hope Przemek got a lift OK and is on his way to Sweden.

Day 242 — 20th August 2011
Sorfold, Norway

We are now past Narvik and on our way to get a ferry from some place whose name escapes me at the moment. We're following the E6, the main spine road that runs the length of Norway. It's pretty much the only road in the north actually, and there's no option but to get a ferry at certain points. There are a few little things grating at me today. For a start, it's raining. There's no chance of getting any exercise either as we need to get some miles under our belt. And the clothes washing situation is getting a bit desperate now.

Oh and the other thing is that Rob keeps asking me to take pictures with his camera while we're driving along. This annoys me for several reasons. Firstly, his camera is so heavy that I struggle to pick the damn thing up. Secondly, I don't really know how to use it, and it's especially tricky to work out which button to press when you're speeding along and need to get the shot before it's too late. Thirdly, and most annoyingly of all, he usually asks me to take pictures of unbelievably boring stuff. Tunnels, for example. He starts going on about the amazing feats of engineering that have made that particular tunnel possible, but I just don't get it. I don't know what he sees that I don't, but to me, a tunnel's a tunnel. Seen one, seen them all.

To top it all off, something has bitten me. My elbow is twice the size it should be, which is a bit worrying. It looks quite comical actually, as if I've got one really muscly arm.

In keeping with our theme of just missing things on this trip, the ferry left a couple of minutes before we got to the terminal. Still, it wasn't long till the next one so we made a cup of tea and had a game of Scrabble. Rob won.

When we arrived at Sorfold we did three sink-fulls of hand washing and hung it all up outside. It rained overnight so Rob had to bring it in at 5am.

Day 243 — 21st August 2011
Somewhere in Norway, the longest country in the world

We went through nine tunnels within the first half hour of our drive today. I counted them. Of course, Rob wanted me to take several pictures of EVERY SINGLE ONE. The man is obsessed!

The Scandinavians must be very patriotic; we have seen national flags flying everywhere. Not just on official buildings but on ordinary people's houses too.

We drank wine and played Scrabble tonight. Rob won, so the score is 8-8 now. Damn.

Day 244 — 22nd August 2011
Lom, Norway

The bloody washing still isn't dry! I'm down to bikini bottoms for pants today.

Another heavy day of driving, but at least the sun is shining now. We are aiming to get to Lom, beyond Otta.

I won the Scrabble tonight so it's 9-8 now. YES! It wasn't looking good at all until I cleverly managed to use all seven letters with 'reality'. I did have a blank, which of course helped a bit. But it's still a whopping fifty-point bonus. I tried not to be too smug. OK, I didn't try that hard.

Day 245 — 23rd August 2011
Juvasshytta Mountain Station, Norway

Yet again I find myself halfway up a mountain. This time it's Galdhopiggen, Norway's highest peak. We are currently 1.14 miles above sea level. This is turning out to be an expensive walk (475kr, which is about £50) as it involves walking across a crevasse field; you need to take a guide with you to make sure you don't die on the glacier. Plus we had to pay 85kr for the toll road to get here.

I was going to do the walk too but when I saw the glacier I decided I didn't like the look of it, so I'm staying in the nice warm van instead.

At least we don't have to drive hundreds of kilometres today. The last few days have been pretty gruelling on that front, not to mention expensive because of all the pricey Norwegian diesel. The good news is that the flipping washing is finally dry.

Rob came back from his walk on a high. He met some people from Stourbridge near Birmingham. I'm unsure whether those two facts are related.

We drove for a bit when he got back down and when we stopped Rob cooked roast potatoes, onions and peppers, with some weird smoked Quorn sausages. All of which was absolutely delicious. It's the first time we've had roast potatoes since we left the UK.

Day 246 — 24th August 2011
Norway, still...
Another big driving day. We are now heading towards a cliff called Preikestolen, which is famous for base jumping. I don't think anyone will be jumping off in this weather.

We are low on water and need to empty the waste water too.

Day 247 — 25th August 2011
Preikestolen, Norway
We drove for ages today but the scenery was special. Dramatic like nothing I've seen before. Every bend in the road revealed a new waterfall, fjord, cliff or mountain ready to amaze us. Some of the rivers were a very strange bright green colour, almost industrially luminous, due to the algae.

As we went over a bumpy bit of road, a fuse blew in the cigarette lighter. This means we are temporarily without music. This is not good.

At 200, Rob gave up counting tunnels today.

We did the cliff walk at Preikestolen, which was pretty hard going and extremely windy and cold at the top. There were loads of tourists on the walk, some sporting completely inappropriate footwear. I saw one woman wearing high heels. The views were impressive, so I'm glad we did it. I was quite scared of getting blown over the top. People (stupid people) kept going right to the edge to have their photos taken, smiling away completely oblivious to the danger. Idiots.

"Look at them Rob, they're mental!"

"Can you hold my rucksack for me? And here's my camera, so you can take my picture when I get over there."

Oh Jesus.

***

There was a massive storm tonight, with thunder and lightning. Not very frightening though.

Rob won the Scrabble tonight, so it's 9-9. Grrrr.

After our walk we slept like dead ones.

Day 248 — 26th August 2011
Deepest, darkest Norway

Blimey, Norway really is quite a long country isn't it. My legs are aching today, thanks to our big walk yesterday. We are heading towards Oslo now.

Only one week to go until the wedding! I'm looking forward to it, especially to seeing my sister and Mark.

We're going to attempt to drive into Oslo tomorrow, in search of a launderette.

There are some very high quality roads in Norway. There are also some exceedingly bumpy roads in Norway. As we drove over one of the dodgy ones, I looked across to Rob.

"Bloody hell, wish I'd worn my sports bra now."

I lost at Scrabble tonight. It's 10-9 now. Rubbish.

Day 249 — 27th August 2011
Oslo, Norway

We got all our washing done at a wee place in the centre of Oslo. I met a friendly Norwegian girl in the launderette, who gave me lots of top tips about where to go in Oslo. Her English was flawless, so good I thought she was Australian at first.

It all worked out OK in the end, but Rob got very stressed driving about in the city centre. Which is totally understandable. Not only are there more obstacles to avoid, but Lara (our satnav lady) doesn't cope well with cities. She often gets a bit confused and sends us in the wrong direction.

We parked up at the harbour, a pretty location nice and close to the excitement of Oslo. The weather is awful, so we haven't been out exploring yet.

The ticket machine for the car park doesn't seem to like our MasterCard, which has been accepted pretty much everywhere else. We had to use our UK debit card. I dread to think how much that will cost.

Day 250 — 28th August 2011
Oslo, Norway

It's absolutely pissing down so we battened down the hatches and spent the whole day in the motorhome. It's raining so much that water keeps thumping up over the harbour side.

Rob got his paints out and tried a few things. He did a kind of modern piece that looked a bit like an army camouflage jacket. I don't think he was entirely happy with it though. He's just ripped it up, declaring, "That's just pish."

He painted quite a nice portrait of me, taken from a photo, so luckily I didn't have to sit in the same position for hours.

I spent hours playing a silly, pointless but quite entertaining game on Rob's phone. I can't remember what it's called now but it was something to do with popping bubbles. I feel slightly guilty for not using my time more usefully or creatively or productively, but not guilty enough to taint my enjoyment. I played it for so long I completed all 163 levels.

I also did a little research on WOOFing (worldwide opportunities on organic farms). I don't know if we'll ever get round to trying it, but I feel a slight need to actually *do* something, rather than just travelling. Maybe this is just my tightly conditioned brain talking, after years of nine-five grind.

Rob got a text from Sven and Jess today. They're going on a whale safari!

"Wow, that sounds amazing! Can we do that?"

Sometimes I forget to say 'shall we' rather than 'can we' when I'm talking to Rob, like he's the parent and I'm the child asking permission.

"Nah," he said dismissively, as if I'd just suggested weeing all over the floor.

"You can do that in Scotland!"

I didn't say anything. But I was thinking, yeah I'm sure you can, but would we? Will we ever get around to doing something that cool back home? Almost definitely not. I must have looked a bit gutted because Rob softened.

"I don't think we have time really, to be honest, not if we want to make this wedding."

I'm having a very bad run on the Scrabble. The score, it pains me to admit, is 12-9. I lost two games today. Rob keeps getting all the good letters. And I know that that's the sort of thing a loser would say. But it's true, I swear.

Day 251 — 29th August 2011

Oslo, Norway

We made it out of the motorhome! In fact, we've had a lovely day in Oslo acting the tourist. First stop was the Vigeland Sculpture Park, as recommended by my Norwegian launderette friend. There were dozens of statues of men, women and children, in beautifully dynamic, realistic poses. So romantic. Groups of Japanese tourists posed beside them, snapping away.

Rob got a puncture but we soon spotted a bike repair shop. It was going to cost an eye-watering £40 to supply and fit a new inner tube, but the kind Italian shop owner, who said he understood how expensive Oslo was for tourists, lent Rob his tools so he could fit it himself. What a nice man.

We rode on up to the National Gallery. We saw Munch's The Scream (it's tiny and not as vibrant as the reproductions) and loads of impressive paintings by Picasso, Cezanne and Manet. We rode over to the Opera House next, a very cool angular modern building that slopes right down to the water. If you cycle or walk to the top (which I didn't) you get a brilliant view across the city.

There were about three million other cyclists in Oslo and generally it was quite good fun joining in. Having said that, Rob is of course much faster and more assertive than me, so I had no choice but to do some dodgy manoeuvres to keep up. I was scared of being hit by a car or another bike, but more scared of losing Rob and having to find my own way back to the harbour.

We have 3G here, thank flip, so we can check the news and emails and generally keep in touch with the world, all free of charge, using the Kindle. A message in my inbox informed me that there had been a recall on my Ridiculously Expensive Bike, something to do with a safety issue on the front fork. There was a bit of toing and froing with the bike shop lady before I found out what was going on, because she'd sent me the official letter as an attachment, and — clever as the Kindle is — you can't download attachments from it.

"Which bit is the front fork?" I asked Rob, who tends to know about these things.

"The bit that looks like a fork, at the front," he said, with that 'silly woman' look on his face. Hopefully we can get the damn thing fixed in Copenhagen.

We are nearly out of food but we're just going to buy the basics until we're back in Sweden and the land of Lidls.

***

I know that, officially, you're not supposed to put cotton buds in your ear. But I do it anyway. Quite regularly. I'm something of a cotton-bud-in-the-ear fanatic. I do it every day. Sometimes twice. Tonight though, when I pulled the naughty bud out, I found that the cotton part was *still in my ear*. I felt a shiver. What a nasty feeling to have something stuck in your ear that shouldn't be!

"Rob...." I gulped, fear on my face.

It was so deeply embedded that Rob couldn't even see it at first. I started to imagine what Norwegian A&E might be like, using sign language to explain what had happened, a Norwegian doctor informing the silly foreigner in perfect English that really, you shouldn't put cotton buds in your ears you know.

I felt my temperature rise as Rob started the removal process with a long, sharp pair of tweezers. I got hotter and a bit sweaty as he delved deeper into my ear, convinced he was about to accidentally pierce my ear drum.

Despite me giggling nervously, which made my ear move in an unhelpful manner, he quickly got it out thanks to his head torch and steady hands.

"Is it out? Have you got it? Is it all out?"

"Yes it's all out," he said this wearily, as if I was always doing stupid things like this.

"Bloody hell, that was horrible. Thank you Rob."

For at least the thousandth time I was thankful for Rob's calm disposition. Not to mention his excellent set of tools. I'm lucky he's thoroughly prepared for all eventualities.

Inexplicably, the Scrabble wars continue in the wrong direction. We're at 13-9. How can this be?

Day 252 — 30th August 2011
Near Moss, Norway

Apart from when we go to cities and have to use official campsites, we usually stop in lay-bys and do what Rob calls 'wild camping'. Sleeping in a lay-by doesn't sound particularly glamorous or comfortable or pleasurable. But what I've learnt is that there are lay-bys and then there are lay-bys. My preferred kind, and they quite often fit the bill, are pretty little picnic stops well off the road. They are usually green with trees and quiet too. We nearly always hold out for one that's well off any major roads, for safety reasons. If we're very tired and just want to stop for the night, we might choose one that's less than pretty but does the job. But they're always safe. In more built up areas, if it's well lit that's a plus.

It's weird when we see other motorhomes parked up. On one hand, it's a good sign if others (especially natives) feel that it's a good place to park. But on the other, we don't like spaces that are too packed. And, while there's something to be said for the safety in numbers idea, just because five other motorhomers think it's a great place to park doesn't necessarily mean they're right.

What's lovely is that we don't have to plan where and when to stop. We have books and websites we can refer to, to guide our basic route. But, in Scandinavia at least, wild camping is such a normal accepted thing to do (and there are so few people around to care what you're up to anyway, as long as you're sensible about it) that we know the minute we get tired of the road, we'll soon find a rest stop. The one we were in last night had lots of lorries in it. This isn't always ideal. Although lorry drivers tend to know where *not* to park, they often set off early in the morning. So your lovely dreamy sleep might get snatched from you by the huge roar of a monster truck engine starting up a couple of metres from your head. At 5am.

One night we made the mistake of parking next to a refrigerated lorry. The driver had to keep his engine running all night to keep his load cool. Which sounds like a dodgy euphemism now I come to think of it.

I've just happened upon a great quote from a French dude called Francois De La Rochefoucauld; 'We are so accustomed to disguise ourselves to others, that in the end, we become disguised to ourselves.'

That is exactly what happened to me at work. What I allowed to happen. I was so caught up in how I appeared to my colleagues (trying to be positive, in my team leader role, when inside I was struggling as the pressure deepened) that I buried the real me. Like the Radiohead song, I lost myself. In the office I covered genuine emotions with jokes, waiting till I got home to cry my eyes out. The public and private faces looked so different, even I didn't know which was real any more.

When I remember that my job was editing a bloody *wedding magazine*, I feel like kicking myself in the head. I am pretty flexible, so could probably achieve this if my self-loathing required. Jesus! If I'd been a cancer-fighting doctor or head teacher at an inner city school or an air traffic controller... something genuinely stressful, it would have made more sense for work stress to bring me down so acutely. My only defence is that although the subject matter — weddings — was undeniably fluffy, that doesn't mean my job was. It didn't feel fluffy. Spiky, more like.

Day 253 — 31st August 2011
Copenhagen, Denmark

Checked my emails earlier and there's nothing from the Danish bike guy who's supposed to be arranging my repair in Copenhagen. Must chase them up.

Once we'd crossed from Norway into Sweden, Rob went into Lidl and spent the equivalent of £50, coming back to the van with only three bags of shopping. Wow, people aren't kidding when they say Scandinavia's expensive.

It turned into quite an expensive day as we treated ourselves to a MAX, the Swedish equivalent of a McDonalds and Europe's oldest hamburger chain. We'd driven past so many MAX signs that I just had to try it, having convinced myself that Scandinavian fast food might be better than the US chains'. I was wrong.

When we were finished eating, I felt like I always do after bad food; really full in a horribly bloated too-much-fat-and-sugar way, but strangely unsatisfied at the same time, because you've digested zero nutrients. I also had a faint but real sense of self-loathing. Never again. We must be getting used to Swedish prices; I thought about £20 for this terrible meal was fairly reasonable.

***

I'm reading 'Dead Souls' by Gogol at the moment. It's about this dodgy Russian guy who, for some reason, starts buying up dead souls, as in serfs who have died but on whom various landowners are still paying a tax per head. It's a bit weird, but pretty intriguing. God I love Russian novels! 'Anna Karenina', 'Crime And Punishment', even 'War And Peace'. I liked them all. Although I enjoyed the peace more than the war. Russian authors are so brutally romantic. Or is it the other way round?

We're very pleased to have reached Copenhagen today, the location of the wedding! But having paid roughly the GDP of a developing nation to camp here last time we passed through, we've opted to park up at the city's man-made beach tonight.

There was a busy VW club rally happening when we first arrived. Everyone looked at us as if to say, hey, what are you doing here? You're clearly a Hymer, not a VW. The place is deserted now though, making us wonder whether it's a very safe place to be late at night.

We've just moved to a spot a bit closer to some lights. There's a beach bar at the end of the strip, which probably explains a lot of the noise and otherwise possibly strange comings and goings.

Plus, we've driven 550km today, so unless I spot a giant crazy-eyed Danish axe murderer in the next hour or so, I think we'll take our chances.

"Do you realise we've been in three countries today?" Rob said over dinner.

Oh yeah. We woke up in Norway, drove through Sweden and settled in Denmark. No wonder I feel tired.

As soon as we got to Denmark we started noticing posters for the upcoming elections. But something wasn't quite right. Almost all the people featured were young and attractive — they can't be politicians, can they?

"Rob, do you think those are the actual candidates?"

"Nah, they're far too young... and some of them are quite good-looking. Must just be people who support those MPs," he said.

"Yeah, that's what I thought at first. But they've got the candidates' names at the bottom of each poster. It would be a bit misleading if that wasn't actually who it said it was, wouldn't it?"

"Hmm. Maybe you're right."

Maybe you don't have to be an old fat unsexy guy to be a politician in Denmark. An image of David Owen popped into my head, the only British politician I can think of who bucked the trend.

I clawed one point back in the Battle For Scrabble Supremacy tonight. Ha! But only just. And only because Rob was left with a 'Q' at the end, which of course equals ten points deducted from his total. So, something of a hollow victory. But a victory all the same! Perhaps this is the start of my comeback?

Day 254 — 1st September 2011
Copenhagen, Denmark

We are staying at City Camp, Copenhagen for the next few nights. It's basically a massive car park next to Fisketorvet, a shopping centre. Bizarrely, the owner of the site has rented out part of his land to a circus group, so as we sat outside eating dinner with Sylv and Mark, who we picked up at the airport earlier, every now and then we spotted a camel or an elephant walking around. We're now on to this evening's third show, which means the same cheesy show tunes are playing for the third time. There's also a pungent animal smell in the air.

As requested, Mark had brought us a load of DVDs. I'll be so happy to have some films to watch again! Even if some of them are quite cheesy. Which they will be, if Sylv has helped choose them.

Day 255 — 2nd September 2011

Copenhagen, Denmark

I have the WORST most evil hangover I've experienced in a long long time. Head throbbing. Feel sick whenever I move. Emotionally and physically wrecked. Beyond repair. Death warmed up in an old microwave and then left to go cold and dark and sad and sick.

Perhaps I am wallowing in self-pity just slightly. It appears I still have my sense of humour, even if in every other sense I am sub-human today. I managed to crack a half-hearted smile when my sister replied to my self-pitiful text with mockery and very little in the way of actual sympathy.

I'm not sure how I managed to get *so* drunk. Except that Danish pubs don't seem to close at 1am like they should, you just carry on drinking until you drop.

The worst part is that I have to try to pull my body and mind at least a little bit more together because I need to leave the campervan. I have to actually get up, get dressed and ride my bike through a foreign busy bustling unfamiliar city full of three million cyclists and drop my stupid potential deathtrap of a bike off so that some Danish guy can fix it. I can barely begin contemplating reaching the bathroom to be sick, let alone doing what I'm meant to be. Will it all go away if I go to sleep?

But what did I do last night? Anything really terrible? Yes! Oh no, it's coming back to me. I got really aggro with Rob on the way home. I think I might have even said a really bad swear word to him. Why would you do that to the nicest guy in the world? I am a terrible person. I would cry over my sins if I wasn't sure it would make my headache even worse. Where is Rob? Surely I wasn't so bad that he can't stand to be near me any more? No no nooooo.

I tried to piece last night together. I remember going to an Irish bar with Rob, Sylv, Mark, Sara, Anders and their friends Brian and Jill. Brian was already really drunk and loud when we got to the pub. I remember finding it very strange that you can still smoke in smaller Danish pubs.

I remember talking about Sara coming over on an exchange programme to live in Dumfries for a year. We talked about how scary the couple she was placed with were. The guy was an alcoholic and when the woman died he became even scarier. She didn't feel safe there so she phoned one of the teachers, Mr Hills. He picked her up and she spent the weekend at his house, before my parents offered to take her in. That's how Sylv and Sara became such good friends. I don't recall the details as I was away to uni by that time.

I remember when we told Sara where we were staying in Copenhagen she said there was a story on the TV news a few days ago, claiming an elephant had escaped from the circus and jumped over a load of cars. In the car park we're staying in.

"But I think it was for publicity because the guy phoned the TV stations before he phoned the police," she'd said.

I remember giggling as I looked over to Rob and noticed how earnestly and intently he was looking at Anders. I nudged Sylv and said, "Look at Rob, the way he's looking at Anders. He's so eager to please isn't he?"

She just laughed at me.

I remember getting so drunk I couldn't speak properly in the pub. I just sat smiling at people and occasionally giggling.

I remember getting aggressive with Rob as we walked home, culminating in me throwing the cashew nuts we'd just bought (and paid a fortune for) down on the ground. I remember getting annoyed because I thought Rob wasn't walking fast enough, then telling him to fuck off when he asked me what was wrong. The weird thing is that even at the time I knew I was being unreasonable but somehow couldn't help myself.

I remember finding the campsite gates locked when we got back. We had to climb through the gap between the ground and the bottom of the gates to get back to the van. Bloody hell.

I remember crying when we got inside and I realised what an absolute cow I'd been.

What an *idiot*.

When Rob got back to the motorhome this morning he was completely nice about my drunken antics. He just laughed at my hungover state and said, "Don't worry about it, we've all been there."

"Rob, I don't think I can take my bike in today," I said pathetically. "I just can't. There's no way I'll make it."

He thought about it for a minute.

"Do you want me to take it in for you?"

"Oh, would you do that for me? That would be *amazing*."

"Yeah, no problem."

"You're a lifesaver, Rob."

"No worries. By the way, I bumped into Finn this morning."

Finn is the owner of the campsite.

"Oh yeah?"

"Yeah. So, remember how we clambered under the gates last night? Well, apparently they weren't locked at all, he just closes them over and puts a chain round them to make them look locked!"

"So we didn't need to....?"

"Nope," he said, laughing.

"For God's sake... "

"I know."

Later on I'd recovered enough to go and help set tables up for the wedding the following day, along with loads of Sara's friends and family. Together we decorated the place. For me this involved moving some chairs and quite a lot of napkin folding.

Day 256 — 3rd September 2011
Copenhagen, Denmark

It's the day of the wedding! We both had a terrible sleep last night as there was loud music coming from one of the flats nearby. The wedding started at 10.30am so we had to get up really early (8am) to make it into town on time.

I wore a red dress and Rob was in his kilt outfit, which attracted a fair bit of attention on the way there. We got a bus from the shopping centre next door to the town hall where the ceremony was held. There was a group of Italian tourists on the bus staring at us and smiling. We all got off at the same stop. An Italian lady tapped me on the arm.

"You going to wedding?" she said, smiling and gesturing towards Rob.

"Yes," I said. The next thing I knew all the tourists were kissing us and shaking our hands. She'd got the wrong end of the stick.

"Congratulations!" they chanted.

"We love the kilt!"

"Enjoy your wedding day!"

"Can we take a photo?"

By that point it was a bit late to try to explain that it wasn't actually our wedding day, so we just nodded and smiled and accepted their good wishes. Loads of cameras clicked at us.

When we got to the town hall Sylv and Mark were already there. Mark was also wearing his kilt and several more groups of tourists asked to take a picture of Mark and Rob together. I nudged Sylv as we watched one group after another taking photos of our husbands.

"Hey, do you reckon they might think Rob and Mark are getting married?" She sniggered.

Sara arrived looking blonde and beautiful in a pretty, understated black and white spotted dress. It was very Sara, very non-traditional. She was already crying.

The ceremony room was tiny but beautiful. The walls were covered with ornate paintings and gold cornicing. Somehow we all managed to squeeze in. The ceremony lasted five minutes, if that. Even in Danish it was pretty easy to follow what was happening: Do you? Yes. Right, do you? Yes. Rings on? OK, you're done. Next!

We trooped out to the courtyard where we drank champagne. When the happy couple kissed for the cameras Anders made a funny mock-disgusted face afterwards, wiping his hand across his mouth, which made me laugh.

The next part of the wedding didn't start until 5.30pm so a big group of us went to lunch while Sara and Anders had their photos taken. Just like last night in the pub, I was completely amazed by how good all the Danes' English was. You could easily forget it wasn't their first language. They even make jokes in English. So impressive.

After a nice but expensive lunch, some of the non-Danes in the subgroup decided to go to the Carlsberg Brewery, which was pretty interesting. Or it would be, if you're into beer and brewing. There happened to be some kind of festival on that day, so it was free to get in.

We headed back to the reception venue around 5pm. There was a double line-up going on, filling me with social dread. I find that sort of enforced socialising a bit stressful at the best of times, never mind in a foreign land. They make me feel under pressure because I can never think of anything to say that's not completely obvious. And I feel obliged to move along as soon as possible because there are bound to be more important people behind me waiting to meet the VIPs. Thankfully it didn't last too long and we were soon sitting down with more champagne.

Before long it was time for dinner and speeches. I found myself sitting with Mark on one side and a Danish guy called Boris on the other. Boris was lovely and, luckily for me, a very skilled and willing translator. Sylv and Rob were at my table too, along with Sara's maid of honour Bettina, who was very funny and friendly. There was also a pretty blonde girl called Anne-Marie, plus Jonas, who was already quite drunk and very handsome in a slightly menacing way. He could play the baddie soldier in a Nazi war film.

There were lots of Danish traditions at the wedding, many of which I vaguely remembered from my time at the magazine. The main thing was plenty of singing. But it's almost impossible to sing along properly when you don't know the tune or how to pronounce anything. Still, it was good fun trying.

The speeches were interspersed between courses. The starter was a little awkward for me as it was just strips of meat with bits of parmesan on the side. Vegetarianism is obviously not big in Denmark. I just ate the parmesan and passed my plate on to Boris, who was happy to help out. Thankfully the next part of the meal was a buffet, so we could pick and choose the veggie stuff. Everything was delicious.

Before we'd even finished the starter somebody started banging cutlery against their plate, and everybody joined in. Boris leaned over and explained that this meant the couple had to kiss. Which they did. Everybody cheered. Often this tradition was followed by everyone stamping their feet. In that case, the couple again has to kiss, but under the table this time.

Another tradition is triggered when the groom leaves the room to go to the bathroom. At this point all the men in the room queue up to kiss the bride. And vice versa when the bride leaves the room. Some guests, I couldn't help noticing, gave the ritual a little too much gusto. I made sure to put on a fresh layer of red lipstick before I joined the queue, leaving a nice red smacker on Anders' cheek.

The Danes say 'skol' instead of 'cheers', but people seem to say it any old time they like; mid-speech, mid-song or just while everyone's tucking into their dinner. They also have a variation on skol. Every now and then, someone will shout 'wah', which is then repeated any number of times before one long 'waaaaaaaaaah' to finish it off.

At a Danish wedding, anyone who wants to can make a speech; they just need to ask the toastmaster's permission. The toastmaster is someone the couple know, rather than a professional who's been hired. The speech rules mean there can be anything from ten to twenty people saying a few words over the course of the wedding meal. Boris very kindly gave me a running commentary on each one.

My favourite speech was Bettina's. She had written a brilliant song about Sara and Anders, the tune to which nobody seemed to know. But the best bit was when she handed everybody in the room a piece of heart-shaped paper and a pencil each (nabbed from Ikea). We were all instructed to write a note for the happy couple. All the notes were put into a wooden box along with a bottle of champagne. We then witnessed the couple jointly hammering the lid down with a nail (Anders narrowly avoiding having his finger nailed too). The box was not to be opened until their first anniversary. Such a lovely idea.

Sara's Dad did almost his whole speech in Danish. He said that when Sara and Anders got engaged, Anders knew he would have to share her love with another man. Everyone looked shocked until he said he was talking about Michael Jackson. Of course. Sara is a massive fan. He made a joke that everybody found hilarious. I looked over to Boris hopefully.

"He said that there's a... statistic, that married men live longer. Or perhaps it just feels that way."

That was mildly amusing, but I was distracted by how good Boris's English was. I can't imagine ever knowing the Danish word for statistic. (I looked it up later; it's 'statistik'.) Sara's Dad swapped into English for a minute.

"I want to say thank you very much to Sylvia and her family, first for coming here for today, but more importantly for looking after my daughter when she went to live in Scotland. I am very grateful to you that you gave her a safe place to live and it was a big relief to my wife and me at the time, to know that she was safe because of you. So thank you."

Sylv nodded an acknowledgement. He said it so simply and sincerely that I got a tear in my eye.

Time for another course before the next set of speeches. I chatted to Boris, who asked how we were enjoying Denmark.

"Oh it's brilliant. Rob is so happy to be back, and I can see why he loves it so much. The people here are always so friendly and happy to help you."

"Ah yes," Boris said, "but they are helpful so that when they get home they can be very pleased with themselves; they give themselves a little pat on the back and say, 'I was very helpful today'."

I laughed at this idea.

"Well, it's very nice to be a tourist here," I told him.

Boris asked about where Rob and I had been travelling so far. I told him where we'd been but that we don't really have a plan for when we get back yet.

"I can hear a lot of fear in your voice, when you talk about the future," he said, looking me right in the eye.

How did he know that? I thought I'd sounded quite lighthearted about everything. Boris must be quite perceptive. Before I knew it I was telling him all about the magazine and how much I'd loved being part of it.

"I liked that feeling of being needed," I told him.

"But what about Rab, and your friends and family. They need you too, don't they?"

"Yes, that's true, but it's not the same as being needed in a professional way, do you know what I mean?"

"I think so. I think it is very difficult to enjoy the moment, but when you get home, maybe two years after you get back, you will look back to this trip you've done and see that it was an amazing thing, that you loved it."

"Yes, I think you're probably right. I hope so."

We stopped talking as the toastmaster introduced three female teenage singers from a local music school, who were going to perform a few songs, unaccompanied. Again Boris translated; they'd never performed in public before so please give them a big welcome as they were very nervous. You could tell they were nervous, but they sounded wonderful. One girl in particular had an astounding voice. She was stunning too. They sang 'Heard It On The Grapevine' and a modern Danish song.

Much later, cake was served. It was the nicest wedding cake I'd ever tasted, so moist and light, with a lovely raspberry mousse layer. Amazing.

Once the food and speeches were finally over, it was time for the first dance and yet another tradition; cutting the groom's socks. This was done mid-air, with lots of men holding Anders up. Usually it's the tie that's cut, but Anders' Dad died recently and he was wearing one of his ties, so the custom had been adapted.

Anders and Sara had made an iPod wedding playlist for the disco, which produced some pretty wild dancing. Probably something to do with the free bar. There was one particularly drunk, quite chubby girl, who made a bit of a show of herself, as my Mum would say. Her skirt, which was way too short anyway, got hitched even higher up thanks to her crazy dance moves. The next time I looked round she was still on the dance floor, launching her face into Jonas' crotch! Oh dear.

When the wedding playlist ended Sara started adding Michael Jackson tunes to the queue. Next time I saw her she was in the middle of the dance floor doing her best Michael Jackson impression. Her moonwalk was particularly impressive. I don't think I've ever seen a bride do that before.

I was sitting watching people dance when Boris came up and grabbed my hand.

"Come on, come and dance!" he said.

"No, I can't. I'm too sober," I protested. But he wouldn't take no for an answer. He pulled me on to the dance floor, not letting go of my hand. Boris twirled me round and smiled at me. After a minute he pulled me closer and put his arms round my waist. I spotted Rob talking to someone on the dance floor, just a few feet away. He looked engrossed in the conversation. I felt awkward and embarrassed (I'm a rubbish dancer, too self-conscious) and also worried about what Rob would think if he noticed. I tried to talk to cover my embarrassment and lack of skill, but Boris just wanted to dance so I gave up and tried not to overthink it. When the song finished he kissed me on the cheek, smiled and said,

"Well, thank you for the dance."

Rob used to get pretty jealous of other blokes when we first got together, but when I looked over he was still well hooked into conversation with one of Sara's aunties. I was glad I hadn't upset him, but *slightly* miffed he hadn't even noticed me dancing with another man.

A couple of hours later, most of the guests were hammered. I was slightly tipsy but not too bad, the memory of yesterday's awful hangover a useful self-defence mechanism.

I sat watching people dance, noticing who was good and who was a bit uptight like me. I saw Rob dancing, laughing and talking with a different auntie now. Aunties tend to love Rob.

Everyone was having a great time but something was annoying me, niggling away darkening the edge of my mood. I couldn't work out what was wrong, until I realised it was Rob. I hadn't spoken to him for hours and hours. He hadn't so much as glanced at me for ages. Is it needy to care that he doesn't need me when other people are around?

I turned to Sylv, who was sitting next to me, with Mark at her side of course.

"Look at Rob," I said, pointing with my head. "He's so bloody... self-sufficient isn't he."

"What, you've only just noticed?" she said.

"It's the double-edged sword thing again, I suppose."

"Eh?" Sylv was struggling to hear me over the music.

"I mean, the things you love about someone can be the same things that get on your nerves too. So I love that he's sociable, but it's hard for a little introvert like me when he takes it too far, you know?"

"Yeah, I think so. With Mark, he's good for me because he's so laidback and easygoing, but when he takes that to the extreme and forgets to do really obvious stuff, it can get annoying."

I stewed over it for a bit, then Rob came over to the table where we were sitting. Not to talk to me, but to get something out of his jacket.

"Rob," I called to him over the music. He walked over.

"You all right beautiful?" he asked, in a way that let me know he wouldn't really listen to the answer anyway.

"Yeah, but I've hardly seen you all night..." I said, trying to not sound like one of those moany clingy women.

"I know Bosal, but we have just spent the last seven weeks together, pretty much talking to nobody but each other, for 24 hours a day," he said with a little laugh, before kissing me on the forehead and walking off. Well, he had a fair point there.

I remembered another wedding, where again Rob and I hadn't really talked all evening. Lots of my best friends were at the party, so it didn't bother me. But I did bump into Rob at the bar at one point. He laughed when he saw me.

"What you giggling at, Bobert?"

"It's really funny, my workmate Scott just came up to me, really serious, and said, 'Rob, you might want to keep an eye on that Al guy, he's getting pretty friendly with Ros.'"

I laughed too. Because Al is... well, he's just Al, one of our best friends.

Rob smiled drunkenly at me and said, "I just laughed, ah told him not to worry boud it. I said, 'Scott, is OK. Me and Ros are just boud as close as izz possible to be.'"

I smiled at the memory. Now, every time I looked to the dance floor Rob was dancing with a different mature lady. It was really funny to watch. They clearly loved the attention and found him very charming.

I watched the dancers enviously, wishing I was as good. The problem is, to look good while you're dancing you really have to just let go, enjoy yourself and not care what you look like. Which I find really hard. Also, as I told Sylv while we watched, I never know what to do with my arms. I'm not entirely sure what to do with my legs either, to be honest.

When the second playlist ran out, Jill and I became unofficial iPod DJs. We chose some great floor fillers and added them to the queue. Our difficulty was, everyone's a critic. And *everyone* tries to butt in with their own suggestions. Which, when we let the more drunken guests take over the controls, often resulted in the worst possible situation a DJ can be in: complete silence!

An hour or so later, the free bar must have kicked in, as I was happily dancing away to Electric Six's 'Gay Bar' with Sylv, Mark, Rob and lots of Danish people. And I didn't really care what I looked like. I was just being silly. When 'Party Rock

Anthem' by LMFAO came on, Sylv, remembering my earlier comment, grabbed my hands, forcing me into some daft arm movements.

By 5.30am, Rob was finding the art of talking rather tricky, so I made an executive decision: it was home time. It took quite some time to leave because Rob insisted on saying goodbye to everyone, starting new conversations because he kept forgetting he was meant to be saying goodbye.

Eventually we escaped and made our way down to the S-train station. Rob was really drunk, so drunk he couldn't remember which train we needed to get. This was bad news; we were now relying solely on the famous Nash Sense Of Direction. Oh dear. I looked at the route maps and eventually thought I'd got it worked out. But the train didn't arrive on time. I asked a few others who were waiting around but they didn't know what the hell was happening either.

"Rob, I want to go home. Let's just get a taxi."

"Whaaat? Nah way, Ros. D'you realise homuch thall coss?" he slurred.

"I know, but I'm really tired..."

"You muss be mental! I'm waiting furra train," he said stubbornly.

This was getting annoying. Rob was acting all lairy, it was cold and draughty on the platform, there was no sign of any train and it had gone 6am. Bloody hell. I kept thinking of that daft song, 'I'm Tired And I Want To Go Home'. But I didn't want to risk us falling out again so I pretended to be patient. Early bird Japanese tourists shyly asked Rob and his kilt to pose with them, providing a bit of distraction. Eventually, a train came that was heading in what I thought might be the right direction.

On the train, Rob was in danger of slumping. I discouraged this, mainly for the sake of the people on the opposite seats.

Amazingly, I'd made the right choice — twice, as we needed to catch two trains back to the circus — and it was only 6.45am as we walked from the second station towards bed.

We saw a jogger out for an early morning run, which made me feel distinctly unhealthy. Still, I was quite pleased to be up this late; it was a long time since I'd pulled an all-nighter. And the sun was coming up beautifully. We stopped on a bridge and admired a glass-fronted building where the pinks and yellows of the sun were reflecting in a very pretty way.

"Love this city," Rob slurred. I took a couple of pictures but Rob ruined them by making silly faces.

I was awfully glad to see our lovely silver fun bus. And happy that this morning we knew not to crawl underneath the security gates. When we got inside I started work on my usual hangover cure; tea and toast. It never fails. Well, hardly ever. It was hard work though; Rob was so pie-eyed he needed a bit of a hand undressing.

"I done unstan' this kild," he said.

I couldn't help laughing when I saw the perplexed look on his face. His eyebrows were furrowed as he put every effort into concentrating on the task at hand. He really couldn't do it, couldn't undress himself. Quite funny really. I thought back to myself a couple of nights ago and wondered, for the thousandth time, why do otherwise intelligent, rational people deliberately do this to themselves?

"Am soy," he said, eyes closed now.

"Eh?" I said, easing his shoes off.

"Said am *zorree*," he repeated, frustrated I couldn't understand him.

"Oh, *sorry,* did you say baby? Listen, don't be daft. You've seen me in worse states."

I tried to reassure him and circumvent any self-pitying stage that might be about to follow.

"Dear oh dear," I said to myself as I got him ready for bed. For some reason this made him laugh and he started saying 'dear oh dear' over and over again in a high-pitched voice.

"I did not say it like that," I said, laughing at his wholly inaccurate impression. Laughing made my task a bit tricky but eventually I got him undressed and went back to the kitchen. He fell asleep sitting upright in bed, mid-incomprehensible sentence, while I made tea. Well, that's booze for you.

I looked over and took him in. He always looks so sweet and peaceful when he's asleep. There was still a hint of confusion above the eyes though.

When I got into bed I briefly wondered whether it was safe to take my usual mirtazapine pill after such a long drinking session. It'll probably be all right.

Day 257 — 4th September 2011
Copenhagen, Denmark

Pissing down today. They were lucky it was so nice yesterday. Tired. Grumpy. Wedding comedown, I suppose. Also, Rob got my hopes up about going to the cinema (which I *love* doing) then decided him and his hangover couldn't handle it.

"I feel strange... and a bit dizzy," he complained.

I didn't feel at all sympathetic. I was in a cool city and I wanted to DO something for flip's sake! But with the memories of my despicable behaviour the other night still fresh, I tried to hide my irritation. Rob had been even nicer to me than usual, after all.

We just about made it to meet Sylv and Mark for food but again, Rob and his dizzy spells couldn't manage it. I messaged Sylv to let her know and she replied telling Rob to "man up". What an offensive phrase that is. Need to buy milk but it's just started raining. A waste of a day.

A bit later we decided to watch 'Ocean's 11' instead of hitting the cinema. The sight of Andy Garcia cheered me up considerably.

Day 260 — 7th September 2011
Copenhagen, Denmark

We had arranged to meet Sylv and Mark at Christiania, the area of the city where hippies live and you can openly buy hash. It was set up as a social experiment in 1971, when the government allowed people to move on to a deserted military base. There have been various attempts to get rid of the community there ever since. Especially because the area would be worth a fortune, several fortunes actually, if it was sold off to property developers. I was keen to see it as Rob had been telling me how amazing it was roughly twice a year for each of the 16 years since he'd lived in Copenhagen as a student.

When we got to Christiania, Rob was disappointed because it wasn't how he remembered it at all. The built-up area is quite small, with a main thoroughfare that has a few clothes stalls and a pub at the end. It was packed with people selling various sorts of cannabis.

This must be Pusher Street then. The people manning the hash stalls didn't look *overly* friendly. Many had shaved heads, hoodies and scary dogs with them. Quite a few of them were pretty beefy, intimidating men. In fact, I didn't see any women at all selling anything. None of them looked the slightest bit like hippies. I didn't see any crusties, hardly any tie-dyed clothes and no white people with dreadlocks.

There was a big poster outlining the nine common law rules in place here; no violence, no hard drugs, no weapons, no bulletproof clothing, no private cars, no bikers' colours, no stolen goods, no sales of fireworks, no firecrackers. And no running. Apparently it creates panic. All fair enough, although I'm unsure who enforces these laws. Another poster explains that the buying and selling of hash is illegal in Christiania, which is odd when you look down the street and see loads of people doing just that. But it seems cannabis sales are merely tolerated by the police here, it's not actually decriminalised. There are a couple of signs making it clear that cameras aren't allowed.

We wandered down Pusher Street. The atmosphere was pretty strange. People didn't smile at each other or stop to chat and although it seemed calm enough on the face of it, there was definitely an edge. It felt like the place could erupt, get edgier, very quickly. The police raid the place every now and then to try to keep the sale of any harder drugs under control. I certainly wouldn't feel very comfortable here at night. On the plus side, there were some cool murals.

Sylv and Mark were having a drink in the bar at the end of the street when we met them.

"So, this is weird isn't it?" Sylv said when we'd all said hello.

"Yeah, I kind of thought it'd be a bit like a permanent Glastonbury..." I told her.

"It's more like a really unfriendly, skanky Glastonbury," Sylv said. "Can't say I'm impressed with all this, to be honest."

Poor Rob looked crestfallen.

"It wasn't like this at all the last time I was here," he said sadly. "It's like... all the hippies have gone."

"And taken the hippie vibe with them?" Mark suggested.

"Yeah, the atmosphere is definitely not the same."

We chatted about the wedding for a bit.

"So what do you want to do, get some food maybe?" Sylv asked.

"Well, I'm not really that hungry yet," I said, looking at Rob. We'd not long had our breakfast.

"I didn't mean get something here!" Sylv said with a derisive laugh, horrified at the thought of buying food here.

"Well, didn't you say there was a nice lake around here Rob? We could maybe go for a little walk," I said. "I don't know about anyone else but now that I'm here I'd quite like to see a bit more of the place."

"Yeah we could do," Rob said.

Surprisingly, considering Sylv isn't really into walking for the sake of walking (walking around the shops is different), they agreed and we all trooped off towards the lake.

The lake itself was quite pretty. But we were a little unsure about the path we were taking. We kept coming to run-down houses with 'Private Property' signs and having to skirt round them to get past. I imagined a massive Alsatian (a big dog I mean, not someone from Alsace) jumping out at us all snarling and toothy, outraged we were on his territory.

Unfortunately, the walk took a little longer than Sylv had imagined when she agreed to it.

"Rob, are we nearly back in civilisation yet?" she called.

"Er, I think so. It's maybe another mile or so," he said.

Sylv and Mark were far enough behind that I could hear them talking, but not what they were saying. I could just imagine how well Rob's estimate went down though. I think I heard some mention of buses. A minute later, Sylv called to us again and we waited for them to catch us up.

"I think we're going to try and get one of those buses back into town. We've had enough walking for one day," Sylv said, pointing over towards what looked like a main road not far away.

"Well, OK, but do you know which number to get? Or which direction to head in from here?" Rob asked.

Because Rob's fit, it doesn't occur to him that other people don't find long walks as easy as he does.

"Nah, I'm sure we'll work it out though," Mark said cheerfully.

"It's up to you, but we'll probably be back on the main street soon," Rob said, "and you can just grab a bus from there. At least I can tell you which way to go from where we were."

They reluctantly agreed to stick with us for a bit. Luckily, before too long we were back in the main throng of Christiania, so we said goodbye to Sylv and Mark.

"I don't think they were very impressed with the walk," I said to Rob when they'd gone.

"No, think you're right there."

We wandered a little more and found a wee buffet-style cafe. There was nobody behind the counter when we got there. But before I had a chance to think, 'Stoners running a business... bloody typical... ignoring potential customers... how do they make a profit with customer service like this?', a lady came to help us. She was mid-fifties with long dyed red hair that needed a trim. She was wearing a long floaty skirt and when she smiled I saw crooked yellowish teeth. At last, a Christiania crusty!

The food looked great. We chose some salad, a veggie lasagne and plenty of creamy potatoes. "What is it with vegetarians and potatoes?" our friend Charlotte always asks. The lady piled the bowls full, charging us a price based on the weight. She keyed in the price and then took a bit off the total.

"You choose potatoes; they are heavy," she explained, "so I charge you less."

"Oh, thank you. That's very nice of you."

We sat outside to eat as the weather was good. I suddenly realised I was starving.

"Ooh, I'm ravishing," I said to Rob, grinning.

"Ha ha," he said. This always makes me laugh, ever since Rob got the words 'ravenous' and 'ravishing' mixed up. The thought triggered a memory of my Mum getting mixed up trying to say 'dado rail'. The best bit was when she paused mid-sentence to say, "Now, I might not get the right word here... do I want to say dildo rail?"

We'd laughed so much my Dad rushed in from the kitchen to find out what had happened. None of us could explain properly until we'd stopped laughing a few minutes later.

"Oh is that all?" Dad had said, vaguely put out that we'd interrupted his dinner preparations for such a silly joke.

It's always mums who do this. Rob's Ma routinely talks about 'erotic vegetables'. I'm pretty sure 'exotic' is the word she wants. I've never quite had the heart to put her right.

"Mmmm, this is amazing," I gestured towards the food. But when I looked over to Rob's bowl it was empty. I just don't get how the man eats so fast. He's a machine!

The food really was lovely, but I found the atmosphere slightly off-putting. The only other place I've seen people openly smoking hash is Glastonbury. Well, I've seen it in Amsterdam too. But at Glastonbury, the festival vibe — the music, the quirky stalls, the costumes, the cider, the holiday feel — puts everyone in a good mood. People are generally friendly and cheerful at Glastonbury. Here though, there were two guys at the same table as us smoking joints as we ate, but they didn't say a word, didn't even smile or nod an acknowledgement. It was weird.

We wandered along towards a bar and ordered two hot chocolates. The barman's T-shirt read, 'Don't drink and drive... smoke and fly!'

I went to the loo and found the most bizarre public toilet I've ever seen. The cubicles were extremely narrow and plastered with flyers and posters — nothing unusual there. But when I looked up I saw a massive fish tank above me, stretching the length of the ceiling. I've never peed below loads of fishes swimming around before. I wonder what the fish think when the music starts blaring at night.

The next morning, after dropping Sylv and Mark off at the airport, we decided to spend one last day in Copenhagen. Rob went over to give Finn some more money and came back with a big smile on his face.

"He wouldn't take any money," he said. "He said, 'Have tonight on me.'"

"Wow, how nice is that?"

"I love Denmark," Rob said for the hundredth time.

I did a little retail therapy today. I bought some lovely denim-style wedge lace-up boots. I also walked past a shop called Athlete's Foot. It's Rob's birthday in a couple of days so I bought him the first four episodes of 'Matador', a Danish drama series made in the 1970s. Bettina had recommended it to him at the wedding. I asked a lady in the checkout queue to confirm for me that the DVDs had English subtitles.

"Yes," she said, smiling politely. She turned back a minute later to say, "You will look forward to this. It's about Danish history, but in a good way."

I also got him a film called 'The Lovely Bones'. Not sure what it's about, but it's meant to be quite decent.

Day 261 — 8th September 2011
Between Hornbaek and Hellebaek, Denmark

We are on the road again, a little bit sad to be saying goodbye to Copenhagen. Before we left we tried to find where Rob used to live, but failed. An address might have helped.

We hit the kerb on the way to this stopover, because Rob was distracted by the satnav. He got very annoyed about it.

I spoke to Mum and Dad today, but not for long as they were off to the vets with Jacques.

Rob beat me in a close game of Scrabble, so it's 14-10 now. Unbelievable.

We heard the waves crashing as we fell asleep. It was stormy but lovely. I dreamt that all my teeth had been bashed in and smashed up. Nice.

Day 262 — 9th September 2011
Gilleleje, Denmark

It's Rob's birthday today. We are north of Helsingor, right by the sea, in a strange little place. It's quite rural but is right next to a big energy plant.

The weather was fine so we decided to go for a bike ride. We'd ridden quite far but were about 12km from the motorhome when Rob got a puncture.

"Oh bloody hell, not another one!"

"On your birthday, too!"

We didn't have the repair kit with us, so I rode along slowly while Rob walked his bike back. We were walking past a farm when someone shouted out to us.

"Sorry, can you say that in English?" Rob answered as I spotted a fifty-ish man with very blue eyes and a rather fetching handlebar moustache. I know handlebar moustaches are extremely unfashionable, but I find them strangely appealing.

"Do you want help?" he said, coming over. Rob showed him the puncture and he went off for a minute, coming back with a repair kit. Soon he'd fixed the hole and was chatting away to us about where we'd been, where we're staying and where we're going next. His wife came out and offered us some lemonade.

"Would you like to touch my animal?"

Rob and I shot each other a quick look and laughed nervously. He seemed so nice, surely he's not some kind of sick pervert? Sick pervert?? As opposed to a nice healthy balanced one?

"Look, I show you," he said.

He grabbed a bucket of grain, opened a gate to an enclosure fenced off with chicken wire and shook the bucket. Four or five deer came running over. Ah, I see.

"Do you want to come in?" he said.

I wasn't too sure, but he promised they wouldn't bite.

"They are like cows, they only have an upper set of teeth, so they can't bite even if they want to."

So I went into the pen and petted them. They were very cute, just like Bambi. My favourite was a pure white one called Bianca.

Afterwards we thanked him profusely and he said, "No problem. Where you stay, it is a short bike ride but a long walk, I think."
So Rob's puncture was fortunate really, leading to a very cool experience. Danish people are so nice!

I cooked fish, roast potatoes and roasted veg for Rob's birthday tea. While it was in the oven we played Scrabble and I felt slightly guilty for beating Rob on his birthday. The score stands at 14-11. For dessert we had wedding cake, which Sara had given us. Delicious!

Rob was very pleased with his DVDs.

"Ah, this is the series that Bettina recommended!" he said when he saw 'Matador'.

"Exactly."

I wondered whether the handlebar moustache man was patting himself on the back tonight, feeling all pleased that he'd been such a helpful citizen.

Day 263 — 10th September 2011
Gilleleje, Denmark

Before we left we stopped in at the farmhouse and dropped a bottle of wine off to the mustachioed man, a thank you for his help yesterday.

A pretty uneventful day really. We drove to a town called Odense to go to its launderette. There were two problems with that. Firstly, it was closed and secondly, it was a cafe, not a launderette.

We drove on, got fresh water and stopped at a lake near Ry. It took us a while to find somewhere to stop as several places had 'no motorhomes' signs, while others had 'no camping' notices. This place is pleasant though.

We are both a bit tired of Scrabble so decided to play gin rummy instead tonight. I was well behind in the card game score, then I had a brilliant round and won 260 points. That's when Rob got extremely pissed off.

"I'm sick of this game, I never want to play it again," he said with a scowl. Fair enough.

We reverted to Shithead after that, our default card game. All three games were so close they came down to the last few cards, which was exciting because you don't get to see your last three cards until the moment you play them. Much more fun than gin rummy.

We had some lovely apple and cinnamon cake tonight. Mmmm. Must do something about my tummy though. Rob's is getting smaller. Mine definitely isn't.

Recently I'd been wondering if my newly increased girth was changing the way Rob felt about me, so I decided to tackle it.

"Rob," I said. He was doing something on the Kindle.

"Yeah?"

"You know how I've… well, put on weight since I started taking those pills?"

He immediately started gurning, puffing his cheeks out in a silly attempt to make his face fat.

"Stop it. Look, I just wondered, you know, whether you… still like me as much, you know, in *that* way?"

I felt stupid, embarrassed, but wanted to know the answer.

"Course I do. Don't be daft. You're beautiful Bosal."

It was good to hear that, and he did say it routinely, but I wasn't sure whether he was just trying to make me feel better this time.

"It's just that…"

"What?"

"Well, you know at the wedding?"

"Yeah."

"Well, a few years ago if you'd seen me dancing with another bloke you wouldn't have liked it, but now you don't even notice."

"Like when you were dancing with Boris you mean?"

"So you did notice?"

"Of course I did."

"Oh. But you didn't mind?"

"Should I have?"

"No, but…"

"Shall we go back to Copenhagen so I can punch his lights out?"

"Ah you're just being silly now."

"You're the one being silly, Bosal," he said, gathering me up in a big hug.

"You've no need to worry. Look, I can still just about get my arms round you."

"Oh you cheeky…" I slapped his behind.

Day 264 — 11th September 2011
Hals, Denmark

Woke up at 11.05am today, nice! We stopped off at Denmark's highest point, Mollehoj. Until 2005 the Danes believed another hill very nearby was the highest point. By the time they realised, they'd already built a tower at Mollehoj, to show off the peak. We climbed up the tower's stairs, although there was a lift option. Afterwards we walked up the hill to the real highest point, only we must have taken a wrong turn at some stage because we ended up walking through fields full of cows. We even had to climb under an electric fence at one point.

After a mammoth bike ride (33km, and some of it was decidedly hilly — I thought Denmark was supposed to be flat?) it was too late to go to Ikea and buy a drying rack, as we'd planned, so we decided to drive on a bit further and get closer to Saeby, where there's, hopefully, a rest platz with a washing machine.

We changed road types on the way, from motorway to coastal, but couldn't find anywhere suitable to stay when we felt like stopping. Rob reckoned we'd driven so far that we might as well get the ferry. The crossing took all of five minutes. It was pissing down but (there's always an upside) I did spot a rather handsome ferry operative, all dark and moody, wearing a jumper that reminded me of the Sean Connery film 'The Hunt For Red October'. I tried to get a good look without staring.

At the other side we drove on until we saw somewhere that looked all right to park in, right on the edge of a forest. When we pulled in we saw a sign that indicated more parking spaces deeper into the forest. We drove for a wee while but, maybe because we'd been on the road for quite some time, the track felt like it was going on forever. And it was definitely getting narrower. Although it was not quite dusk yet, the trees above were so dense that there was no daylight at all filtering through.

"This is starting to get a bit Blair Witchy," I said. There were still loads of parking signs but now we could see a few houses and there wasn't anywhere obvious to stop.

"It doesn't feel quite right does it. I think we should head back to where we were before," Rob said.

"Righto."

We were in a somewhat tight spot by then, so I got out to help Rob reverse without hitting any trees. During the journey I had taken my shoes off, so now I quickly slung my knee-length boots on, with the sides hanging down on the ground because I couldn't be bothered zipping them up. After an Austin Powers-style 200-point turn, we got back down the everlasting track.

We parked in the original spot nearer the road and I started making dinner, quite hungry and massively glad not to be on the move any more. I started taking my boots off and grabbed my slippers, then stopped, thinking I'd spotted a piece of red fluff on my leg.

Then the piece of red fluff started moving.

I yelped (in quite a silly manner, I'm prepared to admit) and immediately flicked the red alien off me in a panic.

"What's wrong?"

"There was something on my leg, something red."

I kept examining my leg for more aliens, imagining I could feel things crawling on me. Now though, we had the problem of a rogue bug loose in the motorhome. Rob got his head torch out and I kept jumping around, freaking out every few minutes when I thought I'd spotted it running towards me. Rob eventually found it, a giant red ant. What a nasty thing!

"Ugh. That's horrible."

"Yeah, they bite as well, you know. Poor thing," Rob said, looking at me accusingly. "He's probably nearly dead."

"Well, I do feel bad for him, but he shouldn't have crawled up my leg should he?"

That'll teach me not to do my boots up. I still felt a bit jumpy. And to make it worse we kept hearing really strange, unnerving noises. It sounded like someone repeatedly tooting a horn of some kind. Not a car horn, more like a Viking hunting horn. I tried not to imagine some kind of crazy Viking human sacrifice ceremony going on in the depths of the forest.

Over dinner Rob asked me how I was feeling.

"All right, I think," I replied, wondering if he was referring to the red ant incident.

"I mean, after Christmas and everything. Because I think you seem a lot more relaxed."

"Yeah. Well, I think I am. I'm definitely trying to be, and I think I'm getting better at being... in the moment. But I still feel I can get emotional quite easily sometimes. And I still feel a bit... sort of wistful when I think about my old job."

"Well, that's all understandable."

Day 265 — 12th September 2011
Vester Halne, Denmark

We got all our washing done at a huge trucker stop in Saeby. It was very cheap but because we picked the wrong settings for the first load, accidentally putting a pre-wash on, it took seven hours to do the whole lot.

I got a fright when a frog jumped out of our washing bag. It's a good job nobody else was in the laundry room at the time, because the fright caused me to utter a very rude word quite loudly. Can't think how he got in there.

The weather has turned nasty and looks set to stay that way for a few days. We've decided to go to the Munich Beer Festival via Berlin, Leipzig, Prague and Dresden. It's going to be a busy, exciting few weeks I think.

We really need to fill up with water soon. I would very much like a shower. Rob beat me at Scrabble, *again*. And only just. *Again*. Damn it.

I stayed up late reading 'In Search Of Adam' by Caroline Smailes. Not because it's so good, because I was waiting for a non-harrowing part where I could stop, a part that wouldn't give me nightmares. In terms of human suffering, this is a book that ticks all the tragic awful boxes; sexual abuse, self-harm, suicide, it's all there.

Day 266 — 13th September 2011

Grindsted, Denmark

We woke up at 8am.

"Why am I awake? And what the hell's that bloody noise?"

Rob looked out the window.

"Oh. There's a vehicle... think it's resurfacing the road."

"Of course it is. Brilliant."

The perils of life on the road. I know 8am isn't exactly early for many people, but I'm really not at my best in the morning.

"Oh look at those lovely flowers Rob, they're so colourful aren't they," I said when we were back on the road, pointing towards them. Rob started laughing.

"What?"

"They're not flowers, they're tags for the trees!"

"Oh. Well I still think they're lovely and colourful, very pretty."

"You daftie!"

Rob kept looking at me and laughing. I had to join in really. Maybe I should wear glasses when we're travelling.

I spotted a female tractor driver, but didn't bother pointing it out to Rob in case it was really a big hairy bloke and my eyes had tricked me again. Actually female drivers of all kinds are quite common in Scandinavia; female bus drivers, truck drivers, everything. I'm starting to believe that Scandis are, in many ways, much more advanced than us.

Something else I've noticed about Scandinavia is that they leave all the swear words in songs played on the radio. Absolutely *all* of them. All I can say is, that Eminem person should wash his mouth out with soapy water and give himself a smack on the bottom. *Immediately.*

We drove to a beautiful beach where we could park just about on the shore itself. We had a slight problem though: violent rainstorms and gale force winds. Which made it a pretty silly place to stay. It was meant to have a water point, according to our little aires book, but the tap had been closed off for the season. So lovely as it was, we had to move on.

In the brief time we'd stopped at the beach, a massive amount of foam from the sea had attached itself to the motorhome. It looked very funny, as if the vehicle had an albino Afro, and as we went off, drivers from passing cars blatantly pointed and laughed. Some of them even took photos. We laughed at the amusement we'd caused.

"This isn't exactly what I had in mind when I imagined rocking up at the beach," Rob said.

"No, me neither."

We headed towards the services at Soby Vest, where we knew there was water. But when we arrived we discovered we didn't have the correct attachment to fix our hose to the tap. We have about four of the damn things, but none of them fit this tap. Which meant we could attach it, but there was ten times as much water spurting out the sides in every possible direction as there was actually going down the hose. Which meant it took ages to get filled up. Which meant we got cold and wet because it was still pissing with rain and very windy. Which meant, all in all, it wasn't the most fun fill-up session.

Because we finally had access to water, Rob took the opportunity to clean the foam off the side of the van. I started laughing because every time he put the sponge on the ground the wind blew it away. Each time he almost retrieved it, it took off again, just out of reach. Didn't Charlie Chaplin do a sketch a bit like that?

"It's not funny, Ros," he said, frowning. It kind of was, but I tried to snigger more quietly. Eventually I offered to hold the sponge. A few minutes later when I got soaked by the dodgy tap, Rob laughed his head off!

"Oh I see, *that's* funny is it? Why you..."

I pointed the hose towards his feet and took my watery revenge.

We treated ourselves to a smoked salmon salad with potato wedges and cheese. Mmm. Plus some wine. We watched 'Point Break' after tea, a surfing film with an utterly ridiculous plot. The laptop was playing up, making the picture and audio out of sync, which was annoying. Still, I did enjoy our little escape from the real world.

Day 267 — 14th September 2011
Near Lubeck, Germany

Another fairly uneventful day, except for leaving Scandinavia. The weather is still awful. It's supposed to get better soon. We will hopefully reach Berlin tomorrow. I find it odd that the Germans have no speed limits on their motorways. They do generally drive quite responsibly though.

Rob usually sets the cruise control to 80kph (50 miles an hour), the best speed for fuel economy. But today we kept getting tooted at by angry German truck drivers, who reckon that's way too slow. One guy even shook his fist at us, so we had to go a bit faster.

Rob won the Scrabble again tonight, making the score 16-11. For flip's sake.

Day 268 — 15th September 2011
Potsdam, Germany

What an entirely pish day I've had.

I went into Lidl and filled the trolley. But when I gave the guy my Caxton card, he shook his head and said something in German. OK, they don't take MasterCard. I got out my Smile card, which is a Visa. He shook his head again. What the...? Shit. I didn't have enough cash on me. I looked at the full trolley, wondering how long the ice cream would stay solid for. I tried to gesticulate the idea of me going to an ATM and coming back but the guy just looked blank. I apologised, but he just shook his head again, looking at me as if I'd just weed all over his deli aisle.

I gave up trying to communicate and walked down the street, but failed to see a cash machine anywhere. I went back to the Lidl car park, remembering that there was a cafe on the corner. After some language difficulties, the cafe guy told me where to find the railway station, where there was a cash machine. I had no idea how far away it was from his description.

I went back along the main street and tried to remember his directions. But I couldn't find the station anywhere. Eventually, after asking yet another German, and still not finding the station, I walked back to the van, dejected, and explained to Rob what had happened. He used the satnav to tell him where the nearest ATM was and headed off on his bike.

He was away so long I started to think he'd been run over. I thought I'd better go back inside to tell them we wouldn't be long. I really didn't want to, but I also didn't want them to put our shopping back on the shelves. Now there was a woman on the checkout. I waited in the queue. When it came to my turn I pointed to my still-full trolley, which was off to the side, and said 'ten minutes', holding all my fingers out to indicate ten.

She started talking to me in German. I didn't get why though. Had it not occurred to her that, if I could speak German, I probably would have done that by now? The woman behind me in the queue started chipping in. I couldn't understand a word of course, but from her tone — and the way the checkout woman laughed along with her — I knew it was something snide about me. I felt like crying when I walked out.

When Rob finally got back, I made him go in. I'd had enough humiliation for one day.

He was smiling as he came out with the trolley.

"Bloody miserable bastards in there," I said, pointing over to the shop as Rob handed me the things from the trolley.

"Ah, he was all right. I managed to get a smile out of him eventually. She was a bit nippy though, right enough."

As rubbish as the former East Germany has been so far (most people look a bit sour-faced to be honest), at least I'm not stressed out on deadline. And at least I'm not manning the Scottish Wedding Directory stall at the SECC wedding fair, which is what I'd be doing this weekend had I not escaped from my editorial prison.

We drove round for ages looking for somewhere to park up for the night. We're now at a stellplatz at the side of a main road, but it's not too noisy.

The only positive thing about today was beating Rob at Scrabble. Yes! I used all seven letters, *twice*, would you believe, putting down 'residual' and 'pervades'.

Rob just set the vehicle alarm off, going outside for some fresh air. Ha ha!

Day 269 — 16th September 2011
Berlin, Germany

Well, ich bin and all that. After a fairly stressful drive into the city centre, and a few wrong turns, we are here. We are paying 17 Euros a night to stay on what is essentially a car park plus showers and toilets. There is space for 45 motorhomes, just. We're fairly tightly squeezed in. I'm glad I didn't have to reverse into our little spot. I'll probably be able to hear the old people in the next van snoring tonight.

On the plus side it's pretty central, in the mitte district. And it's a good job we got here when we did this afternoon because the place is totally full now, we've seen the owner turning people away.

Rob just met a gay couple, one Brummie and one Welsh, who told him about a Berlin club they went to. When you get inside the bouncers give you a black bag to put all your clothes in; everybody completely strips off.

"So what night do you want to go?" Rob said.

"Ha ha."

We made sarnies to go and cycled into the city centre. It was a bit scary because there were so many other cyclists, not to mention cars and pedestrians to look out for. And of course it makes it harder not knowing the road layouts.

We couldn't find the German aires (stellplatz) book that we need anywhere, but we had a good look round and visited all the touristy places. Checkpoint Charlie, the Brandenburg Gates, the Reichstag, sections of the Berlin Wall that are still standing (it wasn't as high as I'd imagined), and The Topography of Terrors, a very well put together open-air exhibition.

We also saw a completely different side to Berlin, an area (I've forgotten what it's called now) that felt quite bohemian and hippy-friendly. There were some squats and lots of excellent graffiti; not just people's nicknames in huge letters, but truly artistic pieces that looked like they should be preserved in a gallery. They had clearly been produced by talented people and I wondered how long they'd been there, hoping nobody would paint over them. Some of the best graffiti we saw was along remnants of the Berlin Wall.

Poor Rob fell off his bike, when his front wheel became wedged in a tram line. It was horrible to see. He hurt his side and his hand, but not too badly I don't think.

"Oh fuck, are you all right?" I said, thinking what an inadequate question this is when a person is quite clearly not all right.

"Yeah I'm fine," he said dully, picking himself up quickly. It was a busy area and a little crowd had gathered round us. People started talking in German, presumably asking if he was OK. Maybe some lucky person had captured the whole thing on video phone, and was quids in after sending it to the German equivalent of 'You've Been Framed'. While I was still trying to get a proper look at his injuries, about ten seconds after he'd come off, he started walking away.

"Rob..."

"Let's just go, OK," he said. I was about to protest and insist he at least sat down for a bit, when I realised he was more embarrassed than anything else. The pain would come later.

Despite all that, I'm pleased to report that Berliners seem a lot happier than Potsdamers.

Day 270 — 17th September 2011
Berlin, Germany
We went to the posh shopping district to look round but after walking a couple of kilometres to the tube, my newly booted feet were already in agony. I'm not generally one of those women who wears unsuitable shoes; my boots had looked comfy enough, but turned out to be stealth blister assassins.

We tried to go to a rooftop bar called the Solar Sky Lounge, but we (very un-coolly, I felt) arrived before it had opened for the evening. So we got a couple of drinks in a nearby cocktail bar first. 22 Euros! 22! For *two* drinks. Two!

I should have just spoken to the barman in English, instead of nervously attempting to ask for a vodka and lemonade in German. Something got lost in translation; when we got outside I noticed I had a vodka and a little bottle of bitter lemon. Which was fine by me, it just wasn't what I'd tried to ask for.

`"Look, I've got a bitter lemon. Quite eighties isn't it. Haven't seen one of these for a while."

For some reason the drink reminded me of 'Only Fools And Horses'. Maybe it was the colourful little umbrella cocktail stick.

"Bitter lemon eh. You must have said please too many times," Rob said with a smirk.

"Eh? Oh yeah, I see what you mean. Maybe I accidentally said, 'Bitter lemon, bitte'."

This made us laugh for quite a long time.

We went back to Solar later but the burly bouncer told us (in perfect English) they were having a special event so we should come back tomorrow night. Darn those VIPs!

Instead of spending half our life savings on another round of drinks, we headed straight to Cookies Cream, a vegetarian restaurant I'd read about on the Lonely Planet website.

Ages later we found it. It's not the sort of restaurant we'd normally go to. In fact, it's a place so hip it insists on being very much hidden from the masses; you have to really make the effort to enjoy the reward of eating there. It's at the back of a hotel service alley. Just as you're thinking you can't possibly be going the right way, you spot an out of place chandelier.

We buzzed upstairs and someone let us in. We walked up a black staircase that went on forever and belonged in a seedy nightclub. Maybe the staircase was black so that the contrast struck you when you finally reached the actual restaurant. It was lovely, all bright and airy and white linen tablecloths. Quite posh, I noticed, having expected something more quirky-hip than high-end-swanky.

It was completely empty apart from a couple sitting at one table, probably because it was still early. An attractive waitress came over with a big smile, quickly but not too subtly looking us up and down.

I didn't bother even trying to speak German.

"Hello, we didn't make a booking… " I said, smiling back.

"Oh I'm sorry, we are fully booked tonight."

She didn't sound very sorry. I actually thought she was joking at first, as I looked around the small but decidedly empty restaurant.

"Er, we could come back later?" I suggested.

"Well… maybe if you come back, I don't know, around 11.30pm, we can find a table."

Yeah right. Thanks a fecking bunch! As I focused properly for a second on the well-groomed solitary couple tucking in at their cosy little table in the corner, I suddenly got it. They clearly weren't fully booked. We just weren't cool or important or well-dressed enough to get in. For feck's sake. We both pretended not to notice what a snooty cow she'd been as we left. Rob started laughing when we got outside, but it wasn't his happy laugh.

"Well, sorry about that. She obviously took one look at me and decided I wasn't getting in looking like this," he said.

"Don't you be sorry! We're both dressed casually, I'd no idea it was so posh."

"To be honest, I probably wouldn't have felt very comfortable there anyway."

"Mmmm," I said. I knew what he meant, but I was thinking my feet, at least, would have been a lot more comfortable than they were right then.

I was on a bit of a downer after our second knockback of the evening. Imagine getting rejected by a bloody vegetarian restaurant! What could be more tragic? And I'd been well looking forward to a lovely veggie meal (and a nice long sit down). Luckily we had the Kindle with us, so we rustled up some free 3G magic and managed to find another veggie restaurant just round the corner. This one had lots of Chinese and Thai dishes on offer and was much more down to earth than Cookies Cream. The staff were very friendly too. I had an aubergine satay curry, which was pretty tasty.

"Well, that was really nice," Rob said after we'd finished our second glass of wine. "And probably a lot cheaper than the other place."

"Yeah, that's true. And I was just thinking, this is definitely the first time I've been to an Asian vegetarian restaurant."

"Good point."

I noticed the restaurant's tagline; 'made with fresh vegetables, love and nothing else'.

After dinner we wandered around for a bit but didn't really find any bars. We overheard some youngsters talking English and Rob asked them where they'd recommend going. They said Berghain, the famous club, didn't even open until 3am, or would be dead till then at least. This was about 9pm. Anyway they mentioned some street or other, where there were lots of nice bars, so we got the tube there.

We found one of the bars he'd suggested, and it was OK, quite busy but the DJ was playing some good tunes. Again the drinks were ridiculously expensive. My big problem was my feet, which by then were so sore I could barely walk, let alone dance at some cool club (where, judging by our track record this evening, we would just get knocked back from anyway). Rob's side was hurting from his bike incident too, so we decided to just go home. Three trains later we got there, just after midnight. In the van we listened to the radio and had some vodka, but my heart wasn't really in it booze-wise. When I suggested going to sleep we had a mini-argument. We don't really have proper rows; we usually just stick to a few tense moments, tutting and dirty looks, a couple of well-directed sighs and occasionally a 'what's *that* supposed to mean?'. Or perhaps an accusing 'Oh and I suppose that's my fault is it?'. This one centred on Rob's disappointment over us not going clubbing. In Berlin, which is famous for its clubs, you know. Apparently this was all my fault for wanting to go out too early in the day. I hadn't realised he was so bothered about it, otherwise I would have suggested going out later. On this rare occasion I didn't blame myself. I blamed my horrific boots.

Day 271 — 18th September 2011
Worlitz, Germany
It's raining today, matching my rubbish mood. The Motorhome Facts website said the stellplatz we're at cost seven Euros a night. Turns out it's now ten Euros, plus two for electricity. What a rip-off. Although, I have to admit, it is nice and quiet and peaceful here.

We watched 'The Fighter' tonight, which was pretty good. It's about some Irish boxer and his bro, a true story. It's funny at the end when you get to see the real-life boxers the characters are based on; let's just say they didn't look much like Mark Wahlberg and Christian Bale!

Day 272 — 19th September 2011
Weissenfels, Germany
It's sunny today and we've been on a leisurely 16km bike ride, through a forest and some old industrial bits.

We finally managed to get the German stellplatz book — which we've been trying to track down for ages — in Dessau. At last. We also spotted an Ikea, so Rob nipped in and got us a drying rack. Now we're heading to Merseburg near Leipzig, to what is hopefully a free parking space, so that we can go and explore Leipzig tomorrow.

I feel much happier now that we're out of the city. I always feel so pressured to go and see and do lots of things in cities. I'm so worried about missing something amazing, especially in the capital. Whereas in the countryside I feel justified in just relaxing and being lazy.

***

Bit of a strange evening. The free parking place at Merseburg was right in the middle of a housing estate. When we got there I wandered down from the stellplatz for a bit just to stretch my legs (which I never normally do) and noticed there was an outdoor table tennis table. I *love* table tennis! I strolled back to the van.

"Oh Rob, I wish we had table tennis bats with us!"

"Why?"

"There's a table down there."

"What, you mean outside?"

"Yeah, just down there, in the park."

"Oh, that's cool."

"Well yeah, it would be, if we had bats with us."

"Do you really want a game then?"

"Yeah of course, I'd totally love a game, but we can't can we?"

"So you'd really like to play right now?"

"Rob, why are you being weird? Of course I'd love to play, but we can't!"

He went to the back of the van and rummaged around for a minute until he found a brand new set of bats and some balls.

"Well, you could have your birthday present early."

"Oh man, this is brilliant! That's an excellent present. Let's go and play now!"

"What, before tea?"

"Yeah, come on, it might be too dark after tea."

"OK then."

Of course, he totally thrashed me. Rob is annoyingly good at just about every sport. However, I got some great shots during our games. If you were awarded points for style, I think I would definitely have won.

After tea we were about to have another game when Rob's Mum phoned. By the time they'd finished talking it was quite dark, and a wee bit windy. But we had another game anyway and promised we'd have one more session in the morning before we left.

After dinner we played Scrabble, but when Rob went out for some fresh air he came back looking concerned.

"What's up?"

"There's a guy sitting outside in a car."

"And?"

"And I don't like the way he was looking at me. He just kept staring."

"Oh. Well I wouldn't worry about it, he's probably just about to buy some drugs or something."

We carried on playing Scrabble but Rob looked distracted.

"I don't like that," he said, looking out the window. "He's still there, still staring."

After a while the guy hadn't budged and Rob suggested moving on. The place did feel a bit different since it had got dark too.

"Ah! But what about the table tennis?" I was so disappointed.

"Ros, we always said if one of us had a bad feeling about a place, we would move on. Go with your gut instinct, there's a lot to be said for that."

This is true. I'd really wanted another game in the morning though. Damn! So we drove to another free parking place 15km away. It was in a big retail park and there were lots of other motorhomes there. Rob felt a lot happier, but of course there was no table tennis table.

I won the Scrabble tonight, so the score is now 16-13. I'm catching him!

Day 273 — 20th September 2011
Leipzig, Germany

I stayed up until about 2am last night reading 'Starter For Ten' by David Nicholls. It's about a geeky student who's well keen to get on the University Challenge team. I hardly ever laugh out loud when I'm reading, but this book is genuinely hilarious. I kept thinking I was going to wake Rob up.

We realised yesterday that we have the wrong version of the stellplatz book; we bought the German one but what we need is the pan-European one. So Rob has gone off on his bike to the Leipzig branch of Thalis, the bookshop we bought it from in Dessau, to see if he can change it.

It is beautifully sunny today. We rode along the river into Leipzig, but failed to find either of the health food shops listed on Google, where we thought we might find some veggie sausages. (Vegetarian cuisine is a speciality food in Germany, we're learning.)

Day 275 — 22nd September 2011
Leipzig, Germany

We've been staying at a rather strange location the last couple of nights, around 7km outside Leipzig. We are basically parked in someone's back garden. The idea was to stay one night and in the morning go and pick up the second half of the stellplatz book (turns out the book comes as a set of two, only the shop in Dessau didn't realise this and just gave Rob one half). The Leipzig branch annoyingly didn't have a copy, so we're now waiting on the second half being posted from Dessau to Leipzig. When Rob went in yesterday morning it hadn't turned up. So we're currently waiting on a phone call to confirm that it's arrived this morning. The post is meant to arrive by 12pm. It's now 12.37pm and no phone call yet.

When Rob was getting dressed this morning I noticed a very strange-looking insect bite at the top of his leg. It had a kind of black head.

"Oh, I think that's a tick bite," Rob said, getting the tweezers out and twisting it off. "I hope it's not infected."

"Infected? What with?"

"Lyme disease. That can be pretty serious. If you don't catch it early enough it can cause paralysis. And it can send you round the bend."

"Blimey, let's hope you don't get that then," I said, after making the obligatory 'how will we know the difference' joke.

"It's quite disgusting what they do really, these little buggers. They burrow down into your skin and then suck your blood until they're full."

"Mmm, lovely."

We thought we may as well do something fun while we were hanging around in Leipzig, so we went to the Leipzig Panometer, a 360-degree panoramic depiction of the rainforest. I'd been a bit moany about paying ten Euros each to get in, but it was well worth it. We learnt lots and it looked amazing; it was brilliant the way the sights and sounds changed as it progressed from daylight through to nightfall.

But the best part of the day was finding an outdoor table tennis table in a Leipzig park. We managed to get a good few games in, even though it was quite windy. Rob completely whipped my ass again. The final score was an unbelievable 13-2. Games that is, not points. Anyway, I did make some fantastic shots, and we both enjoyed it, which is the main thing. Isn't it.

We watched 'The Wrestler' tonight. It's about an old past-it wrestler struggling to adapt to a normal (ie non-wrestling) life. It wasn't half bad, although I do find Mickey Rourke's plastic fish face a bit off-putting.

Rob is in Lidl at the moment. And if this damn book ever turns up we'll be heading off to somewhere near Dresden later.

Last night and yesterday afternoon we played three games of Scrabble. I caught up a bit but during the last game Rob made a seven-letter word on his very first shot, which was fairly demoralising. The score is now 17-15.

Day 276 — 23rd September 2011
Dresden, Germany

We have the blooming book at last! When the second part of the book still hadn't turned up (on our third day of trying and waiting on the post), we just got our money back and bought the two parts in another shop. The lady at the original Thalia bookshop gave us some lemon bonbons as a thank you for our patience. Most of which I snaffled.

The not so good news is that the place where Rob had the tick bite now looks a bit weird. Actually it looks like a target, with a red bit in the middle then a big red circle going halfway along his torso and down his leg too.

"Rob, what the hell is that?" I said when I saw it.

"Oh, that doesn't look very good really, does it..." he said, looking at the area but sounding completely unconcerned.

"Does this mean you might have Lyme Disease do you think?"

"Yeah, possibly."

"Well, should we try and find a hospital?"

"Nah, we'll leave it till Monday eh."

Despite the 'eh', he said this not as a question, but a statement.

"Rob," I said, putting a hand on each of his arms and making him look me in the eye, "didn't you say Lyme Disease could be pretty serious if you don't catch it early?"

"Er, yeah, that's true."

"So don't you think it's quite important that we get this sorted out as soon as possible?"

"Well, yeah-"

I cut him off before the 'but' kicked in.

"Come on then, let's go to the hospital."

Rob was extremely reluctant — why are men always like that with anything health related? But I was adamant, unusually so, that it needed to be dealt with. Twenty minutes later we went out to find a doctor.

We located a hospital using the Kindle and walked there straight away, wondering how close we'd get to seeing an actual doctor on a Saturday afternoon. When we got there the hospital looked a bit quiet. I wondered if it was the wrong type of hospital.

Having explained to a guy behind a glass screen what the problem was (luckily we'd thought to look up the German word for tick bite, 'zeckenbiss', before we left), we were immediately dispatched to another hospital.

It wasn't too far and the weather was good, so the walk was quite pleasant. At the second hospital we struggled to find the right department. When we finally got there, Rob explained to the receptionist what was wrong. She asked Rob to show her his European Health Card and pay ten Euros, which he can claim back when we get home. She asked (in perfect English) whereabouts the bite was. Rob almost started to explain, then apparently thought it would be easier to show her. But as he started pulling his jeans down a bit, the lady laughed and raised her hand to stop him.

"That's OK," she said. The look she gave said hey, I work in admin, don't need to see any flesh thank you.

We waited for a couple of hours. I was relieved that this appeared to mean someone could see us today. There were loads of people waiting. A nice German doctor in her sixties prescribed a three-week course of antibiotics.

After Rob had picked up his prescription we went for a look around Dresden. There are beautiful, dramatic buildings dotted around and there is an obvious openness to the city. We found a health food shop stocking loads of different veggie foods. We bought two different kinds of sausages and some schnitzel burgers. They were quite pricey but I don't care. In fact, we are ridiculously pleased about finding such things. Finally, something to eat other than potatoes, eggs and cheese.

There is a hotel next to our parking place where our stellplatz book indicated there was a launderette. However, when we went inside to ask about it this morning, we found out it's a laundry service offered by the hotel itself, rather than a self-service launderette. Tonight we went back to the hotel and picked up our massive bag of washing; they'd washed, dried and neatly folded the whole lot for the measly sum of eight Euros! And we didn't have to lift a finger. Brilliant! I wish it was always so easy.

Following my recent great run on the Scrabble, I've just encountered a very unlucky run of crappy letters. The score is now 20-15. So unfair.

Day 279 — 26th September 2011
Marktleuthen, Germany

We are in a nice quiet little town where we're going to stay until Rob's feeling better. The big red and blue bruise/target where he was bitten is getting bigger and bigger and is extremely sore to touch. Poor Rob. Mind you, the stellplatz we're at is perfect for recuperation; it's totally free and you can stay as long as you like, even the electricity is free. As is drinking water and waste emptying. They just encourage you to make a donation when you leave. Pretty good. There are lots of trees and a play park next door.

A man came round last night to explain how it all works here. When he realised we didn't speak German he went away and came back with his wife, who did speak our lingo. They gave us a bundle of info on the town. You can order rolls to be delivered for breakfast each day, fresh from the local bakery right to your doorstep.

Like most of the places we stay at, there are only a couple of other motorhomes here, and they're both owned by silver-haired Germans.

It was misty this morning but since we left Berlin every day has been sunny. It is about twenty degrees today.

After dinner we watched 'The Bourne Identity', which we enjoyed, even though I don't generally like action films. It's to do with this guy who can't remember anything but is ridiculously good at fighting. I must have been drunk or something last time I saw it because I remember being really confused by the plot.

We just played Scrabble. It was looking good for me until Rob got 'oozy' — on a triple word — and scored 74 points. Oozy!? What kind of a word is that? Although it might describe Rob's rash quite well. It's 21-15 now.

Day 280 — 27th September 2011
Marktleuthen, Germany

Rob is starting to feel a bit better.

"So what do you want to do next?" he asked.

"Well, the plan was to go east, into the Czech Republic and Poland maybe, is that right?"

"Yeah, but I'm wondering if we should leave eastern Europe for another trip."

"OK."

"Thing is, I'd love to see those places, but I don't think we've got time to do them justice and they're not as well set up for motorhomes, so it could be quite stressful too."

"Well, you could be right then. Especially as you're not 100% yet."

"That's the other thing. The doctor did advise not leaving Germany until I was better."

So we've decided to go to Oktoberfest tomorrow. Oktoberfest sounds so much cooler than the Munich Beer Festival. Despite it mostly taking place in September. What's that all about? I'm quite excited. And I don't even like beer.

Day 281 — 28th September 2011
Munich, Germany

Well, here we are in Munich then. It's a bit of a shock to the system, I must say. Usually we stay in very quiet places with a couple of pensioners, if anyone, for neighbours. Now though, we're in an absolutely humongous car park, normally used as parking for a sports stadium. And there are hundreds of motorhomes, maybe even thousands, from all over Europe. They are all here for Oktoberfest and most of them are under forty! Actually, most of them are probably under 25. We're the old duffers here. At the moment there is some quite loud music playing, and there's a food stall and bar open. Lots of people are sitting outside their vans drinking. It basically feels like a festival vibe, except that everyone happens to be staying in campervans and motorhomes. Tomorrow we're going to go to the actual festival, which is a train ride away.

Rob's big red mark has gone down loads, but he's still quite tired, either from the disease itself or the antibiotics.

"So, let me get this right. We decided that, because you're not well, we should take things easy, yeah?" I asked Rob as he went for a little lie-down.

"Yeah."

"But then we thought we'd take it easy by going to a huge festival that's all about drinking beer? Clever..." I said, starting to laugh.

"Mmm, I see what you mean. Probably not the most sensible thing we could have done. It'll be fun though."

I took the opportunity to have a lovely long shower earlier, seeing as endless hot water is included in the nightly price. It was smashing, amazing even. Except that I caught sight of myself in the mirror as I came out. I was disgusted by the size of my stomach. I look about five months gone! I will have to start doing something about that.

We've just had a beer and a joint with Rico and Michaela, two young Italian blokes from the motorhome next door. Even though I don't like beer, I thought I'd better get in the spirit of things. When in Munich... Rob told them it was my birthday (it's actually tomorrow but it was past midnight by then) and they gave me a birthday kiss, one on each cheek (I mean four kisses in total, I'm not saying each bloke chose a specific cheek). I was a bit embarrassed really. Especially because one of them was quite good-looking.

Rob is now having a whitey. I can hear him retching in the bathroom. Oh dear. Who would have thought that antibiotics, beer and cannabis don't mix?

Day 282 — 29th September 2011
Munich, Germany

It's my birthday! And we're going to the beer festival! We woke up pretty early due to the *very* loud music one of our neighbours was playing, so we got ready and walked the short distance to the tube. There was a nice atmosphere on the train, with loads of people in fancy dress. We spotted lots of lederhosen and blonde pigtail wigs. Rob had decided to wear his kilt.

When we got there we wandered around for a while. It was basically like a massive amusement park, with rides, food and drink stalls and ginormous official beer tents. Our first stop was the Fischer Vreni tent, where we bought a one-litre beer each.

An old guy sitting nearby showed us how to hold the tankards properly, with all your fingers on the inside of the handle. There was another old bloke leading an old skool type of band at the front of the tent, which must have held at least 500 people in neat rows of tables. The band leader looked just like Leslie Nielsen. I felt like I was on a cruise ship and the captain had decided to take the mic. As we walked past, Leslie smiled right at me and gave me a little wink. We had another beer (I hadn't quite finished my first so Rob polished it off for me) and then ordered food. We both had lovely fish dishes. I got redfish and Rob had coalfish. Both came with deliciously creamy potato salads.

We got chucked off at 3pm as there was a reservation at our table, so we just moved a bit further down the tent. We were about to head outside for another wander round when I spotted another couple of guys wearing kilts. We went over and had a bit of a chat with them. They were from Edinburgh and invited us to join them for a drink. They were nice to talk to but after a while I said to Rob we should head off; I didn't want to outstay our welcome.

Then we went on the dodgems, which was brilliant fun. I haven't done that for years. In fact, I think I cried last time; the violence was too much for me when I was five. Rob took a video on his phone and when we watched it back later, all you could hear was me giggling and Rob saying things like, "Out my way!"

"Well, that was great fun," I said afterwards.

"Yeah, it's really the only way to do drink driving isn't it."

We wandered around some more and eventually ended up in a completely packed out beer tent, wedged between some lovely older ladies from Munich (we were wedged that is, not the tent). They were very nice and friendly and quite funny. There was a Russian guy at the table too, who seemed a little strange and didn't appear to be with anyone else.

When the barman came over with a beer that had a huge head on it and tried to hand it to Rob, the ladies all started shouting "Nei, nei, nein!" and made him take it away. They tutted and rolled their eyes at the guy, who looked half-sheepish and half-oh-blimey-why-me about it. He came back with a much better-looking drink.

Again I couldn't manage a whole litre of beer so I gave Rob the end of mine. How do blokes drink so much of this stuff? I lost count of the number of times I had to pee. Vodka is so much easier.

Rob told the old ladies it was my birthday. They all congratulated me and one even gave me a bag of smoked chicken as a present. I thought it would be rude to say, 'actually I'm a vegetarian', so I just thanked her and gave it to the Italian boys when we got home.

Each of the older ladies told me how lovely Rob is. I find it amusing when people who've just met him tell *me* that; me, the person who knows him better than anyone! At the same time, I'm pleased he makes a good impression.

I happened to look round at Rob at one point and was surprised to see immediately that he was extremely drunk. I thought we'd better make a move. With Rob off his trolley it was up to me to negotiate our way back to the tube station, which somehow I managed no problem. I must have subconsciously paid attention this morning.

I even managed not to pay, which gave me an 'ooh you are naughty' little thrill. If anyone asked, my plan was to present them with this morning's ticket and play the dumb tourist.

Day 283 — 30th September 2011
Sulzemoos, Germany

I didn't sleep too well last night. Think I was a bit hot and also kind of needed a wee but didn't want to disturb Rob by waking him.

Spoke to Mum and Dad today, as I was a bit too tipsy to talk to them on my birthday yesterday. They seemed OK.

We've just arrived at a parking place. Much as I enjoyed Munich, it's nice to get back to the quiet life again.

I noticed my fingers were sore this morning. I looked at my hands. I had bruises on my fingers from holding those massive tankards yesterday. What a big jessie! I literally can't hold my drink.

"So. You were pretty out of it last night eh," I said to Rob, who claimed not to feel too bad. "You're lucky I managed to find our way home."

"Yeah, I suppose drinking on antibiotics isn't the best idea."

"No. Probably didn't help that I kept giving you my drinks to finish either."

"That's a good point. There was probably about a pint in every one of those!"

"Sorry about that Bobert."

We watched a terrible Robert Redford and Jane Fonda film called 'Barefoot In The Park'. Probably one of the oldest, most cringe-worthy rom coms ever made. So cheesy it made my cheeks tingle. That was our third choice after starting 'Apocalypto' (looked great but my eyes felt too tired for subtitles) and 'District 9' (load of rubbish about aliens, we got about four minutes in and then turned it off). Rob fell asleep during Barefoot but I felt I'd invested too much time not to see it through.

Rob just beat me at Scrabble in the most annoying manner possible. I was leading all the way through, having scored eighty points with 'creased'. He started saying things like, "Oh there's not much point carrying on now, I don't think." But not actually conceding the game of course. Then he just happened to put 'haj' (which doesn't even sound like a real word to me) on a triple word score, with the damn 'j' (which is worth eight normally) on a double letter. All of which jamminess won it for him. How irritating can you be? The score is a horrendous 23-16. I feel quite sad about it. To be more precise, I can't begin to describe how annoyed, irritated and hard done by I feel. Well I can, but I won't.

And yes, I am aware that it's just a game. And that it doesn't really matter. And that Scrabble is supposed to be fun. And, yes, I have heard the phrase 'don't sweat the small stuff'. But still.

Day 284 — 1st October 2011
Kisslegg, Germany

Got stuck in traffic for an hour today, the first time that's happened in ages.

While we sat frustrated and motionless, something made me think about being a kid, when you're little and have that list of things you think or hope will happen when you grow up. You get married to a cool bloke. Tick. You get a good job doing something you enjoy. Tick. And you live in a nice home. Tick, tick! With everything I wanted, how could I have been diagnosed with a *depressive psychotic episode*? What the hell did I have to be depressed about? I had everything I'd always wanted. OK, we didn't have kids yet. But I didn't want them yet. So I don't think that sent me to the dark side.

It still shakes me up, that I lost the plot so badly I was in a psychiatric ward. Not just for a few days either, for three entire weeks. It's very weird to look back on it now, like a long, particularly vivid dream. I was heavy with a guilt that thumped through me, so conscious of my family and friends' distress. In some ways it was worse for them, because they remember more about it. My memories are very fuzzy. And for much of what I do remember, I'll probably never be certain what was real and what was imagined.

As time moves further and further away from my stay on the ward, I feel safer. Not complacent, not oh-that-will-never-happen-again certainty, but definitely better, further removed from insanity.

***

We have had two whole proper actual weeks without rain now. Amazing.

There are no facilities on site here — water and electric hook up are available, but only in summer — but it's nice enough.

I am quite into the book I'm reading, 'David Copperfield' by Dickens. Like most Dickens books I've read, there's plenty of death and dismay and the main character has a bloody tough life. I'm looking forward to — hopefully — some riches after David's abundance of rags.

I had a sore tummy this morning (due to the curse) and Rob currently has a pain in the neck (no it's not me). We're hoping his pain is nothing to do with the Lyme disease.

Rob made me actually cry with laughter earlier. He got his wedding ring and the other one he wears, inherited from his Grandpa, and put them on his eyelids, screwing his eyes and face up to hold them on there as if they were tiny glasses.

"You look like... a German... maths teacher," I said, between gulps of laughter.

"It is I, LeClerc," he said, although I'm sure the 'Allo Allo' character he was alluding to is French, not German. I kept trying to take a photo but I was laughing so much the camera wouldn't stop shaking. Every time I finally got it together, Rob would laugh, which made the rings fall off his eyes.

I keep laughing every time I remember the dodgems too. *Out my way!* I like how Rob's intelligence doesn't stop him being really quite daft sometimes too.

Just won two games of Scrabble so I'm only five games behind now, yaas! And we played outside. Double yay. We're hopefully going for a bike ride tomorrow morning, if Rob's feeling up to it. He's still pretty knackered.

Day 285 — 2nd October 2011
Rielasingen-Worblingen, Germany

Bah humbug all round this morning. Rob's neck is too sore for a bike ride and I've just tried to buy Mark's thirtieth birthday present but the Kindle's not working properly so I was thwarted. And another thing... my fringe looked really stupid when I woke up this morning. Trivial troubles, I know. But that hasn't stopped them grating on my nerves. At least it's not raining. It was very misty, or foggy, last night and this morning.

We're in the south west of Germany at the moment, on the way to the very famous Black Forest region. I'm still trying to think of a good joke about cakes for when we get there. After that we'll go to Switzerland and Italy.

***

After a pretty drive through the Black Forest, we turned up at Singen. We handily chose the one day of the year they have some kind of festival there. The stellplatz car park was completely rammed. After a tricky bit of reversing (tricky for Rob that is, all I had to do was hold my breath and keep an eye out for run-overable children in his blind spot) we headed to the nearest rest area, at Rielasingen-Worblingen. And actually we're glad about the festival now, because it's much nicer and quieter here and isn't just a car park in the town centre, like the Singen one. There are six pitches and electricity costs fifty cents a kilowatt hour. The only downside is that we can't get 3G on the Kindle here, not even Edge, which is almost as good as 3G.

The sun came out in time for our cycle (Rob decided he could manage one after all this afternoon). We cycled 15km to the next town, where it was well busy. The streets were very full with people and push chairs, thanks to some kind of harvest festival. Not the easiest place to wheel your bike around. There were all sorts of stalls selling lovely-looking jams and honeys and mead. Oh and meat. Lots of meat.

I felt a bit emotional today. I don't know why. It's not PMT time. Maybe I'm having a delayed Oktoberfest hangover? I started thinking about work again, about what went wrong. I wonder if I should have just been more honest, should have been confident enough to simply be myself. Every morning I'd fake it, hiding behind a mask that said 'I'm coping'. I used humour to keep the atmosphere light and friendly, when in fact I felt like shit. That pretence was probably more tiring than all the extra hours, more tiring than the stressful busy nature of the job. Pretending to be someone I wasn't was exhausting, not to mention soul-destroying. And if you pretend for too long, you forget who you really are.

I should have been more open. Maybe my role wasn't to keep everyone else motivated, to keep the team upbeat. Maybe I'd have been better sticking to my role as natural born worrier; worrying about little details nobody else noticed (or cared about) was actually one of my strengths! And unless you're a convincing actor (which I'm pretty sure I'm not), putting a brave face on things is pointless. The truth was probably written all over my sad wee face. I thought of Alan Partridge talking to his downtrodden PA Lynne. "I can read you like a book, Lynne. And not a very good book."

Anyway, that's in the past and doesn't matter now, as long as I don't make the same mistakes again.

My mood today might be something to do with the harrowing film we watched last night, 'The Lovely Bones'. It was pretty good but I thought it might have been a tad more feel-good seeing as it's a Hollywood film. It's about a young girl who gets murdered. Not what you'd call a barrel of laughs. Weirdly, the actor who plays the murdered kid's younger sister looked way older and absolutely nothing like her.

Had the most annoying game of Scrabble so far. And God knows, that's saying something. Rob got literally all the good letters and mine were worth one each, nearly all the way through. So it's 24-18 now. So unfair. I'm almost too sad about it to be irritated any more.

Day 286 — 3rd October 2011
Rielasingen-Worblingen, Germany

It's really annoying that the Kindle won't work here. I really could do with buying Mark's birthday present soon.

Quite a lazy day today. I went for a walk into the town and managed not to get lost. I felt much better after a bit of fresh air. I feel that my hour on foot justified the choc ice I scoffed afterwards. Apart from that, we've mostly just spent the day sitting in the sun reading. I've managed to avoid Scrabble so far, but I don't think there'll be any escape tonight.

"This must be what it's like being retired, don't you think?" I said to Rob this afternoon.

"How do you mean?"

"Well, we just sit around reading or playing Scrabble, we have our tea at 5pm, like old people do... we listen to the wireless, then we go to bed ridiculously early."

Rob started laughing.

"We've even been for afternoon snoozes a couple of times," I pointed out, warming to my theme.

"It doesn't help that you're sitting there like that!" he said, pointing at the tartan blanket I'd draped over my knees.

"Well, it gets chilly in the afternoons."

"Now you sound really old."

Now that the weather's turned around, I felt a bit strange to be sitting doing nothing. Fair enough reading books and lazing about all day while you're on holiday, but we're not technically on holiday, we're travelling, which is a bit different. I can't get it into my head that I'm not skiving while we're on this trip. I quite often find myself wondering what I should be doing next, rather than what I feel like doing next. I think I've not only been institutionalised by the Scottish Wedding Directory and its funny little ways, I've also become conditioned by years of working too hard. I keep telling myself to relax, that I deserve a bit of fun after what I've been through, but I'm not really convinced. I'm all for other people relaxing, though. So I was pleased that Rob was very much enjoying

'Starter For Ten'. He kept laughing out loud so that I had to stop the book I was reading to ask him which bit he was at. Then I got to enjoy it all over again.

Day 287 — 4th October 2011
Rielasingen-Worblingen, Germany

I've just been for a run and I'm not exaggerating when I say that my face is luminous pink. I look ridiculous! Anyone who sees me like this must think there's something terribly wrong with me. Still, it felt good to be running again.

I was thinking about the empty feeling that not having my old job gives me. It's a bit like the moment you finish the best book you've ever read — there's a wistfulness about such a good story ending and a future that feels blank as you wonder 'what next?' You feel the chances of finding a *second* equally compelling story are slim to feck all.

We each won a game of Scrabble tonight. 25-19.

Day 288 — 5th October 2011
Scheidegg, Germany

We were all set to go this morning, until a German guy called Milco rocked up. He started talking to Rob about motorhomes and his business, something to do with using agitation to clean things on an industrial scale. Rob ended up speaking to him. On an industrial scale.

At first when I saw him chatting to Rob I thought, oh good, someone around our age. Not that I mind talking to older people, but it had been a while since we'd spoken to anyone without grey hair. Milco's was still brown, although receding, and he looked forty-ish. He was quite short and stocky, and looked very confident. His English was excellent.

We soon learned that Milco had some pretty unusual (OK, let's just say mental) views. He's completely sexist for a start, not that that's what made him mental. He said at one point, "Look at her," gesturing to me, "she goes crazy every month because of the moon."

What I should have said was, "Actually it's a surge of quite powerful hormones, not the moon, that causes PMS. And women don't 'go crazy', they just get a bit emotional or moody. How do you think you might behave if you had painful cramps, felt like shit and bled for a week every month?"
But of course I only came up with that answer afterwards. Instead, not wanting to sound like a bitter angry old feminist, I made some fairly rubbish little joke along

the lines of 'at least I've got an excuse, I don't know what Rob's is when he's a moany cow'. Ha ha.

This isn't what alerted me to the sexism, though. There were just too many not-very-subtle messages; references to 'when she makes you coffee', for example, and 'her cooking you some eggs for breakfast'. (At which point I felt compelled to inform him that Rob is the "egg chef" in our partnership.)

These references were not made naturally, unselfconsciously, as I've heard old-fashioned men do, without meaning any offence, within the realms of normal everyday conversation. Milco's were more deliberate and didn't quite sit naturally with the rest of the topic, as if he'd only said them to test our reactions to the idea that the female would naturally carry out these menial tasks, this woman's work.

Apart from the casual sexism, he was OK to talk to. I made an effort to get on OK with him despite the chauvinist attitude. A policy that worked. Until he started going on about cancer.

"Did you know there is a cure for cancer?"

"Right," I said slowly. "No. Must have missed that story in the news. What's the cure then?"

"You can look it up, it's all documented. There is a doctor who found a cure for cancer, but it's all been covered up."

How to frame this question politely...?

"You don't seriously believe that do you?"

He looked at me sadly, as if to say, here's another one who refuses to see the plain truth of the matter, a truth so obvious to me.

"If you can open your mind to this, you don't ever need to worry about having cancer again, and you can tell your families this and then your mother, your father, your sister, everyone in your family and who you love, they can all be free of disease for all their life."

It sounds lovely. I would love to do this for them. It's a shame he was talking absolute bollocks.

"OK," he said, "let me explain it like this. When you go to see a doctor, and he tells you you have cancer, does he know what has caused it?"

"Well, no. Because no one knows what causes cancer yet. I mean, there are loads of theories-"

He cut me off with, "Ah! So let's say you have a car engine, it doesn't work, and you go to a mechanic. Imagine if he tells you he will try to fix it, *without understanding what is causing the problem.* Would you have much belief that he could... cure your car?"

I tried to humour him by going along with his logic.

"OK, what does this doctor think causes it then?"

"The same thing as all other diseases, it's an emotional trauma."

"Riiiight... so how does he cure this emotional trauma? And why would anyone want to cover it up if someone had proved this to be true?"

"OK, when you go and see the doctor, you think he wants to help you, right?"

"Yes of course," I said, trying not to get annoyed.

"But he doesn't. He wants to stay in a job. If they admitted we know the real cause of cancer, doctors would not have a medical industry to give them a job. They say we can try chemotherapy, or radiotherapy, but they know this doesn't usually work."

I thought about what he was saying, but really I was only looking for ways to tell him it was bollocks without being rude. A lot of people question the effectiveness of conventional cancer treatments, but this guy had taken it too far. He reckoned the "rich elite" all believe the theory and treat their families accordingly, in secret, of course.

That bit reminded me of the Dad in 'So I Married An Axe Murderer', my favourite comedy film, the bit where he goes on about a secret society of the five wealthiest people in the world. *It's a well-known fact, they're known as the Pentaverate, they run everything in the world, including the newspapers. So who's in this Pentaverate? The Queen, the Vatican, the Gettys, the Rothschilds, and Colonel Sanders before he went tits up. Oh, I hated the Colonel with 'is wee beady eyes! And that smug look on his face, 'Oh, you're gonna buy my chicken! Ohhhhh!'*

"I'm sorry, I just don't believe much of this."

Any of this, actually. He kept saying it was well documented so I asked, several times, for the name of the doctor he reckons cured cancer. He seemed reluctant to give it to me but eventually did. I got him to spell it so we could Google him later.

"This was thirty years ago he found the cure. The authorities, the elite, they use his methods but the mainstream have ostracised him because it's not in their interests to admit the truth. They say he hates the Jews but that's not true."

Hmmm.

We carried on talking for a while, and there were some topics we found common ground on, for example the link between oil money and the most recent Iraq war.

He was an interesting person and quite skilled at reading people. For example, as we were talking I kept thinking, we should really get going now. I didn't express it though, didn't want to be rude. Just then Milco pointed at my shoes, which I'd subconsciously shifted towards the motorhome, and said, "But she wants to leave now, I think."

Top marks for interpreting body language, Milco. Not quite a Derren Brown level of spookiness, but lots of people don't notice these things.

"Well, he was certainly a character," I said when we'd waved goodbye and driven off.

"Yeah. Bit of a nutter eh."

Poor Rob had two terrible games of Scrabble so it's 25-21 now. I say 'poor Rob', but of course I was barely able to contain my jubilance. YES! I got a fifty-point boost with my seven-letter 'brainier'. The 'b' was already on the board so I was pretty brainy to get that one, I reckon.

Day 289 — 6th October 2011
Scheidegg, Germany

Wow, yesterday felt like a really long one. After our mammoth mental morning with Milco, we set off at lunchtime. The road we were meant to take was closed. When we got to the aire we were aiming for, where we'd planned to stay a few days, it was €6, not including lecky, per night. Which might not sound that much, but it was more than it had said in the book. And the place wasn't even that nice. So we decided not to stay after all. The next aire along the road was in a town centre, which Rob doesn't generally like. This one actually looked OK, ie safe, but was packed. So we moved again.

The place we eventually ended up in is very pretty, with plenty of space (and only one other motorhome) and trees as well as — big bonus — a Lidl right across the road. It's nothing fancier than a big car park, but it's a good-looking leafy one, so you don't notice the concrete. And it's about a five-second walk from a river, which is handy for walks. There's also a swimming pool nearby; I'm determined to use it, mostly so I can snatch a lovely long free shower where the hot water isn't in danger of running out. This aire costs €5 a night, but that includes electricity, so we're quite happy. I'm glad we're staying at least a couple of nights. I'm sick of being on the road day after day. I just want to chill out for a bit really.

The Kindle is working again, thank flip.

Rob has, of course, already made friends with the people in the other motorhome. He's so sociable! Which is definitely a good thing. But it's a bit like when you fancy a couple of drinks, then you meet a few friends who've been out all day and you realise you're playing catch up. You are drunk, you know you are, but because they're so much more so, you eventually go home unsatisfied because, in comparison to their merriment, you feel like a great big boring sober party pooper. Well, it's a wee bit like that.

Rob hasn't relayed the whole story to me yet, but it sounds like the Austrian guy, Michael, from the other motorhome, has quite an interesting history. All I know so far is that he has a Hungarian wife, called Agota, who's a bit younger than he is.

Rob is quite impressed by the spec of Michael's Winnebago-style vehicle (maybe a little envious too). It has a dishwasher and a toilet tank so big you only have to empty it once a month (ours is more like every two or three days). All its tanks are about three times as big as ours; their water tank holds 450 litres rather than our 120. Which is lucky because Agota likes to have two showers a day!

Rob is most interested in the technical spec. My favourite fact about their van, though, is that it's big enough for *two* tellies, so he can watch Austrian TV and she can watch Hungarian! And people think you're roughing it living in a motorhome.

After dinner Rob and Michael bonded as they chatted outside and once I'd put some insect repellent on (the mozzies here are awful) I joined them, a wee bit shy at first.

There's something quite lovely about Michael, I decided as I listened to him talking. He's not wildly handsome exactly. He's about forty, completely bald, with quite a solid beer belly. He rides a very cool moped and wears a diamond stud in one ear — but somehow the earring adds to the manliness of his demeanour. His eyes twinkle with what I'm pretty sure is mischievousness. And he has that quiet sort of confidence — he seems very comfortable with himself, without being overbearing or arrogant — which is always attractive in a man.

Another thing is his dog. He looks just like the kind of guy who would own a Rottweiler or an Alsatian. Definitely a scary-looking hound. But no, Michael has a tiny little Chihuahua. The most unmanly dog you could imagine! It even has one of those daft little dog coats on. It says, 'My daddy loves me'. Usually I'm vehemently opposed to any instance of animals wearing clothes. It's not cute or funny, just wrong. But in this case the dog, Bean, looks so tiny, skinny and generally pathetic (it's not cold right now but when I bent down to say hello I noticed his puny twiglet legs shaking), I'm inclined to think he probably needs the extra padding.

"Before I was engineering with Mol Group. It's a company in Hungary for oil and gas," he was saying when I tuned back in, "but I was made redundant from there when, you know, the company liquate. So then I was engineer with another Hungary oil company. But it also went, how do you say, went under?"

We both nodded yes.

"So then I think, maybe it is safer for Agota's country that I am not engineer any more," he said with a smile. We laughed. I got the feeling he had made that joke before.

"Agota and me decide with the redundant money, to buy a place in Indonesia, a beach bar."

"Oh right," Rob said.

"It was devastated by the tsunami, you know, before we buy it, but we decide we can build it up again."

"That sounds cool," I said, not because he was waiting for a response, but because I'm conscious I haven't said anything at all since I came out.

"Yes," he said, looking me in the eye.

"But then we make it a success and when we do there is a group of Indian guys who always want to buy it. They come every one or two months; 'How much do you want for your bar?' I tell them, 'No, thank you, we don't want to sell'.

"But they keep to asking all the time. So one day I say, just to be, you know... to have them gone from asking me all the time, I say a silly price. A really silly price. I think, ha! This will make them leave me alone. And the man goes away but he comes the next day and he says, 'Yes I pay you this much'. So we talk and we say, yeah, why not?"

I was still mulling this over when Michael started explaining the job he had had between being an engineer and owning the beach bar.

"I make holes," he said. Rob and I both looked at the ground.

"No," he said, laughing. "I don't know the English word but I make holes in people, small holes," he said, pointing to his earring.

"Ah!" me and Rob said in unison, "body piercings!"

"Yes! That's the word, piercings."

Interesting as Michael was, I went inside then as it was getting cold and I could feel things biting me.

Later I asked Rob how old he thought Michael might be.

"Oh he told me he's 52," he answered.

"What? Bloody hell, I thought he was about forty!"

I was shocked.

"And he smokes!"

"Yeah. I suppose he does look a bit younger."

We did some washing today. It's such a pain doing it by hand. It takes ages and squeezing isn't nearly as effective as spinning. Plus it makes your hands ache after a while. Hopefully it will be sunny tomorrow so we can get it dried. I think it's meant to be wet the next few days though.

Rob just tried to get the satellite TV working. It was very frustrating. It took a lot of positioning and rotating and 'anything? / no, nothing' conversations. Miraculously he eventually tuned in to something. For a whole precious hour we had Channel 4! And Film4. Amazing! Then it got cloudy and all the good channels disappeared in a puff of smoke, never to be seen again. We were left with porn and god-botherer channels again. And badly dubbed German film channels.

I went for a long walk along the river today. So long that Rob thought I'd got lost. Actually it's quite easy not to when you have a river to walk beside. As long as you keep it on the right (or left) of you and keep going in a straight line, it's almost impossible to take a wrong turn.

When we were out talking to Michael tonight (I say 'out', I was inside the motorhome with the mozzie net firmly set across the door, while the two blokes stood outside), he said to wait a second as Agota had a present for us. I had a slight mini panic while he was away because I find presents extremely embarrassing when you have to react properly while the giver is watching. Rob and I looked at each other, wondering what it would be. Two minutes later he came back and handed us a massive coned-shaped joint.

It turns out that Michael met his wife when she was just 15. He said they weren't allowed to get married until she was 16.

"So we had a baby while we were waiting, because, you know, you can't just do nothing," he said, grinning.

I thought he was joking for a second. But there was no punchline. Blimey. This guy gets more interesting every day.

I just lost at Scrabble. It's 26-21 now. Damn! Rob got *two* seven-letter words, so I didn't stand much of a chance.

Later. Just played *again* and I lost. *Again.* And this time I lost in the most annoying and stupid manner. I stupidly opened up the triple for Rob. I think I was panicking about the time (we inflict a ten-point penalty for every minute you go over the 35-minute game limit) and just put any old thing down. Unfortunately Rob chose this moment to use his 'q', on a double letter, on the triple word. Which gave him a whopping 75 points. I didn't give up though. I even caught him up and heroically overtook him, despite a definite deficit of good letters in Rob's favour. Until right at the end. He then asked one of the most irritating questions I've ever heard in the history of Scrabble Wars: "Is there such a word as 'pangs'? There's not is there?"

I couldn't believe it. Is there such a word?? I can actually remember *using* the word 'pangs' *in a conversation with Rob* just days ago. When he'd won the game by getting a horrendous number of points from the word 'pangs' (the 'p' was on a triple letter, the word on a double), I happened to casually mention the fact that I'd said the very same word to him recently. A word he'd just questioned the existence of. His response?

"Oh, I must have thought you said 'pans'."

Pans?! I can't believe that I've lost at Scrabble, to someone who doesn't know about the word pangs. Pans!

Day 290 — 7th October 2011
Scheidegg, Germany

Damn, we'd got the washing almost dry but it started spitting, so we had to drag it all inside. Serves me right for feeling so smug about getting it done and not being somewhere windy and rainy.

It was raining when we went across the car park to fill up with water too. The water flows ridiculously fast here so we had a good comedy moment when our hose nozzle flicked off and the water started going everywhere. Had even more fun trying to get the hose attached again. That was after a mini-panic caused by us tripping the electricity; something to do with the point we're using being only eight amps, according to Rob. Lovely Michael came to the rescue and helped us get it going again.

I have at least 13 new mozzie bites on my legs. They look disgusting and are incredibly itchy. Well sexy.

We were talking with Michael this afternoon about how being in a motorhome is brilliant for not getting hassled by the police. We've been through quite a few places where police had set up temporary checkpoints, often at roundabouts. Officers stop various cars, asking the drivers questions. But as soon as they clock the motorhome, they always wave us through.

"There was only one time I was stopped by the police, in the motorhome," Michael said. "When Agota and I were passing through the border between Albania and Macedonia. We had all correct papers, of course, but there were two policeman and a... how you say, snifter dog?"

"Sniffer dog, yeah," I said, trying not to grin at the thought of a little dog delicately holding a brandy glass in its paw.

"They are suspecting us; they look at the papers, the visas and they say 'Why are you going to Macedonia only for one night?' We say, 'We don't have any more time than one night.'

"So the police dog is barking, bark bark bark; he is scaring our little doggie. But the police say, very polite, but he says, 'Please can you get out of your vehicle?' So Agota and me get out.

"The police say, 'Is there anything you want to tell us about, before we search your vehicle, sir?'. I say, 'No, of course not'. The dog is still barking at our dog. The police are two hours, looking at everything in the van. *Every*thing."

"Noooo," we both said. Nightmare...

"Yes. They even take... what's the word? It's like the inside walls... to check underneath."

"The panelling? Seriously, they took all that off?"

"Yes, seriously. Two hours they spent. All the time the dog is bark bark barking away. The police find my tobacco and my rolling papers. He says, 'Why do you not smoke a normal cigarette? Why do you need to roll your own cigarettes?'

"He is narrowing his eyes at me. I just stay relaxed, I am still very polite and cool with him. I just say, 'The price of normal cigarettes is very expensive, the price of tobacco is much much cheaper.' He says OK. Then the police dog, he still barks.

"My dog is scared, his leg shakes, so I ask the police, I say, 'Is it OK if my wife takes the dog for a walk? He is a little afraid of your bigger dog.' He says, 'Yes, no problem. You need to stay here while we check your vehicle, but it's no problem for your wife to take the dog.'

"So Bean goes walking with Agota, he has his little coat on so he is nice and warm. And finally the police say, 'OK, thank you very much sir. I'm sorry to take your time. Have a nice trip.'"

I was thinking, wow, how unlucky. But the punchline hadn't been delivered yet. The sparkle in Michael's eyes was more prominent than ever. Just before he said it, I guessed. But of course I didn't steal his thunder, managing to look really surprised when he said, "It was lucky they only want to search the van; we had two kilos of grass hiding in Bean's clothes."

Later. Just got beaten *again* at Scrabble. Guess who got all the good letters? Not I. So unfair. 28-21.

Day 291 — 8th October 2011
Scheidegg, Germany

It was raining today so we've had a lazy one. Just looked up Dr Hamer and his 'German New Medicine', Milco's cancer cure guy. I've never read such a load of old rubbish! According to Wiki (due to my journalism training I am compelled to verify this information with at least two independent sources next time we get the proper internet) Dr Hamer has been struck off in a number of countries, his work has been widely discredited (in more than one case his dodgy theories have even, reportedly, led to unnecessary deaths) and aside from all this, he's accused of being a *nazi sympathiser.

Rob tried to get the satellite telly working again. He spent *ages* doing it. But we could only get the worthless channels. And the worst film channel ever invented, Movies For Men. We watched a really bad Rob Lowe film on there. I feel disgusted I just wasted two hours of my life on that. Even though Rob Lowe is very very attractive. On the plus side, we do currently have BBC 6 Music and Radio 4.

We've bought some red wine to drink tonight. If Rob doesn't hurry up his conversation with Michael, I might have to start drinking on my own.

Sylv sent a picture message of herself dressed as She-Ra at Mark's 30th birthday party. She looked absolutely fantastic and I got a tiny bit homesick when I saw it, plus a wee wet eye (only one, mind). Mainly due to the red red wine (can anyone say that without wanting to sing it?) I'd consumed by the time it came through.

Day 292 — 9th October 2011
Scheidegg, Germany

Must have slept for about 12 hours last night. Brilliant.

It's still raining. Went for a walk into town earlier. Didn't find much of interest, except a shop that *might* sell veggie sausages, which we're pining for once more. I'll pop back when they're open tomorrow. I didn't get wet on my little trek. Or lost. So quite successful really.

I have become quite obsessed – I mean quite in the old-fashioned sense of the word, ie completely – by a game called Bubble Blaster 2, on Rob's phone. You have to burst lots of bubbles as quickly as you can. It's a lot like Puzzle Bobble, a game with which I have a history of addiction.

---

* I don't think they deserve a capital letter.

Day 293 — 10th October 2011
Scheidegg, Germany

I went for a lovely long walk along the river. It took well over an hour. I bet Rob was starting to wonder whether I'd got lost.

We half-listened to the football on the radio. It was Scotland against Lichtenstein. I say we half-listened because we actually missed the only goal of the match; Rob was fiddling with the satellite settings at the time. He had been planning on going to see the game in Lichtenstein but didn't feel up to it because of the Lyme disease.

A massive motorhome just turned up and Rob and Michael are busy chatting to the guy who's in it. Sounds like a very strong Midlands accent to me. I know I should probably go and be sociable and say hello, how are you etc. But I just can't be bothered. Should it bother me more that I can't be bothered?

Michael told us he makes €200,000 a year from his 'third' business. Nudge nudge. What I can't understand is what motivates him to do it. He told us that he could have retired early on the proceeds of the beach bar sale alone, so why risk it? I also find it strange that neither Rob nor I have seen Agota yet. I know she's a massive stoner (Michael said she just smokes smokes smokes all day long) but still. I'm starting to wonder if she's really in there at all.

Went to the health food shop today and bought lots of lovely-looking veggie sausages and schnitzel burgers. Mmmm.

Beaten again. The rubbish letters all clung to my hand as I delved into the bag looking for some good luck. Too depressed to even note the score.

Day 294 — 11th October 2011
Scheidegg, Germany

We're preparing to leave Scheidegg and, in fact, Germany. Germany was starting to feel a bit chilly. All the autumn leaves had fallen and you could almost smell winter in the air.

We decided to get south of the Alps before the snow kicked in. After a very short drive through Austria, we will go across the border into the breathtakingly expensive but disgustingly beautiful Switzerland. Or is it the other way round?

That kindly soul Michael has just romantically ridden off into the sunset with Rob on the back of his moped. Or is it a scooter? What's the difference anyway? OK, the sun wasn't really setting and I'm almost certain there's no actual romance involved.

They've gone to an office somewhere so that Rob can get the right papers to make sure we're all legal and above board once we get to the Swiss border. The entry requirements are slightly different because it's not in the EU. So nice of him to take Rob. Michael's been to Switzerland a few times and said it would be easy to show Rob which forms we need.

I bet Rob wants to buy a moped when they get back.

Day 298 — 15th October 2011
Verbania, Italy

Well, Switzerland was as gorgeous as everyone would have you believe. But in a slightly clinical, unreal way. It has an 'orderly ruggedness', as Rob put it. We only stayed one night, in a lay-by-type stop, so we can't quite claim to have experienced Switzerland properly, but I'd definitely like to visit again.

We've been in Verbania for the last couple of nights. The aire here is packed out (we got the last space and we've seen loads of people turned away since) and costs €10 a night. This includes electricity but no 'tip out and top up' water services, so we're mildly outraged — if that's possible — by the price. But somewhat pacified by the weather, which feels distinctly summery for October. It was 28°C when we arrived and the sky has been blue since we got here. Today is cloudy but with an undercurrent of potentially bright sunny loveliness. And having visited an aire that looked nothing like its picture in the book and was €12 a night without electricity, and wasn't even pretty, we decided this was fine.

Watched 'Trading Places' last night. Classic.

The Scrabble wars continue, and the last few battles have been good ones. Good for me that is, ha! I'm only seven games behind now. Yes!

Day 300 — 17th October 2011
Monzambano, Italy

We're staying at a lovely little site 8km from Lake Garda. The top part of this place looks just like a car park, although quite a green leafy one. But when you drive down to the lower level, where we were last night, it's just beautiful, thanks to even more trees and a massive duck pond in the centre. They close the bottom bit when they're not busy so we're back up at the top now. It costs €10 a night here, but that includes water and waste emptying, electricity and, best of all, proper actual wifi. Real live internet access! There is also a laundry in the town so we're definitely going to go and use that.

"Do you fancy going for a bike ride to Lake Garda?"

"Yeah OK, it's meant to be quite nice isn't it?" I replied. I'd heard of it through the honeymooning couples I'd interviewed at the magazine; they'd all said how romantic it was.

"How far is it though?"

"Well, not too far I don't think..."

"Humour me with specifics," I insisted, using my favourite line from the Michael Douglas film 'The Game'. I like to know what I'm letting myself in for.

"About 8k," he said, having consulted the map.

"Right, so 16k there and back. OK, I can cope with that."

We started out following a national cycle route that followed a river.

"This is lovely," I shouted to Rob ahead of me.

But a few kilometres in we noticed loads of fishermen blocking our way. Then a sign informed us that the cycle route was closed today because of a fishing competition. Bugger.

We were forced to cycle along what turned out to be a major road, ridiculously busy with cars, lorries and motorbikes. And because they were Italian almost every driver came far too close and there was a lot of highly inappropriate overtaking. We had a few scary moments, but made it to the lake unscathed.

"Well, that was fun," I laughed, a bit shaky from the fear of being squished all over the road.

"Bloody typical of our luck!" Rob said.

"I know. At least the lake's pretty though..."

After we'd eaten our sandwiches and done a spot of people-watching, Rob managed to find another route back so we didn't have to risk our lives again.

I've finished 'The Life And Adventures Of Robinson Crusoe' by Daniel Defoe. Serves him right really, getting stranded on a desert island. I mean, every boat trip the guy took ended in disaster, even before he got shipwrecked and had to live on his tod. Plus, the whole point of the cruise was to go and get slaves from Africa. I know, I know, you can't judge him using a modern moral compass, but still, I wasn't exactly full of sympathy for the main character. The page-turn-ability factor wasn't bad I suppose, although I did cringe at his descriptions of "local savages". On to 'The Gambler' by Dostoyevsky now.

The Scrabble score is 34-27. That's all I'm going to say on the subject.

Day 301 — 18th October 2011

Monzambano, Italy

We did a 20km cycle to the Lidl at Peschiera Del Garda today. No fishing comps to thwart us this time!

Ours is the only motorhome at this site now.

Day 302 — 19th October 2011

Monzambano, Italy

Rob downloaded a good dose of British TV today, 'Have I Got News For You' and 'QI'. Really enjoyed those. Love having the internet!

We also Skyped Sylv and Mark, making the most of the internet. It was lovely to see them and talk properly, even though there was a bit of a frustrating delay and we couldn't hear them very well.

Day 303 — 20th October 2011

Monzambano, Italy

Oh dear. I was just reading Rob's notes from my descent into the abyss. Blimey. Had a bit of a cry and feel quite shaky now; there were so many scary bits I'd either forgotten or never knew about in the first place. I'm shocked by it.

I was just thinking the other day that I hadn't cried in a while and wasn't feeling quite so emotionally fragile! The whole hospital episode still seems like a protracted bad dream, but Rob's notes made it real again. The bit that hurt most to read about was Rob coming home to find blood all over the bed and the bathroom. I was so out of it I didn't even realise I'd got my period. What a terrible sight to come home to.

"I'm sorry, I didn't mean to upset you," he said.

"It's not your fault," I said, the emotion of the eye-water making it hard to talk normally. "I... I just can't believe I let myself get in such a state."

Rob held me tight and stroked my hair.

I'd been feeling so happy the last few days! But that's what always happens, a high then a low. Sometimes I wish I was one of those steady dependable types who is always somewhere in the middle.

When I'd finished crying I went for a walk round the park. I stopped by the duck pond, listening to them quacking away as if they'd just heard the funniest thing. I noticed a black swan I'd never seen before, and another with a bright red fuzzy mohican-style bit of hair on the top of his head. How simple life must be if you're a bird. No getting sectioned or getting over psychotic episodes.

Reading Rob's notes shines a different light on the experience. When I first got out I was almost embarrassed that nothing more serious than overwork had caused my downfall. I feel more accepting about it now. I still believe that, as far as human suffering goes, my anguish was at the lower end of the scale. But you could say that about most situations. It was painful enough. Painful enough to leave a shadow. What I need now is to forgive myself.

A couple of hours later, I thought about that again. Wait a minute, why do I need to forgive myself? I'm not a criminal. If I'd broken my leg in a skiing accident (how middle class) or been run over by a bus (careless), I wouldn't think forgiveness was relevant. I suppose it says a lot about the way my brain works. Mike The Psych was right when he said I was driven by guilt. I do feel guilty that I let myself go mental. Maybe I'm not quite at the acceptance stage yet. And maybe it would help to work out why I'm so hard on myself. Even if the breakdown was my fault, shouldn't spending three weeks on a mental ward be punishment enough?

This afternoon we opened the wine that our German friends Jess and Sven gave us back in Denmark, justifying it (the clock read 3pm at the time) by telling ourselves we hadn't drunk much for a while, and anyway, it was only 5.5%. And we are kind of on holiday. Still, it felt very naughty.

Rob went to the local launderette and did all our washing. It's lovely to have nice clean bed clothes again.

Later on Rob did his good deed for the day by helping a Slovenian family fix the boiler in their motorhome. He spent ages doing it. Maybe he will pat himself on the back tonight...

I won at Scrabble tonight so it's 34-28 now.

Day 305 — 22nd October 2011
Monzambano, Italy

Rob went to get bread this morning and came back laughing his head off.

"What's so funny?"

"The locals! They all think I'm mental!" he said, still laughing. "All the old people were laughing and pointing at my bare arms; they kept saying 'Fredo! Fredo! [Cold! Cold!] ' So I said, 'No, Scozzese [Scottish], this is caldo! [hot!]'. They were falling about laughing," he said, grinning away.

We just Skyped Mum, Dad and Adam. It was great fun.

Day 307 — 24th October 2011
Monzambano, Italy
I've had another really bad run at the Scrabble, losing three in a row. The last one was incredibly, annoyingly close. 38-29. So pissed off.

Day 308 — 25th October 2011
Monzambano, Italy
It has rained all day. We were meant to go to Venice today. Rob was using the internet on the Kindle.

"Oh, there's not much point going to Venice today. It's flooded."

"Yeah, very funny."

He looked at me.

"I'm not joking. It happens all the time there. Honestly."

"Oh come on, I'm not that daft. I suppose you're gonna tell me the streets are full of water now?"

He was always pulling my leg. He started laughing, which didn't help his credibility.

"Look, if you don't believe me..."

He showed me the Kindle and it was true, he wasn't lying at all.

"See, you shouldn't doubt me Bosal."

"Yeah, that'll be right."

There is a German couple in a motorhome across the way. They have a dog who they left outside in the rain all night. Poor thing. How cruel can you be? We were tempted to invite him into ours.

I've clawed one back so it's 38-30.

Day 309 — 26th October 2011
Sernaglia Della Battaglia, Italy
Bit of a stressful day. First problem was the satnav behaving very strangely. We eventually figured out we'd accidentally left it on the bike setting rather than the car one. Idiots. We were also both very hungry as we'd only had a slice of cheese for breakfast, having decided just to get going and eat properly later.

When we got to our planned stop the place looked absolutely lovely. Unfortunately it was also closed for the winter. So we stuck the next set of coordinates into the satnav, which led us through a beautiful town that had ridiculously narrow cobbled lanes, not motorhome-friendly wide streets. People kept staring at us as they breathed in to let us pass, as if to say, 'What the hell are you doing here?' One young guy smiled and mouthed the word 'wow' in our direction. It was *very* tight. I don't know how Rob kept his cool. There was literally an inch either side of us, and there were plenty of telltale scrape marks along the medieval walls. We only just made it through the village, and even after that the satnav took us on a few more narrow steep windy roads.

Just when I thought our day couldn't get any worse, we stopped for diesel and the self-service machine ate our €60 but didn't give us any fuel! There was no one around so we'll have to go back tomorrow and see if we can sort it out. At least we have a receipt.

The aire we're at now is called Le Grave. It's a lot nicer than it sounds. The lady who came to collect the money used the actual words 'mamma mia'.

The rain was consistent to the point of stubbornness today.

I lost TWICE at Scrabble tonight so the score is 41-32. Every time I feel like I'm catching him he wins another three or four in a row and I'm right back where I started. I'm unbelievably pissed off that he always gets the good letters!

Day 310 — 27th October 2011
Sernaglia Della Battaglia, Italy

What a beautiful day. It's 20°C, sunny and the sky is blue. We did some washing this morning and some of it's dry already.

We have just been for a bike ride through some nearby towns, along a river and into a forest.

"Was that a gun?" I asked Rob, when I heard a loud cracking sound.

"Mmm, maybe," he said, unconcerned. I heard a few more disturbing noises and hoped we weren't about to get shot. A few minutes later I spotted a guy coming towards us along the path. As he got closer I could see he was out hunting; he had a dog and a huge shotgun with him.

"Buongiorno," he said, giving the customary head nod.

We smiled and mumbled the same back.

Day 311 — 28th October 2011
Cavallino-Treporti, near Venice, Italy

A good day. The guy at the petrol station was very nice and smiley and had absolutely no problem giving us our money back for the petrol that never appeared. His English was almost as limited as our Italian, but through sign language we gleaned that Rob had somehow managed to press the wrong button on the machine, one that didn't correspond to the pump we were trying to use.

Whoops. He reminded me of Bruce Willis. Such a nice man too. As we left he gave us the peace sign and wished us well on our journey.

Drove round for *ages* looking for some discount sports outlet where Rob could buy cheap ski boots. Well, not cheap, but cheaper than usual. Which is still flipping expensive. Anyway we just didn't have any luck finding it. Eventually Rob took the wholly desperate measure of actually asking someone. Again through sign language, we gathered that the guy was telling us to follow him. So we did. And we found it perfectly easily. Another thoroughly lovely Italian man! My perception of these continentals is vastly improving each day. Not that I was ever anti-continental, but I find these small kindnesses very touching. Rob has bought some ski boots.

Went on some pretty narrow roads again today, but it wasn't too scary.

Just parked up. It's beautiful here. We're staying on a long strip of a car park that looks out over the water, just a few miles down the coast from Venice. There are a couple of other motorhomes here and we're just metres from the beach. There are signs up implying, well stating really, that we should be paying €7.50 to park here. Not even per night, per 12 hours. Unfortunately, the restaurant where you're supposed to buy the parking tickets appears to be closed for the winter. And nobody has come round to take money off us so far. Result!

Venice tomorrow!

Day 312 — 29th October 2011
Cavallino-Treporti, near Venice, Italy
We're not going into Venice today as Rob didn't sleep too well last night. Going to try a bike ride on the beach though.

Later. Riding a bike along this beach didn't work. The wheels sank into the wet sand.

We have run out of proper tea so we're on to the last resort cheapo brands of Darjeeling and Earl Grey lurking at the back of the cupboard. Not good. They taste weak and slightly soapy.

Lost at Scrabble. 43-33. Extremely annoyed.

Day 313 — 30th October 2011
Cavallino-Treporti, near Venice, Italy
Woke up feeling a bit perturbed, after an unsettling dream. At first I was just relieved it wasn't really happening.

"Had a weird dream..." I told Rob, as the dream memories came back to me.

"Yeah?"

"Mmm. I dreamt we'd cooked loads of food but it'd fallen into the sink by accident and got washing up liquid all over it. Then I looked round and there was this short Indian guy standing at the front of the van, dancing. It was really strange."

"I had a bit of a funny dream too," Rob said after a short pause.

"Really?"

I was intrigued; Rob very rarely remembered anything of his dreams, whereas I'm always boring him with details of mine.

"Yeah, I dreamt I had terminal cancer."

"Oh my God, that's awful!"

"Yeah. I only had a few weeks to live. People kept asking what we were doing for Christmas and it was really awkward because we kept having to explain that I'd be dead by then."

"Jesus, that's horrific. I can't believe you never remember your dreams, but the one time you do, you dream *that!*"

We were both quiet for a minute, then I started giggling.

"I'm sorry baby, but that's just awful!"

Rob started laughing too. When I saw his shoulders shaking, it made me laugh even more.

"That would put a bit of a downer on the holiday wouldn't it," he said.

"Yeah, just a bit."

Although we've been staying right on the seafront for free, Rob reckons he'd feel better about leaving the motorhome all day, while we go to Venice, if we took it somewhere more legitimate. Somewhere less likely to get broken into. So we headed to a motorhome zoo just down the road, where you park so close to the next van you can probably hear your neighbours turning the pages of their holiday reads.

It was so busy Rob found it tricky to park, but he managed. It cost €20 to park overnight but it's a weight off Rob's mind.

We got the ferry into Venice and wandered round for a while. It was just as beautiful as I'd imagined. I felt like I'd been here before, probably because I've seen so many films made here. I'd been prepared for really smelly canals, but we must have picked a good day as I haven't noticed any whiffs. Apart from Rob's 'man smell', but I'm used to that.

The place was completely packed out with tourists, amazing for this time of year. It must be a nightmare in summer.

We'd brought a packed lunch because we read online that the restaurants in the centre of the city were extremely expensive. We found a bench in St Mark's Square and started tucking in.

"Oh look, Rob, we're breaking the law."

We were sitting right next to a sign, in Italian and nothing else of course, but with helpful diagrams to tell you in no uncertain terms that you mustn't eat food here. Drinking coffee was also a no-no. Other forms of uncivilised behaviour, such as scoffing ice cream, were forbidden too.

"Bloody hell," Rob said.

"What's that all about then? Is it in case you make a mess?"

"Maybe they just want to make sure you buy from the local food places, rather than bringing your own."

We weren't exactly worried by the sign, but we did start eating just a little faster, throwing the odd furtive glance around in case the Food Police were looking our way.

We were lucky the weather was so nice. It felt like the height of summer in Scotland. We walked around admiring the gondolas, the precarious-looking buildings and the smartly dressed people. It may be a cliché but Italians really do know how to dress well. They're not so much uniformly fashionable (in fact, we saw plenty of that ultimately uncool combination: white socks and shiny slip-on shoes), but generally, regardless of age or wealth, they really make an effort to look smart. Clothes look high quality, freshly ironed and as if some thought has gone into them. I didn't see anyone you could describe as scruffy.

Despite the wide selection of beautifully decorated masks and endless pieces of Murano glass on sale, our own tourist spend was pretty much limited to two delicious ice creams. It would have been rude not to on a day like this. The portions were huge and the total price was only three Euros. Who said Venice was a rip-off?

When evening arrived and we'd had enough of walking around, we found a cafe that didn't look too expensive and sat down to enjoy the sunset and a bottle of red wine. We did some people watching and as the wine took hold it all felt rather lovely. A massive boat came in to dock and I tried to capture the spectacle on my camera phone. It amused me to imagine all the people on board, what they might be up to. I wondered if it was like 'Carry On Cruising'.

It was getting colder but the sunset was so beautiful I didn't want to leave our table outside the cafe. Rob chivalrously offered me his duck. (His body warmer is filled with duck feathers, which isn't very good vegetarian behaviour really, but that's why we call it his duck.)

We were hungry when we got home and decided to eat at a seafood restaurant just a few metres from our motorhome zoo. It was quite busy for a weeknight in October.

"Blimey Rob, look at these prices!"

It was incredibly cheap. A one-litre carafe of wine was only €5. Because we'd had our second dose of wine by then, we weren't shy about ordering. Pronouncing things badly and pointing at the menu to prevent misunderstandings is perfectly acceptable isn't it? Better than just speaking English anyway.

I ordered a seafood pizza. I was very impressed by the look of it; half the creatures in the sea — mussels, octopus, non-chewy squid and more — seemed to have made it on to this piece of dough.

There was a slightly awkward moment when the waitress said something we didn't understand. Rob stared, his face blank. I frantically replayed the phrase in my head, trying to make sense of it. It sounded like, "Dee-zet for you?"

She repeated it, looking a bit annoyed that these stupid, slightly drunk foreigners couldn't understand her perfectly decent but thickly accented English.

I suddenly realised she must be asking if we wanted *dessert*.

"Do you want pudding Rob?" I said quickly, my tone implying that I had, of course, understood all along and was just waiting on my thicko husband catching up. Ahem.

"Oh, no, thank you," Rob said with a smile designed to cover our embarrassment. She walked away with a smile of her own, one that didn't reach her eyes.

Day 314 — 31st October 2011
Cavallino-Treporti, near Venice, Italy

Back to the free camping spot by the beach this morning. The sky has made itself blue again today. It's 15°C at the moment and it's only 10am.

We watched 'Crash' tonight. It's about a load of people who don't know each other but some bad stuff goes down that links them together over a couple of days. They're all, in different ways, a bit racist. It wasn't bad but was pretty heavy, not exactly uplifting.

Day 315 — 1st November 2011

Cavallino-Treporti, near Venice, Italy

We went for a nice bike ride (20km) before 'enjoying' a mammoth Scrabble sesh. We played four games, winning two each. A most annoying result because in effect nothing has changed. The score is 45-35.

We still don't have any proper tea; it's all about the coffee in Italy. The situation prompts a sigh of irritation every morning when I wake up and remember. I decided to try a new technique today, combining 'proper' Tetley decaffeinated tea with cheapo-nasty-foreign-bought-but-readily-available Darjeeling bags. The experiment failed. It still tasted a bit funny. Actually, it was pretty disgusting. I couldn't ignore the soapy edge. We'll be forced to take drastic action, switching to coffee maybe, if this carries on.

Day 316 — 2nd November 2011

Cavallino-Treporti, near Venice, Italy

The warm weather continues, as does the Scrabble carnage. I think Rob's getting bored of winning. Four games today. I lost them all. Two were extremely close, a single point between us in one game. I'm so pissed off about it I've suggested a Scrabble amnesty; when Rob reaches fifty wins, we'll start again. Something needs to change because morale is dangerously low. My Scrabble mojo is curled up in a foetal ball in a dark corner somewhere, licking her wordy wounds.

I think I may be experiencing the opposite of success breeds success. The more I fail, the harder I try to grip the tiles of success, and the faster any potential inspiration slips out of my clammy hands. Something like that anyway.

In a bid to do something other than lose at Scrabble, I suggested starting the jigsaw of a tiger we brought with us. It was fun, quite relaxing, a nice quiet form of escapism. Rob's visually astute brain made him very good at finding the right shaped piece at every turn. I had the odd moment of brilliance, and we made a good team, because I was more inclined to match pieces by colour and pattern. Still, I couldn't help thinking, if this was a competition, Rob would win. It's annoying being married to someone who's so bloody good at everything! Right now I can't think of anything, with the exception of swimming, at which I can beat him. And that doesn't really count because he never goes swimming. The only other thing I'm better at is the board game 'Articulate'. I'm quite nifty at that.

Day 317 — 3rd November 2011
Classe, Italy

Today we left our free spot near Venice, got some LPG and stocked up at Lidl. We bought a bottle of vodka for less than five Euros! And four bottles of red wine, for about €1.50 each, two of which were 1.5 litres!

We drove to a place where we could fill up with water and empty our waste and are now at Classe, close to Ravenna. It looks nice enough, but there are no facilities. The motorhome battery is down to 55% (this is not good at all, according to Rob) so we'll soon head somewhere with electricity, perhaps San Marino.

Rob's parents, Rosie and Barry, are hopefully flying out soon to meet up with us and have a little break. They're both good fun and I'm looking forward to seeing them. The prospect of sharing the motorhome with two extra people sounds a bit too cosy for comfort. But with a bit of luck we'll be able to find them a lovely cottage to rent.

We finished the jigsaw tonight, all 500 pieces are in position. Enjoyable as it sort of was, I'd be happy never to see another tiger whisker again.

Day 318 — 4th November 2011
Brisighella, Italy

This aire is on the edge of the town and has plenty of trees. There was a police car here when we arrived at lunchtime. The policemen were talking to a crusty-looking couple who had a campervan. We had no idea what they were saying of course, but we got the feeling the crusties had been victims of some kind of crime, though not a particularly serious one going by the looks on their faces.

Tonight a guy from the local council came over to ask us if everything had been OK since our arrival. But as we'd only been here a few hours, we couldn't tell him much.

We went for a bike ride this afternoon and although we didn't go far it was totally knackering, because it was mostly uphill. However, we did enjoy some amazing views from the clock tower and the top of the castle. It's a very pretty town, with neat lines of cute little trees, cobbled streets and a skyline packed with flat sand-coloured roofs.

Rob decided to wash the top of the motorhome this afternoon. My extremely boring but important job was to hold the bottom of the ladder.

Rob reached fifty Scrabble wins so we've started afresh. I feel like a weight has been lifted from my word-weary shoulders. And guess what? I've just won the first two games of the new set! During the second, I got *two* seven-letters, 'partied' and 'victors'. I have to say, it was quite funny to be the pleased-with-myself player (OK, the smug player) for a change, and to look over and see Rob's disgruntled expression. Ha ha!

Tonight we drank wine and watched one of my favourite films, 'American Beauty'. It's about a bloke who has a brilliant midlife crisis.

Day 319 — 5th November 2011
Brisighella, Italy

Rob has a mozzie bite on the outside edge of his ear. It's swollen right up. He must have got it when he cleared out the guttering yesterday.

"No offence, but you look a bit like the Elephant Man," I said, not bothering to stifle a laugh. "Ha, you've literally got a thick ear."

Rob tried to look offended but was soon laughing too. It just looked so silly, especially from the back. It made me laugh even more when I saw his shoulder shake coming on.

I didn't sleep particularly well last night. We went to bed a bit later than usual (after three games of Scrabble, all of which I won — mwahahaha!) and I didn't do any exercise yesterday. The book I'm reading, 'Sectioned: A Life Interrupted', is pretty good too, so that didn't encourage sleepiness. It's the true story of a guy who gets sectioned five times. He manages to make it funny as well as serious, for which I'm very grateful.

I was just sitting quietly, reading my book, when Rob burst into the motorhome.

"For some reason, I really feel like watching 'Poirot'," he said decisively. I laughed.

"Is this some kind of homesickness, a craving for old British TV?"

"I dunno, maybe. Although that would be weird, as Poirot is Belgian."

Rob didn't get his fix, but I felt brand new after showering.

We went for a walk in the rain this afternoon. It was quite nice, although some parts were a bit jungly. I kept thinking David Bellamy was about to pop out from the undergrowth.

I've just measured my waist. It's 38 inches! Or 37.75 if I hold the tape measure a bit closer. Jesus. That can't be right can it? Must try harder to stay out the larder.* A lot harder. Can that measurement really be right?

---

* I only used that word for rhyming purposes, we don't have a larder in the motorhome.

Our tape measure is a piece of string with a marker on it, because the only actual tape measure we have came out of a cracker and is only about 15 inches long.

"Blimey," Rob said after he'd told me how wide I was. "Reckon the old prenup's gonna kick in soon..."

"Oi! That's not very supportive."

"Sorry. You'll need even more support if you get any bigger you know."

"Rob! That's not very nice."

Loads of Italian motorhomes have turned up. They all appear to know each other, so it must be some sort of club or rally meeting.

Day 320 — 6th November 2011
Brisighella, Italy

Finished 'Sectioned' last night. So glad it was a happy ending! I told Rob how much I'd enjoyed it.

"There's a lot of painful stuff in there, but he tells the story in such a beautiful way..."

"I take it it's called 'Sectioned' because the guy was actually sectioned?"

"Yeah, not just once though. Five times."

"Bloody hell."

"I know. Imagine going through what we did another four times."

"I'm not sure how well I'd cope with that. I mean, I was so relieved you got better... it'd be so demoralising to go through it again."

"Too right. Did you ever think I might not recover?"

"Well you know the doctors warned me you might not?"

"What? No, I didn't know that. That's not very encouraging!"

"Well, I think they were trying to prepare me for the worst, you know. They said some people don't, they just snap and they're never the same again."

"Oh man. That must have been horrible for you to hear."

"Yeah it wasn't the best."

Jeez, I suppose I get the whole 'preparing someone for the worst' idea, but it's not very helpful. Whatever happened to the power of positive thinking, don't psych docs believe in that? I wonder how many people don't recover.

We spent quite a pleasant day wandering around a local 'meat festival'. There were lots of non-meaty things to look at too.

"Blimey, I stick out a bit here, don't I?" Rob said.

"What, being ridiculously white and blue-eyed you mean?"

"No, look how tall I am compared to everyone else."

I looked around and right enough, Rob was towering over even the tallest of the Italians.

Spoke too soon about having a pleasant day. Just had a row with Rob after he stood on my foot. I wasn't exactly in agony, and he didn't stamp really hard or on purpose or anything, funnily enough. What offended me was that I didn't hear him say sorry. He swore he said it of course.

A little while later, we'd kind of made up. Having said that, I'm not sure a game of Scrabble is the best road to reconciliation. Rob has just spent *ages* on one shot, because he was convinced there was a seven-letter word there somewhere. Which means he's now in a bad mood with himself because he's hardly got any time left. In fact, he's so down on himself I actually wish he'd get it together and win. Compassion has eclipsed my competitive spirit. And I was so bored waiting for my go that I've eaten about 25 chocolates. Now waiting for the self-loathing to kick in. So we're both in a great mood.

We were feeling sleepy pretty early tonight so thought we might as well not fight it. Just as I was falling asleep Rob said he thought he'd just heard someone trying the door latches on both sides of the motorhome. I felt torn between sleepiness and alarm.

"Don't worry about it," he said.

"Not *entirely* sure that's possible now…"

I must have dropped off though, because a bit later I woke up feeling slightly anxious. As I came round I realised it was all the noise that had woken me up. The locals were still celebrating their meat festival; I could hear rowdy, drunken laughter and shouting, and a hell of a lot of fireworks. There was a party going on in the park just next to us. Bugger.

I couldn't believe Rob was sleeping through the noise. I wondered how late it would go on. Surely they'll all want to go to bed soon? I checked the time on my phone. Oh. It was only 9.45pm!

Day 321 — 7th November 2011
Brisighella, Italy

Dreamt I was still working at the wedding magazine last night. My subconscious hasn't caught up with reality yet.

Feeling the need to get out of the motorhome, I put my brolly up and ventured into town. There were a few nice-looking shops to browse. Or there would have been, but as usual I'd coincided my trip perfectly to fit in with siesta time. I can't get used to shops closing for a few hours in the middle of the day.

There was one shop open though. I was so happy to find it I practically ran inside, singing "Buongiorno!" before the owner could change his mind and pull the shutters down in my face. The guy must have been pretty pleased to see a customer while the rest of the world slept, because he launched into three or four paragraphs of super-fast Italian as soon as I got in the door. When he finally paused to take a breath I said, "Parla Inglese?", giving him an apologetic look. He just laughed and shook his head good-naturedly.

Through a combination of pointing and sign language, I soon had what I wanted, a black mascara. Not before coming across as a flash foreigner by offering him a fifty Euro note, which, of course, he couldn't change. Still, we got there in the end.

Day 322 — 8th November 2011
Brisighella, Italy

Still trying to sort out accommodation for Rosie and Barry next week.

It is sunnier today, as is Rob, who has been a bit down just lately. He probably needs to interact with someone other than me for a change.

Day 323 — 9th November 2011
Barga, Italy

Left Brisighella today. We're on our way to a wee place near Siena where there's a farmhouse for Rosie and Barry to hopefully rent next week. So far it's proving difficult to find somewhere we can park outside in the motorhome.

Started 'The Trial' by Franz Kafka last night. It's quite intriguing so far.

I felt a bit sick as we drove across the windy mountain roads today. It probably didn't help that I was texting Francesca, the property owner (in Italian, with some help from Google Translate) as we were zooming around. No reply yet.

***

What a good day. The cottage was lovely, as was Francesca's Dad, who showed us around. He hardly spoke any English but everything was pretty self-explanatory so it didn't matter. At one stage he started pointing at his house and saying "Berlusconi!" over and over again. We didn't understand what he meant until we spotted a little ironwork of a pig that was hanging from the wall.

"Ah! Yes," we said, laughing as we caught on. "He is a pig," we agreed, nodding away.

We're not leaving Barga for a whole week, which is a brilliant thought. Rob made a mistake with the ticket machine when we arrived so we had to phone some council guy for help. He is coming to sort us out in the morning.

I've just won a game of Scrabble.

Day 324 — 10th November 2011
Barga, Italy

28°C! Another good day. Barga is absolutely beautiful in the daylight.

I went for a run round the car park we're in this morning. I am really enjoying running at the moment. It makes me feel good for the rest of the day. It also makes me think my tummy is at least going in the right direction.

The guy came to fix the problem with the ticket machine and wouldn't take the extra €5 we owed, so we are paying a discounted rate of €45 for seven nights. There are loads of mountains round here so we're going to climb one in a couple of days. I hope it's not too gruelling.

Things are going crazy in the Eurozone. One country after another plunges towards financial crisis, like economic dominos. Berlusconi has resigned. Francesca's father will be pleased, along with quite a lot of other people.

We went for a look round the town and its cathedral, from where you can enjoy great views across Barga. Barga bills itself as the most Scottish town in Italy; the connection goes back to the early 1900s, when loads of Tuscans left Barga for Scotland to try to get work. There is even a Scottish museum here. We didn't see much evidence of Scottishness as we walked around today. But that could be because it was all closed up for siesta by the time we went out. We'll have to pop back out later.

We were going to watch 'The Girl With The Dragon Tattoo' this evening but the DVD was scratched and didn't work properly, so we went with 'Dogma' instead. It's about a couple of angels who are trying to get back into heaven, having been chucked out. That tells you all you need to know about how much sense the story makes. We don't have many films left to watch now.

Day 325 — 11th November 2011
Barga, Italy

It's 27.5°C out there. Amazing.

Had some red wine from cartons last night. It cost sixty cents per litre. That's cheaper than water! It tasted surprisingly all right.

I dreamt I was Steve Coogan's PA last night. I'm a massive fan of his, but I wasn't star-struck in the dream; we had a great connection and I knew he really needed me. It felt brilliant. I was quite disappointed when I woke up.

We're going to walk up a mountain tomorrow. I can see it from here, and it doesn't look too bad. By that I mean that it looks, from this angle at least, fairly rounded, rather than sharp and pointy. I feel slightly nervous about it, though that's probably silly. Rob has bought a local map and knows what he's doing, so I'm in safe hands. I suppose I'm most worried I won't be able to take the pace.

Day 326 — 12th November 2011
Barga, Italy

We got up early and left the motorhome at 8.30am. The walk was quite civilised at the beginning; there were some steep bits, but nothing I couldn't handle and I felt good thinking about all the calories I was burning. I was relieved to see that the walk was very well signposted, with easily spotted bright red markers on trees every 200 metres or so. No need to worry about getting lost then.

A few hours into the walk Rob said, "Right, we need to make a decision. Do you want to carry on and try to reach the summit, or turn back and go the way we came?"

I'd just assumed we'd make it to the top, and although I could feel painful blisters starting to form where my boots were rubbing, I said, "Well, to be honest I'd quite like to make it to the top."

"The only thing is that the scale is a bit bigger than I'd realised and I'm slightly worried about the lack of daylight. I'm not sure we'd have time to get back down before it gets dark. And we don't really want to be walking down when it's pitch black. Especially because I've forgotten to pack the head torch."

I soon caught on; this was one of those times when Rob asked my opinion having already made up his mind what we'd do. But his hillwalking knowhow outstrips mine in every sense, so I didn't mind.

"Well, whatever you think best."

In light of my pre-walk trepidation, I now felt slightly cheated, disappointed that the hardest part was over so easily. That the physical test wasn't just a tiny bit more challenging. Rob showed me another path on the map, one that, handily enough, led straight back down the mountain. I don't really get maps, so I just nodded and pretended I was taking it in. Really I was just thinking about the very old-fashioned swirly font the map was written in. I hoped the typeface wasn't an indication of its age. What if the paths had changed since it was made?

The start of the new path was fairly obvious, but after ten or fifteen minutes it didn't really feel like a proper path any more. More an overgrown path. Or an ex-path. We had to make a bit more effort to wade through increasingly coarse undergrowth. I kept thinking of David Bellamy and his beard.

Twenty minutes later I was finding it really hard going. Not only did I have to concentrate on what I was stepping on, or in, so that I didn't slip on a branch, but I also had to stay alert as to what was happening at eye level. Several branches had already nearly taken my eye out.

"This is pretty difficult," I called out to Rob, trying my best not to sound moany. He was miles ahead and had been totally silent for what felt like a very long time.

"What, this? This isn't difficult!" he shouted back with a derisive snort, as if I'd just said the most ridiculous thing he'd heard in years. He turned round long enough to give me a bemused look that said, who is this mad woman I'm married to? I felt like saying, 'Oh sorry, did I say difficult? I meant to say fecking tedious and bloody hard work!'

But I stayed quiet.

The words of psychologist Mike came back to me: *Our circumstances aren't always ideal.* Got that right, Mike.

The ground got tougher and tougher to walk on, the nice little path we veered off from nothing but a distant memory. Eventually even Rob conceded that the second path we'd chosen must have become overgrown.

"This fucking map, it's *shit*! Why don't they have OS maps here?" he said, almost shouting. It was so unlike him to not be calm and level-headed that I immediately felt a bit scared. Bloody hell. Until now I'd just been pissed off. Now I was worried. Maybe we were really in trouble here?

"It would be a hell of a lot easier to work out where we are without all these bloody trees!" he said. "OK," he went on, clearly trying to stay focused, "the best thing to do in these circumstances is to follow the stream. That always guides you towards the bottom of the hill."

Of course. It sounded obvious now he'd said it, but I'm glad he knows about these sorts of things. I spent a second marvelling at what an intelligent husband I had. Then I remembered that he'd forgotten the head torch. The daftie.

We gave up on the non-existent path and started walking by the stream. But we progressed horribly slowly. It was very slippy, the undergrowth was still thick and we kept having to swap sides depending on which way was less tricky to walk along. It was tough, and made tougher by several random trees lying in our way. They must have fallen in the storms they've had in the area over the last few weeks. As we trudged along, the same thought kept coming back to me: what if we reach a point we can't get past?

I was really hungry but Rob wanted to make more progress before we stopped to eat our sandwiches. Especially since he was worried about the rapidly diminishing daylight.

A bit later we parked ourselves on some huge stones and wolfed our food down. I instantly felt loads better for the sustenance and a little rest, but just after that we hit a big problem. Rob was up ahead of me but started walking back in my direction. He shook his head.

"There's a ravine. There's no way we can get past it. It's way too dangerous."

I tried to remember exactly what a ravine was. When it came to me I tried not to think of the ravine involved in the really gruesome bit of '127 Hours'.

"So what are we going to do?" I tried not to sound panicky.

"We'll have to go up and over instead. We'll scramble up the bank and find another way."

I looked up and my heart beat a bit faster. The bank was *very* steep. I didn't like the look of this at all. But I tried not to look like a big scaredy-cat.

"You go in front of me," Rob said. "Don't think about it, just do it."

I started making my way up, but it was exhausting. I kept putting my feet down on what I thought was solid ground, only to find myself knee-deep in sodden leaves. The wet leaves made it really slippy. This was not good. And to make it even trickier, there was nothing to grab on to, to help pull me up. I said so to Rob and he told me to head to the right, where there were a few trees we could use for leverage. I headed in that direction but I was struggling. I felt really weak.

"Rob, I can't do this. It's too steep."

"Just keep going. Don't stop and think about it. You're doing fine."

By the time we reached the clump of trees, my arms were killing me and I was breathing heavily.

Our circumstances are not always ideal.

Again I went first, trying to control my fear, trying not to think about how steep it was and how easily I could fall back down to the bottom. I was shaking, with fear and exertion. Rob told me where to put my feet, but my spindly arms were having trouble heaving the rest of my newly-bulky body up. I kept thinking, how the hell did we get into this stupid situation? I thought we were just going for a nice walk. Finally I was within reach of the trees and I quickly grabbed the nearest one, a big thick solid-looking tree, so I'd have something to hold on to at last.

"Not that one!" Rob shouted. But it was too late. The tree snapped off at the root and toppled over falling right on top of me. I put my hands up to protect my head but with nothing left to grip, I started slipping down the bank. Rob grabbed my calves and steadied me.

"It's OK, it's OK, I've got you," he said.

My next worry was the tree hitting Rob on the way down. But luckily it got wedged between us, until Rob freed it, sending the damn thing spiralling down the bank. It made a loud thwack-splash sound as it hit the ground and tumbled into the stream.

"Are you OK?" Rob asked.

"Yeah, I think so. I suppose that tree must have been rotten then."

"Yeah, that's what I was trying to tell you."

I noticed a cut on my hand, though I couldn't feel it yet. My joggy bottoms were ripped too. I was even shakier by then and only just holding back the tears. We weren't anywhere near the top yet. Even though I felt awful and wished it was over, it did occur to me that (assuming we survived) at least I would have a good story to tell afterwards.

"Fuck's sake, fucking hell," I muttered, as I started replaying what had just happened.

"You're OK, you're all right," Rob said in his reassuring voice. "Just get your breath back and we'll get going again."

Rob encouraged me to keep going, but it was so tiring. Finally we made it to some even ground at the top. I checked out the cuts on my hands and legs, but still couldn't feel them. That'll be the adrenaline then. I was breathing hard. Rob hugged me and I showed him my war wounds.

Not long after that, we found another path. I was extremely happy about that. Thank God, we're going to be OK now.

"We have to get a move on Ros," Rob was saying. "I'm really worried about the lack of light."

"I know, Rob. I'm going as fast as I can here."

"I know, I know you are."

But after five or ten minutes, the path seemed to be going uphill. Which was definitely not supposed to happen. Rob studied the map.

"I think we're at this point here," he said, pointing. "You see where the river starts to fork? I reckon that's down there," he pointed towards where we'd just been. I looked at the map (I was actually looking this time) but there were about five different places where the river forked, so I was pretty sure what he'd just said was an educated guess, at best.

"So rather than risking this path taking us back down to the river, I think we should head up the hill and hopefully we'll meet the point where we left the first path we were on."

Hopefully!? Hopefully really isn't what I wanted to hear just then. I deserved a definitely after what I'd already been through. What if we don't find the first path again? Then we've just wasted a whole load of energy going back up the bloody hill!

But I didn't say that, of course, because it wouldn't have been very helpful. And I didn't have any better ideas. So I just steeled myself for the climb ahead.

Going back uphill was physically punishing; we'd already been walking for five hours pretty much non-stop and because it was steep I had to keep stopping every hundred yards or so to get my breath back. It wasn't too brilliant psychologically either, considering we had twice thought we'd already finished the ascent before that. At least the ground was solid here. I was worn out, dead on my feet. I kept thinking, that's it now, I can't go any further. But there was no choice really. At one point I suggested phoning someone to come and rescue us, but Rob just laughed. Well, I suppose the laughter was quite reassuring anyway.

"Ros! I think I can see the top now," Rob shouted a few minutes later.

Well, thank fuck for that. Of course, it was ages before we actually reached it, but the thought of being nearly there gave me a much needed mental boost.

Rob must have been right about the fork because a little while later we found the original path. I never thought I could be so happy to see some little red way markers. What a relief!

There was still a long way to go. We were quite literally not out of the woods yet. We made good progress for a while but when the light levels dropped, making our way down became a lot more arduous.

"I don't remember seeing that house on the way up, do you?" Rob asked.

"No, I don't. But maybe we weren't paying attention... or p'raps it looks different from this angle?"

I was desperately hoping this was the case, but I knew we were almost certainly going in the wrong direction. As we walked past the unfamiliar house two huge dogs came steaming up to us, barking fiercely and snapping at our heels. Rob had to repel them with his walking poles. Bloody hell.

We decided to go back to the house to ask the owner for directions. Which made one of the dogs even more excited about the prospect of eating us. Naturally, he didn't speak a word of English (the owner, not the dog). While we were failing to understand each other, the guy's wife appeared. We must have looked a bit of a state because she gave us a wide-eyed bewildered look.

The man, who was in his fifties and had a handlebar moustache, was kind enough to leave his nice warm home and accompany us down the correct path, pointing us in the right direction before he left. We thanked him as best we could. But it wasn't long before we took another wrong turn. Bugger. At least there was another house, so we stopped there for further guidance. We rang the doorbell but before anyone had a chance to answer, a young guy appeared out of the darkness. Where the hell did he pop up from? He was carrying some kind of rifle or shotgun and his forehead was sweaty. I looked down to his waist and saw an ammunition belt full of cartridges. Apart from that, he looked pretty friendly.

Could today get any more bizarre? Disappearing paths, trees that come away in your hand, scary dogs and now a lone huntsman of some kind. He said he spoke English and then proceeded to talk to us in pure Italian. The only word I caught was Luigi, which reminded me of the character from the computer game Mario Kart. We could at least tell from his sign language that we were to turn right when we got to the house further down the hill. Luigi's place perhaps? Once again, the guy was happy to go out of his way to physically show us the right path, coming part of the way down with us. How kind and helpful Italian people are!

It was properly dark by then but Rob had a light bulb moment: his smartass phone had a torch app! It wasn't the same as a real torch, but at least we had some light to guide us. He didn't have much juice left in his battery, so we knew it would soon cut out.

We kept thinking we were going the wrong way again but eventually spotted more houses and more lights. Both were very good signs! Then, in what almost felt like an anticlimax after everything that had happened, we made it to the main road into town. Having said that, I was very happy indeed to see the signpost for Barga. It was now more likely than not that we wouldn't die today after all. Unless we got run over by one of the cars speeding by. Actually there was no pavement on this road, and we were in the dark, in Italy, so the prospect wasn't totally implausible.

Our next mission was to make it back in time to go to the local shop before it closed at 7.30pm. We made it, just, picking up a pizza, wine and a couple of other bits and bobs. After our long strange day it felt weird to be in such a normal everyday environment again. I was dazed by the bright lights. We didn't have a purse or wallet with us, just a twenty Euro note. I looked in the basket.

"Do you think we have enough to cover this?" I asked Rob as we stood waiting in the queue.

"I hope so."

The final hurdle of the day was not having enough cash for all our gubbins. We kept putting things back, red-cheeked, until we could afford our little bundle. Even then we were ten cents down, but the kindly cashier let us off. So embarrassing. Five minutes later we were back at the motorhome. I'd never been so pleased to see the dream machine.

Once we'd eaten I checked the pedometer, which had counted my steps during our mammoth ten and a half hour walk. The display read 38,838! Blimey.

We both laughed but Rob suddenly turned serious.

"I feel like I've let you down," he said.

"Don't be daft. It was nobody's fault, just one of those things. I'm just glad it's over."

He looked really sad so I tried to make him laugh.

"You do realise you've put me off hillwalking for life, don't you?"

He was horrified. "Oh no!"

"Rob, it's OK, I never really liked it anyway!"

He finally managed a little smile.

"You did good today, baby," he said, looking serious again. "You really dug deep, you know, physically and mentally. I was impressed."

"Well, I was crying inside most of the time, but thanks."

We were so shell-shocked we barely managed a glass of wine before hobbling to bed. It wasn't even 9.30pm. Rob's breathing changed almost immediately to the heavy kind that signals imminent sleep. I'm always amazed how quickly he drops off. Before he drifted away completely I gently nudged him in the side.

"Just so you know, you owe me a new pair of joggy bottoms."

Day 327 — 13th November 2011
Barga, Italy

We didn't do much today. Except fail to find the local festival that was apparently on in town. Rob put some cream on my cuts and gave me blister plasters for my poor wee broken feet.

Day 328 — 14th November 2011
Barga, Italy

Played a few games of Scrabble today. The score is 9-6 now. To me, of course. Ha, how quickly I've gone from desperado to smug git!

Day 329 — 15th November 2011
Barga, Italy

Spent ages cleaning the motorhome in preparation for the in-laws' arrival on Wednesday. Rob took a long time sewing up the black material we use as chair covers. It looks so much better now. I spent quite a bit of time reading 'The Case Of The Missing Boyfriend' by Nick Alexander. It's about a fag hag type of bird who, as the title suggests, is single. It's pretty entertaining, and well-written, if a wee bit lightweight.

Day 330 — 16th November 2011
La Salvia cottage, near Siena, Italy

Went to Lidl and spent €105 on supplies for the week, before picking Rosie and Barry up from Pisa Airport. There was a slight misunderstanding when we attempted to find them. Rob had told them to stay at the pick-up point, logically enough, but for some reason they started walking towards the exit.

"So where are you now?" I asked Rosie on the phone. Rob was shaking his head and swearing under his breath.

"Er, I'm not sure Ros. We seem to be in a bit of a pickle, I'm afraid. I can see a coach…"

I looked around. I could see at least twenty coaches just from where we were. There must have been hundreds of them in the whole airport.

"Right. What else can you see?"

"There's a big sign, I think it's for a supermarket," she said. "Oh and there's an elf."

"An elf?"

"Yes, you know, a what do you call it… a garage, I mean a petrol station."

"Ah! Right, stay there. We can find that. Don't move!"

"OK."

We checked for Elf under the list of petrol stations on the satnav and soon found it. Rob spotted them, not staying put as instructed, but walking along a busy road with no pavement. They looked lost, like refugees who'd got off at the wrong stop.

"Why the hell didn't they just stay where we told them to?" Rob said.

"I don't know, but don't start shouting when they get in, OK?"

The cottage was just as lovely as I remembered. I especially loved the amazing power shower and the presence of a washing machine. The only slightly weird thing about the place is that there is a whole load of flying beetle creatures that we seem to have awoken from hibernation. They look a bit like very athletic ladybirds, but they're larger, longer and sleeker, with a more metallic reddish black sheen. They are coming in from one of the window frames and there are hundreds of the little blighters. I'm glad I'm not sleeping in the cottage!

Day 331 — 17th November 2011
La Salvia cottage, near Siena, Italy

Rob and his Dad have purged the beetle things. Well, most of them. Every now and then one of us spots one or two crawling along the wall as we sit at the dinner table.

The house was freezing when we arrived but we worked out how to turn the thermostat up on the pellet stove thingy, so it's nice and toasty now.

Day 332 — 18th November 2011
La Salvia cottage, near Siena, Italy

I'm sitting outside reading, Rosie is painting in the garden and Rob and his Dad are playing boules. All this, in the middle of November.

We were sitting quietly in the living room this afternoon when Rosie started screaming her head off and flapping her arms around. She stood up and stamped her feet.

"Whatever's the matter Rosie?" Barry asked.

"It's OK, it's OK, I think it's gone now," Rosie said breathlessly.

One of the beetles had flown on to her chest. We all had a good laugh about it once she'd recovered.

We are still spotting the odd beetle on the wall every now and then. We're getting a wee bit jumpy too, imagining we can see them when there's actually nothing there.

It took a while but Rob finally got the splinter out of my index finger tonight. It had been there since the dreadful walk last week. Ouch.

Day 333 — 19th November 2011
La Salvia cottage, near Siena, Italy

I've just had a dream that the nurses and doctors were trying to make me go back into hospital. They tricked me, making me think I was just going to a meeting. There were lots of doctors and other medical staff there and the basis of their decision was that even though I looked and sounded and acted OK, they — the professionals — could tell that, deep down, I was very unbalanced. I was pretty upset that this was happening against my will. None of the usual doctors or nurses was there. At that point I realised it was a dream and woke up.

When I went back to sleep the dream was still going on but I had more control over it. It's so weird when that happens. In the second part I was about to go home. I was better and thanking Nurse James for his help in getting me to that point. I was making tea and it seemed like we were in the kitchen of my parents' house in Dumfries, rather than in a hospital. Nurse James was standing behind me and he put his arms around me and hugged me for a long time. At first I thought he was being nice and I was quite enjoying the hug. But the longer it went on, the more I started to think how inappropriate it was. I tried to get away then because I was feeling uncomfortable but he held on tight. Eventually he let me go, but when I turned round to face him it wasn't Nurse James at all, it was Jim Robinson from 'Neighbours'! A man I've always found quite attractive to be honest.

Last night the Egertons reminisced, mostly about cars they used to own. I didn't mind though. That was our third night in a row on the wine. Must give it a miss tonight. Or at least go on to vodka — far less calorific.

I had just put my boots on when my leg started to feel a bit itchy. I scratched it but it didn't do any good. So I took my boot off to have a look. I threw the boot away in fright when I saw one of the little beetle things on my leg. What I thought was an itch was actually one of the little buggers crawling up my leg! Nasty little thing. He must have got in my boot while I wasn't looking. Ugh.

Francesca was here when we got back from a day out in Siena, so we stood out in the cold talking to her for a while. She's funny. She didn't stop talking the whole time. We heard all about her boyfriend and the things he does to annoy her. She's a bit mental really, but nice.

"Do you want to come in for a cup of tea?" Barry asked her.

"Ah no, I have to go now because it's getting dark and I don't have my glasses with me. If I don't go soon I won't be able to see when I drive home," she said.

Day 334 — 20th November 2011
La Salvia cottage, near Siena, Italy

Woke up this morning thinking about Stobhill and the mental ward. It still shocks me sometimes, the fact that it really and truly happened. Was it inevitable or just bad luck? There are a lot of 'what ifs' when I go down this path, to do with whether it could have gone differently. What if I'd been better at expressing myself, like Madonna? What if Rob hadn't been made redundant? What if I'd had a different job, a different boss? What if we'd never moved from the south coast of England? What if the weather had been better? It sounds silly to link something as huge as the weather with my tiny personal downfall, but the relentless snow and ice did make it exceptionally difficult to get around. My usually reliable stress relief method — walking off my worries, which always helped me sleep too — wasn't available. I don't allow myself to wallow in these 'what ifs' for too long though, because what's the point? I can't change it now, I can only concentrate on not letting it happen again.

***

I've finished 'The Trial' by Franz Kafka. No idea what that was all about.

Rob and his Mum have been arguing about religion. I don't know why they don't just agree to disagree. Order is now restored; Rosie is painting and Rob and Barry are playing boules.

Day 335 — 21st November 2011
La Salvia cottage, near Siena, Italy

Off to some medieval town whose name I can't remember at the moment. Just started 'Candide' by Voltaire. It's OK so far.

Measured waist. Not good.

It's Rosie and Barry's last day here tomorrow. I'll be sorry to say goodbye to the nice cottage, and I'll miss Barry and Rosie's company, but it's been a lovely experience and I'm happy they've had a nice holiday.

Day 336 — 22nd November 2011

La Salvia cottage, near Siena, Italy

Quite a nice last day really. Rosie painted; a teapot, which was excellent, and a portrait of me, which was not so excellent. That was my fault really. The sitting didn't go very well, mainly because I got fidgety and couldn't sit still for long enough. We had a good laugh about it though. When I realised I couldn't manage to keep my face in one position I started being deliberately silly, so that every time she looked up from the easel I had a different daft expression pasted on.

"Oh Ros, you are funny sometimes," she said with a smile. "That must be why you fit in with this family. You're just as daft as us."

I took that as a compliment.

Rob made a lovely tea of jacket potatoes, fish, gorgonzola and broccoli. We all laughed at Barry when he pronounced it 'broccolie'. We laughed again when he said, "OK then, I'll just have to re-programme my pronunciation of that vegetable." Now there's a sentence you don't hear very often.

For dessert we had stollen and other cakes *and* half a choc ice each. Good job I went for a run this morning.

Day 337 — 23rd November 2011

La Spezia, Italy

Sunny and warm again today, 21°C. Amazing.

We're both quite tired after an early start this morning and a bit of wine last night. We had to get up at 7.23am. Most uncivilised.

We said goodbye to Maris, Francesca's father, and made a quick stop at the Leaning Tower of Pisa, before dropping Rosie and Barry at the airport. Despite having seen lots of photos, I was still surprised by just how much it leans. It was good to see the tower, but very, very busy for November.

We are at La Spezia now, a coastal town. Though you wouldn't know it from the strange place we're in. It's a massive aire full of stored motorhomes, giving it a slight ghost town vibe. Bizarrely, there's an ambulance depot just inside the entrance. A man on reception took our passport numbers when we came in. We just pay a donation when we leave tomorrow. It's not exactly picturesque and there is quite a lot of graffiti, but it's fine for one night. Need to play Scrabble now to keep ourselves awake.

Can't believe we only have 26 days of our trip left.

Day 338 — 24th November 2011
Genoa, Italy

We both had massive sleeps last night; 11 and a half hours for me! I felt like a new woman after a run and a shower this morning.

I won the Scrabble yesterday but we were so tired neither of us enjoyed it.

Beautiful sunshine and blue skies today. Lots of tunnels. Decided to head vaguely in the direction of Genoa and forget about Florence for now.

***

We've had a frustrating day, driving round places looking for snow chains for the tyres and a protective cover for the windscreen, which will help with condensation and keeping the motorhome warm as we move north during the winter. Rob reckons we will need both items when it starts getting colder. Actually you can get fined for not having snow chains on certain roads in France. It felt like wherever we went they either didn't have the right things for our vehicle or we weren't even able to find the place where they might sell them, or we found the right place but couldn't park anywhere near it.

We are in Genoa now, at a free stop with electricity that's at the back of a motorhome accessories company. Rob is going to try them in the morning to see if they have either of the things we need. I really hope we can get everything we need tomorrow so we can get back to enjoying ourselves again!

Some water from the toilet bowl splashed up into my eye this afternoon. I think that was the low point of the day.

Covered loads of miles today, although we did see some pretty towns and villages. Didn't get here till 8pm. Had two glasses of wine and crisps *and* chocolate tonight. Slightly disgusted with myself now.

Only 24 days left.

Day 339 — 25th November 2011
Borgo San Dalmazzo, Italy

Blue skies and completely sunny again this morning.

Today is already going better than yesterday. We have just got the snow chains for €94! Apparently this is cheap. Rob is now checking whether we need two pairs.

"Right, shall we go and find a McDonalds so we can find out where to buy the screen cover?" Rob suggested. You can pick up a free wifi signal at McDonalds.

"OK, let's go. We can take a look at French aires to stay at on the way back too."

"Good idea."

Did I mention that I hate McDonalds? Passionately, vehemently hate it. I always *thought* I hated it, then I read a book called 'Fast Food Nation' by Eric Schlosser. Which detailed exactly why I was right to despise it (as well as all the other massive fast food chains — I may be a hater, but don't accuse me of prejudice; I hate fairly). Unfortunately I read this worthwhile book so long ago that I can't remember precisely why I hate McDonalds. Just that I definitely do. Something to do with cows? How they treat them maybe. Oh and workers. They don't treat those very well either. I'm pretty sure they're bad for the environment, corporately aggressive and produce food with a nutritional value of zilch, too.

Having said that, the depths of my contempt don't extend to, for example, not taking advantage of McDonalds' free wifi service. Because free internet access is The Best Thing Ever when you're not at home. You don't even have to buy anything at McDonalds; you just hang around close enough and the wild wild world is at your oyster-tips.

So free wifi at McDonalds was a good plan. In theory at least.

"This can't be right," Rob said, glancing at the satnav with a frown. "We're going round in circles."

I can't say I'd noticed, but that was hardly surprising.

"It can't be down here..."

Rob was about to make a right turn, but carried straight on at the last second. The car behind gave us a long hearty honk.

"For fuck's *sake*! She was trying to take us down a one-way street the wrong way! *Fuck*ing hell."

I knew it was best to keep quiet in this situation. After several more false turns, the pishy-coloured arches came into view.

When we stopped I made some sandwiches while Rob set the internet up. Five minutes later his brow was still furrowed.

"What's wrong, baby?" I was almost scared to ask.

"I can't pick up the signal."

Rob kept moving the lightsabre thing around outside the skylight (I think it's a booster or something, but it looks just like a lightsabre) at the back of the motorhome, quietly swearing as he did so, but it just wouldn't work. That bloody thing is useless.

The next frustration was not being able to find the aire we'd picked out to stay at tonight. Back on the road! We couldn't find the next one along after that either, but finally stopped at Borgo San Dalmazzo. We're parked on a big car park at a sports centre.

Just played two games of Scrabble. I won both, the first easily, because I had two seven-letters. Rob had nae chance. I'm still not sure how I won the second, except that Rob went over his time limit and couldn't get rid of the 'q' he got right at the end. It's 12-6 now.

I'm reading 'Silas Marner' by George Eliot at the moment. It's about a weaver dude whose life falls to bits when he's accused of a crime he did not commit. I'm now thinking about the start of 'The A Team'. It's OK but a little dull in places (the book I mean, not 'The A Team'. That was never dull).

Day 340 — 26th November 2011
Borgo San Dalmazzo, Italy

We're surrounded by mountains, which we can see a lot better than when we arrived last night. A few other motorhomes have turned up.

I'm about to break my 12pm caffeine rule. A moment of wild abandon.

Rob is currently using the SIM card from my mobile, to access the internet through his computer. It costs £2 per day but the download limit is quite low. So I hope we get what we need before it runs out. The reason he's doing this is that the Kindle wouldn't load the map image we need from the Motorhome Facts website. Oh and the database of stopovers that we'd downloaded to the computer has somehow been wiped. So Rob is in an excellent mood.

Today I thought I would write a list of stuff I started doing when I went mental, so I would know if it ever looked like it was starting again. Here goes then;

I thought anything and everything was my fault, whether it was things that have gone wrong for friends or family, or bigger things. For example, thinking something I'd accidentally done had led to a massive riot or to a bomb going off. Or else I thought someone I knew was a criminal and had done all the abominable things. For example, I might convince myself that my brother was Richard Reid the shoe bomber. This tied in with what I call 'personal conspiracy theories', for example thinking people were not who they said they were: they were other (potentially criminal!) people.

I talked in riddles, rather than speaking properly. 'We're all in the same boat' was a favourite. I found meaning where there was none. I spotted non-existent patterns too. I saw symbolism in everyday things. A cup, for example, became more to do with 'a cup of human kindness' than a vessel you have a drink from. Or I thought to myself, there must be a particular reason why that person has left that particular object lying around near me. That person is (obviously) trying to tell me something!

I counted a lot. 1, 2, 3, 4... Or went through the alphabet. 'A' is for such and such, 'b' is for... oh, what's 'b' for again?? Nightmare, I can't remember. Panic!

I replaced normal thoughts with colours. So red equalled stop/danger, green equalled go/sickness/green-eyed monster, that sort of thing. I didn't believe stuff could just be random. Another similar madness trait was where my thoughts and speech revolved solely around film and song titles. For example, if someone mentioned cider, I might automatically answer 'With Rosie.' This made even less sense to sane people when they wouldn't have got my cultural references anyway.

I started saying weird stuff. (For example, "I understand now... we're all in the same boat." Or "There are two sides to every story.") Which wouldn't have been so weird, except that was all I was saying. Rob looked worried and said, "You're starting to say weird stuff."

I thought I was a terrible, evil* person who'd done abominable things to the people I love best. I believed I was everything awful; greedy, selfish, ungrateful... whereas actually I'm quite a nice person most of the time.

I believed I'd always been mad and not realised it, people had clearly been covering for me for years (but at least I knew now). This was often linked to another feature of my madness; that is, taking a memory that's real and warping it, so that it bore no resemblance to the truth. For example, I could take my wedding day (which normally I'd think was a good thing) and twist the whole thing inside out and upside down until it became a macabre nightmare.

I imagined that people were keeping big fat secrets from me, especially big fat family secrets. For example, someone's sister/brother is actually their mother/father. So and so was gay and was in a marriage of convenience. (That phrase always made me snigger a little bit, because it must be really inconvenient

---

* I don't really/normally believe in good and evil at all when it comes to people. I think acts described as evil are probably just down to chemical imbalances in the brain. Everyone is a mixture of good and bad, so you shouldn't demonise people. At least that's what my Mum told me once. And she's pretty wise. Usually.

to be married to someone you didn't love. Ha ha.) Or so and so is so and so's secret love child. And of course, everyone else had known about this secret for years, I'd just been blinded...

I had to be prompted to do stuff you normally do without thinking. Eating comes to mind. Mainly because I didn't feel hungry. I didn't notice or realise when I should have done other obvious stuff. Like washing. Or putting my face on.

I thought everything was a test or a trick or a joke. I could turn a medical examination into a scene from 'Carry On Doctor', for example. The joke was usually on me.

I believed the opposite of what I normally would. In other words, my world went topsy-turvy. A person I couldn't stand, for example, became simply misunderstood; I became the bad guy for not giving them a chance. Believing in God was another example of this.

Day 341 — 27th November 2011
Caille, France

Things have gone slightly wrong today. Not disastrously wrong, not catastrophically wrong, just annoyingly, nerve-gratingly wrong.

We drove to what was supposed to be an aire in Monaco. It turned out to be an underground car park where you're not allowed to sleep overnight. Not that you'd want to; the sports cars whizzing round and the overwhelming smell of petrol wouldn't be conducive to a good kip. Also, you have to turn off your gas, so we wouldn't have even been able to have a cup of tea in the morning. Which is of course completely unacceptable.

Before we even got to the non-aire, we drove around Monaco's narrow streets for ages trying to find the place.

"The co-ordinates must be wrong," Rob said. "It's trying to tell us to go over there to that underground car park."

Soon we realised that that, in fact, was very much it as far as Monaco motorhome stopovers go.

"Well, we might as well go and have a look," I said. After several hours on the road, I was pretty keen to get out the van.

The dude manning the booth at the entrance barked an instruction at us in French and gestured where to park up. Rob answered him with a confident

"Merci, monsieur." And then drove off in the wrong direction. In my mirror I saw the guy come out of his wee booth and start waving us back the other way.

The look on his face was fairly blank, with a hint of 'bloody tourists'.

"Er, Rob, I think I heard him say 'dernier sur la gauche' or something. Doesn't that mean last one on the left?"

"Ah bollocks."

It was early evening by then and once we'd parked up, I asked Rob what he wanted to do.

"Well, we're here now. I suppose we could go for a look round and then head to the nearest aire once we've at least seen the place."

"Cool, Monaco by night!"

Monaco was amazing, and surreal. The first thing I noticed was how incredibly clean each and every street looked. There were posh cars, hotels, apartments and yachts on every corner, making it look more like a film set than a real living breathing place. Actually, posh doesn't really do it justice. Opulent, flashy and lavish is more like it. There were tonnes of exotic plants, brightly lit fountains, high end (stupidly pricey) designer shops and beautiful old buildings. Nearly every shop had a photograph of Prince Albert II, Monaco's main man, as well as his wife Charlene. He looked very ordinary, with a big baldy slaphead, but the princess was stunningly beautiful.

The whole place radiates extreme wealth. We stood at the harbour speculating just how much the plushest boats might have cost. Every now and then Rob pointed out that we were walking along parts of the famous Grand Prix track.

We got back to the motorhome around 11pm, resigned to the fact that old Albert and his pretty lady didn't want reprobates in motorhomes lowering the tone by staying in his nice little principality too long.

It was gone midnight when we arrived at the next aire. Unfortunately it was full. So off we went again, driving for another hour — along some very narrow, dodgy roads — towards the next stopover. This one was in a town called Caille.

"Oh bugger," Rob said as we arrived.

There were only two spaces and they were both taken.

"Oh man… I can't be bothered going anywhere else."

We decided no one would much care if we just parked up close to the aire, got some sleep and hoped that one of the other motorhomes left early in the morning, allowing us to slip into their place.

The plan worked perfectly, except for a slight palaver with the service machine. Rob went to all the trouble of going off into the town to swap two one

Euro coins for a two Euro coin, because that's all the machine accepted. This wasn't particularly easy in itself, because 'the town' was a tiny village with hardly anyone out and about at the time. When he came back and put the coins in, the electricity worked for about five minutes and then stopped.

Electricity was already a bit of a sore point after a slightly unfortunate incident yesterday. It's been buggered ever since I touched the electronic display inside the motorhome. I got an electric shock (something to do with the static produced by my Slanket or slippers, Rob said with an accusing look) and the display got all confused and started saying 'charge +?'. Usually it tells you how the battery is doing, in percentage terms. So we don't actually know how charged, or otherwise, it is now. Which is a bit worrying. Whoops.

All of which means that, rather than just enjoying a nice relaxing day after our mammoth driving sessions yesterday, we have to head elsewhere yet again, to find electricity. Humph.

"Oh great!" I heard Rob saying outside, as I packed things up.

"What is it?" I said, opening the door tentatively, hardly wanting to know what else had gone wrong.

"We've hardly got any gas left either!"

"Oh dear."

Rob looked raging. But I was thinking, oh come on, it's not *that* bad you big drama queen! Not compared with our electric problem. Gas is easy, we just go and fill up somewhere.

We managed to get the LPG fairly quickly. Then we stopped in Dignes Les Bains and Rob used the Kindle (not the stupid lightsabre thing of course) to get on the internet, checking the forums and finding out a bit more about exactly how badly I'd messed up the electronic display. According to those who know about these sorts of things, it should magically go back to normal once we're fully charged.

"Really?" I said. "Well that's good then. Isn't it? I mean, it's not really as serious as we thought maybe?"

I might be off the hook here...

"Possibly," he admitted.

Rob reckons the Hymer needs servicing. I wonder if tourists get ripped off at garages even more than locals. Probably.

We were just starting to feel better about things when we got stopped by the police. They had sniffer dogs searching people's cars at the side of the road. My heart started beating very fast. But the French police lady who came over was quite nice.

"Parlez-vous Français?" she said, having clocked our Scotland sticker.

"Un peu," I said, with an embarrassed laugh. She smiled and switched to English, asking where we'd been and if we were tourists. Rob told her we were on the road to Grenoble and this seemed enough for her. Grenoble is where we're planning to get the screen cover from. I looked back to the cars being searched, wondering what they were looking for.

It felt like we'd already had a long day by the time we got to our parking place for the night. I was well looking forward to getting the kettle on and relaxing for a bit. Then we spotted a middle-aged guy standing next to a transit van, trying to hitch a lift. He had a petrol can in his hand, so we assumed he'd run out.

"What do you think?" Rob said, looking across to me. I was thinking I felt sorry for him; it looked cold outside.

"Go on then, let's do our good turn for the day."

Luckily it was only ten kilometres to the petrol station up the road, so our French oral skills (stop sniggering at the back) weren't tested too thoroughly. Actually I quite enjoyed talking to a real live Frenchie. He spoke a wee bit of English too, and explained in a mixture of the two languages that he was waiting for his daughter ('mon fee') to pick him up but she was stuck at work ('trav-eye'). At least I think that's what he said.

When we stopped again the gas supply was making a funny sort of clack-clack noise. Rob went to check the gauge outside. I tried not to imagine it blowing up in his face. He came back with a furrowed brow.

"It's showing red," he said.

"What? How can it be empty? We only filled up this afternoon."

"I don't know."

Neither of us said it, but I think we were both worried we had a gas leak. We went back to the petrol station to try to fill up again, but it only put a tiny bit in before the machine claimed we were full.

"So what do you think that means then?" I asked Rob.

"I don't know yet, I need to investigate. But I'm wondering whether the gauge is broken."

Later, Rob went on the forums and discovered our gas problem might be to do with buying LPG that had too much butane in it. As opposed to propane-rich LPG. Obviously...

"Butane is useless in cold weather," Rob explained, "which is why you find it on sale in warmer countries. And according to what I've read, it can also confuse the gauge. What we need to do now is run it down and fill up with propane once it's completely empty."

And hope it is that and not something much more dangerous, I thought.

"Hopefully it doesn't run out in the middle of a really cold night," I said.

"Yeah. And hopefully the butane won't freeze either."

I think my French is improving. We were just getting set up at our stopping place for tonight when a lady came up and said something in French. It was dark and I couldn't see her very well but I knew she'd come from one of the other motorhomes. I was about to apologise and say I didn't speak French when I realised that I had understood her question perfectly well. Or well enough, anyway. She'd asked if we knew where the toilet was. So I quickly said 'oui' (making the obvious, very immature joke in my head) and pointed her in the right direction.

When she walked away I wanted to call her back and add 'C'est là' (which I'd remembered means 'it's there') but I think she got the idea. Rob ran off after her to lend our head torch, so she could see her way OK. What a nice helpful couple we are. We can pat each other on the back tonight!

Day 342 — 28th November 2011
Saint Pierre de Chartreuse, France

We found a Hymer dealer where we can get the vehicle serviced but it's Monday today and (just our luck, as Adrian Mole would say) they don't open on a Monday.

The width of my waist appears to have decreased by about an inch. However, I'm not sure I breathe in or out exactly the same amount each time I'm measured, so there is a major question mark hanging over the accuracy. The same way the excess belly fat hangs over my jeans. Disgusting really.

I feel like we've been trying to find a Decathlon shop for weeks now, but it's really only a couple of days.

Later. We finally found a Decathlon! I am the proud, hopeful owner of a new Slendertone Abs System belt. It uses electrical impulses to stimulate your tummy muscles into working overtime. Each throb you feel is the equivalent of around 1000 sit ups. Or something like that. I just tried it. It's quite good, although it is a slightly weird sensation.

It's been a very expensive day; the Slendertone belt was €123 and Rob's skis and poles were €280. Ouch. Rob had to pay with our UK debit card, so God knows how much extra that will cost us. Double ouch.

Managed almost a whole conversation in French today. OK, I was only in a little cafe where we bought chips and chocolate ice cream so that we could legitimately use their wifi network. But still, I was quite pleased with myself. Not that it did much good, because the stupid lightsabre let us down yet again, putting Rob in a bad mood. As did the crazy route the satnav took us to get to the motorhome dealer place; we thought we would check it out before turning up tomorrow.

Later on, Rob said sorry for being such a moody git.

"You're still not allowed to touch anything in the motorhome from now on," he said, half-amused but still slightly annoyed.

"Ah, this again…"

He was referring to a few unfortunate incidents over the last few days. First I broke the hinge thingy that allows the table to move into different positions. Whoops. Rob tried to fix it but didn't manage it, which is unusual for him and made him even more annoyed.

Next I flooded the bathroom. In my defence, I do think that had more to do with the fairly steep angle we were parked on than anything I did wrong. Oh and did I mention giving the electrical (or is it electronic?) display such a big electric shock that it doesn't work any more? I've actually done that twice now.

The more minor annoyance is that we're nearly out of water and we're in some crazy mountain village aire where the tap doesn't work. Excellent.

To top off a brilliantly fun day, some bloody annoying French bloke started shouting at me this afternoon. The rude git threatened to phone the police because he thought we were going to hit his car. We had got ourselves into a bit of a tight spot, with a bus on the other side of a fairly narrow road, and he must have thought we'd got too close to his precious Renault (I've no idea if it was really a Renault). He was sort of half-smiling towards the end of the encounter, but not before he'd started pointing to a bit on his car where someone else had obviously hit the side. He looked so flipping French, sipping his coffee while he chatted to somebody. When he noticed we weren't French he shouted, "I phone police when you hit my car! You understand?"

"Yes, yes, it's OK," I said, with my arm out the window, holding the palm of my hand out in what I hoped was a 'shut up and stop putting Rob off and he'll be less likely to hit your precious car' gesture.

"Well if you didn't park in such a stupid bloody place..." Rob muttered.

"Yeah. What a twat. And he had a face like a pie."

Rob burst out laughing.

"A pie? What kind of pie?"

"I dunno, one that hasn't risen properly," I said, laughing myself now.

As we drove off, I wished real life was more like a film. If it was, I'd have been quick-thinking enough to come up with some kind of brilliant sarcastic French put-down, a retort so clever he'd just stand there open-mouthed, amazed by my wit. Even if I'd known the French for, 'You have a face like a pie!', that would have done the trick.

All in all, life on the road could be going a wee bit more swimmingly just at the moment. Hopefully we can get some of these niggles sorted out tomorrow. Rob didn't sleep well last night for thinking about all the problems.

Can't wait to increase the intensity of my Slendertone belt tomorrow. What a saddo thing to get excited about! I'm also quite excited about buying Christmas presents. And even more excited about making jam, which we'll give away as mini Christmas presents. I love Christmas. I'm slightly anxious about approaching the anniversary of my psychotic episode, but I'm sure it will be OK.

Day 343 — 29th November 2011
Grenoble, France

Well, we have been to Expo Clavel, the specialist motorhome company based in Grenoble that we thought might be able to solve all our major vehicular problems. It was somewhat anticlimactic. They didn't have a couple of the more important things we need, including the windscreen cover. What's really annoying about that is that they do stock them, but can't supply one to fit our particular model. They have ones that fit Hymers from 2008 and later; ours is from 2005. Grrrr.

The guy at the counter was nice, helpful and spoke decent English, thankfully, but couldn't suggest any other manufacturers who might be able to help. He did give us the name of a garage where we might be able to get a service, but in the end Rob decided to wait till we get back to the UK for that. On the plus side, the Expo place had the French version of the aires book, so it wasn't a total waste of time hanging around an extra day for them to open.

We're now off towards somewhere near Chancery, to an aire that has water and electricity, we hope. We're also hoping the gas and electricity problems sort themselves out eventually.

Day 344 — 30th November 2011

Near Chancery, France

Rob popped out early this morning and bought me flowers as a peace offering, a sorry for being a bit of a moody git recently.

"Ah, they're beautiful Rob. Thank you," I said.

As a general rule, red roses aren't my favourite flowers. Not that I'm ungrateful, it's just that they're such an obvious choice. Having said that, they do look very nice. And I definitely appreciate the sentiment.

We got to the aire near Chancery OK last night, but the machine wanted to charge us a frankly extortionate €1.50 per *hour* for electricity! An hour! Our 'leisure battery' (which makes everything except the engine work) is still only about 60% charged and we've spent €19 getting it that high. Desperate times... Rob read somewhere that you shouldn't let the battery charge go below 50%. Ever.

On the plus side, Rob has a shiny new idea that may solve lots of problems.

"I think we should get a generator."

"OK. So we don't have to rely on the battery so much, you mean?"

"Yeah, we'd be so much more self-sufficient. We wouldn't have to find somewhere to plug in all the time... we'd be producing our own power."

"Mmm, I see what you mean."

I thought about it for a second.

"Aren't they quite noisy?"

"Yeah, they can be. I think the latest ones are a lot better in that respect though."

"OK, sounds a good idea... how much do they cost then?"

Rob started laughing in a way that made me slightly nervous.

"Well, the one I think we should get is about €700."

I made a high-pitched sound.

"Ooh, that's quite a lot isn't it?"

Rob talked then about how we could buy a cheaper one, but I knew from experience that once he'd got his mind set on a certain product, there was nothing I could do to dissuade him. Not that this bothered me. If he'd chosen that particular model it was probably the right thing to do. Anyway, gas, water and services, they all fell firmly into Rob's department.

I did the tummy belt thing again yesterday. Went for a run this morning, for the first time in three days. The belt instructions are very clear on the fact that it cannot get rid of fat, it can only strengthen the muscles underneath. In other words, don't scoff tonnes of pies and expect a miraculously flat stomach just because you've bought a belt. But with any luck I'll be a right Slim Jim by the time we get home for Christmas.

There's a shop right next to the place where we're parked tonight. Quite handy. I popped in to get some milk and on the way out spotted a wallet lying on the ground of the shop car park.

"Look what I found," I said to Rob back in the van.

"Blimey, where did you find that?"

"Just outside the shop."

There was a €50 note inside, as well as some bank cards and a photo ID card, which I think all French peeps carry. The picture showed a guy in his sixties with a good head of white hair and a square jaw.

"This feels a bit wrong, doesn't it, going through somebody else's wallet?" Rob said.

"Yeah but we have to…" I answered, enjoying the compulsory nosiness rather than feeling funny about it.

"Wait a sec, what's this?"

I pulled out an A4 piece of paper that looked like it had been folded and unfolded hundreds of times. It was a handwritten note to Jimmy, the owner of the wallet, written in what looked like green felt tip. The lettering was fairly large.

"This is getting exciting! Do you think it's a love letter?" I asked, wishing my translation skills were slicker. The writer was certainly keen on old Jimmy; the phrase 'je t'aime' cropped up several times.

"I don't know… the whole thing looks kind of childish, doesn't it? I wonder whether it's from his daughter or something."

"Yeah, that would explain the huge letters and the green felt tip."
We took a photo so we could translate the whole thing properly later, and then got down to trying to locate Jimmy online.

"Not a very French name is it?" Rob said.

We typed the name on the ID card into the French equivalent of The Phone Book and luckily there weren't too many people with the same name. And there was only one Jimmy LaCroix who lived anywhere near the place we'd parked.

"Yes! We've found him," I said, feeling triumphant and contemplating a new career as a private investigator. "Right, here's his phone number," I said, passing a piece of paper to Rob.

"What? Don't you want to do it? Your French is far better than mine!"

"No, I don't want to. You're better at talking to people than me. Anyway, they'll probably speak English."

Rob reluctantly agreed. Next we looked up the French for wallet on Google Translate; there were a few different options but the easiest to pronounce was 'porte-monnaie'. I was slightly concerned it would come across as door-money, but I kept quiet in case Rob got cold feet and made me phone.

"I think I remember the French word for 'found', Rob. It's 'trouvé'. So you could say 'J'ai trouvé votre porte-monnaie'."

"Blimey, you're good aren't you. OK, here goes. Please don't make me laugh."

I put a suitably serious face on as Rob carefully dialled the number. I had to stifle a small snigger when Rob started out with 'bonne nuit' instead of 'bon soir'. Rob did his best to explain, but he'd barely started when he took the phone away from his ear and looked at the display.

"Oh. She's hung up on me. I don't think she understood..."

"Oh well. Good on you for trying," I said.

I should have known he wouldn't give up so easily. When he tried again it rang for a long time before anyone answered. This time he started with a 'désolé'. But just a few seconds later the woman, presumably Jimmy's wife, cut him off again.

"I think I've just been sworn at in French. She sounded pretty annoyed."

"What a cheek! We're trying to do them a favour here!"

Rob was about to redial but I stopped him.

"Rob, why don't you leave it a while? Maybe Jimmy's still out at the moment... if you get him on the phone you might have more luck. Anyway, this'll be costing you loads."

We decided to have dinner and then give it another shot.

"Right, if this doesn't work maybe we should just hand it in at a police station or something," I said after we'd eaten. Rob murmured agreement but I knew I'd be willing to give up a lot sooner than he would. I'm a nice person, but Rob's nicer.

Thankfully it was Jimmy who picked up this time. I listened as Rob repeated his little spiel for the third time. But Jimmy didn't seem to understand the word Rob was using for wallet. Rob tried different ways to explain, 'pour monnaie', 'pour l'argent'. Eventually, just when I thought old Jimmy was never going to get it, something clicked.

"Oui! Oui! J'ai trouvé!"

Rob was laughing his head off when he came off the phone.

"What did he say?"

"I've no idea really!" he said, still laughing away. "I think he said he was on his way to pick it up and that he didn't even realise he'd lost it."

Given Rob's level of conversational French, I was impressed he'd picked all that up.

Sure enough, an hour later old Jimmy turned up, parked in almost exactly the same spot he'd dropped his wallet and got out of his car. Rob dived out to meet him. They chatted for a few minutes before Rob came back grinning.

"He was really grateful. He said it's very unusual in France to get your wallet back if you've lost it. Most people take the money and throw the wallet away. And look," he said, holding up a €50 note and looking very pleased.

"Wow, he gave you that?"

"Yeah, he insisted I took it. I tried to argue but he pressed it into my hand."

"Cor, that was nice of him. Did you mention the phone calls to his wife?"

"Oh yeah, he brought it up himself. He kept apologising for her."

"I should think so."

"He said she thought it was a sales call and apparently she gets them all the time. I think he was quite embarrassed about it actually."

"Well, that's our good deed for the day anyway."

"Yeah, and we're fifty Euros up."

"Yeah, pretty quick karma eh. Well done for persevering baby."

Day 345 — 1st December 2011
Bray Sur Seine, France

Bag o' shite, as Paul Calf would say. I am completely sick of driving around places looking for bloody electricity. Got to an aire yesterday where they charged €3 for 55 minutes. Not even a full flipping hour!

Next we drove to Thuret (I think), where there were loads of lovely electricity points, none of which worked. I've just been down the road to the town hall to see if they could help. This was after a very confusing conversation, conducted in French (it was inarguably my turn to do the deed), during which a nice French lady kept going on about some bird called Marie. The penny dropped when Rob, surprisingly, told me what 'mairie' means; town hall. Aha! That's why she kept saying 'la mairie' then. But the slackers who work there only bother opening between 4pm and 6pm every Wednesday. Today is Thursday, so that's just swell.

At least we are €50 up. And we talked to Mum, Dad and Adam on Skype last night, which was good. Polished off a 1.5 litre carton of wine last night too. I'm inclined to think Rob had the lion's share though, because although I don't exactly feel great, he has a splitting headache and has been for a lie-down.

The plan now is to get to Paris — quite a long way from here — by tomorrow afternoon, to buy the generator. A stockist in Paris has the cheapest one Rob can find. It's still pretty expensive, but he's always very thorough at researching the best deal. Rob is just off the phone to the Paris shop to check they have them in stock.

Day 346 — 2nd December 2011
Cormeilles, France

We drove for ages yesterday, nearly all the way across France. We have just booked our Eurotunnel tickets for the journey home, so it really feels like the end is looming. In some ways I'm sorry to be going home already, but I'm looking forward to Christmas with my family and friends.

Last night we stayed in Bray Sur Seine, which is about 120 kilometres from Paris. We're off to (fingers crossed) get the generator this morning. Then all our troubles will be over! Well, most of the practical ones at least.

It was dark, grey and miserable this morning. The sun was notorious by its absence. Just like waking up at home.

I did fifty minutes on my tummy belt last night, at strength forty. It felt OK but I'll need to crank it up a bit to get anywhere near Slim Jim status.

Later. After a slightly stressful trip into the centre of Paris (I don't think there's any other kind when you're a huge beast of a Hymer battling among silly little mopeds and badly driven French cars), we are now the proud owners of a top of the range generator. We haven't tried it yet. We've stopped at a quiet wee place called Cormeilles, having spent the rest of the day getting things we need for the generator; oil, jerry can, petrol etc.

The terrible weather reminded me of Glasgow. I thought back to an incident at work, way before the recent trouble started. One of the reasons I was so surprised I went mental is because I'd already been through (or so I thought) the whole 'work stress' thing, 18 months earlier. It started when I asked Lorna for an off-site meeting, which was the only way you could guarantee a properly private chat. I was all fired up about a whole load of work issues, things I was going to make better, fix or at least acknowledge. I can't even remember what most of them were now. Basically there were lots of things that various workmates did that pissed me off and I didn't know how to deal with them. Everything was very informal at the magazine, and I'd got used to that. My request for a meeting was triggered by a conversation I had with my sister. She was the manager at an Edinburgh branch of the chicken restaurant Nando's, and happened to mention a disciplinary issue she was dealing with. Wow, I thought, Sylv actually had procedures in place for this kind of thing! Whereas if someone did something wrong in my office, or didn't do their job properly, I just got pissed off; nothing was done about it. Unless I chose to have a quiet word. But I wasn't sure I had the authority to do that. I was definitely in charge of the words in the magazine, but staffing issues weren't really my department. So what was the alternative, go running to the boss? Then I'd just look like a sneaky snidey person who didn't have the guts to deal with it herself. The workplace equivalent of telling tales to the teacher, or 'singing like a canary' if we were in prison.

Maybe the criminal world was relevant; we always joked that working at the magazine was a bit like working for the mob – a lot of information seemed to be on a 'need to know' basis. The actual print deadline, for example, was a closely guarded secret. What happened was I'd work my arse off, having been told I had to get everything done by, for example, Tuesday, only to find out afterwards that the pages hadn't been sent off until Friday. I could sort of understand the logic of building in a time cushion, but it made me feel foolish and cheated when I found out. Plus, the fake deadline strategy could only work once or twice, unless you had a very short memory.

Anyway, Sylv was saying that it was very frustrating being the boss, because sometimes her subordinates didn't tell her really important things that were going on at the restaurant.

"What sort of stuff?"

"Well, quite often when someone gets sacked, afterwards people start telling me all the stuff they were doing before they left. And I'll say, 'Well why didn't you say anything earlier? I can't deal with it if nobody lets me know.' And they're all like, 'Oh I didn't want to get them in trouble.' It's so annoying!"

That was definitely a problem in my office. But at least Nando's had a structure in place to deal with problems when they did crop up. We had nothing. Right, I thought, I must talk to Lorna about this! After all, Nando's always came out well in those lists of the top companies to work for; they must be doing something right.

So my meeting with Lorna seemed like a great idea at the time. I was going to change things, put procedures in place, and everyone would be much happier.

Problems would be dealt with efficiently, not swept under the carpet. I requested the meeting on Monday and it was due to take place that Friday. The problems started when I built it all up in my head. It got way out of proportion and soon became The Most Important Meeting Ever. I stayed up later and later each night writing notes on what I would say. I barely took any notice of Rob, I was so het up about it. As the meeting approached I got increasingly stressed out and sleep-deprived. I probably didn't eat very well. At work I didn't get much done for thinking about the big meeting. I made the mistake of mentioning it to someone in the office. I probably said something cringingly clichéd like, 'Things are going to change around here!' Of course, within about ten seconds everyone knew about it. I think a few people were worried about what I might say. Lesley, one of the salespeople, said to me, "Well I hope you're not going to mention my name!" No no, I told her, I was just going to "make things better".

At home I had hundreds of Post-its strewn all over the shop, scrawled with phrases that wouldn't make much sense to anyone except me. Even I didn't get some of them. What started life as a great idea for a meeting got warped until I no longer recognised it. All the little things people had done to piss me off over the years, they were all there on the Post-its, some in angry capital letters and underlined in red pen. People being lazy, taking credit for other people's work, playing mind games, acting like a model employee in front of the boss and skiving around the rest of the time... it all came out. Instead of being philosophical about it, thinking, 'Yeah, a few of my workmates are pricks, that's life eh', or even confronting people directly when they behaved badly, I'd kept all my resentment and petty grudges bottled up. I tried not to bitch. Because a) that wasn't nice and b) I was The Editor! I felt like I had a responsibility to appear impartial, above all that office gossip, a fair and benign sort of managerial angel to all the people who helped the magazine come together. Even if I couldn't stand them. There was no outlet, no valve to expel my contempt. Not healthy! Which is why there was such a gush of rantiness spewing on to the Post-its.

By Friday morning I was a nervous wreck. I'd gone a bit loopy with the lack of sleep. What was the point of this meeting again?? Something to do with disciplining people? But what the hell did that have to do with me? That was nothing to do with my job! I'd thought about work so much (the relationships between people, the different roles we played, who pulled their weight and who didn't), that the points I was eager to make just a few days ago had gone all topsy-turvy in my head. What a dick! I kept crying and Rob seemed a bit worried about me. He couldn't understand why I was in such a panic. "It's just a meeting," he said at one point. I'd arranged to meet Lorna at the CCA, a nice cafe on Sauchiehall Street not far from my flat. But I was so tired and strung out I couldn't cope with the idea of leaving the flat. What was I going to do? I couldn't think straight. I know, I thought, as if I'd just found a cure for cancer, I'll go for a shower! That always made me feel better. In the shower I had another light bulb moment; I'd ask Lorna to come to the flat, and then I wouldn't have to go outside. Genius. The meeting was at 2pm and after my shower I phoned work. Beth answered and said that Lorna was out. So I had to explain that I wanted Lorna to come to my flat because I was really stressed out.

"What are you like?" she said, not unkindly, before promising to pass the message on.

When Lorna turned up it felt surreal. The sleep deprivation made everything feel weird anyway, and it was strange to see my boss in my home. I offered her a cup of tea but was too distracted to actually make it. In the end she told me not to worry about it. Great start, really smooth, said my sarcastic inner critic. Lorna looked quite worried.

"So, what's going on? And if I don't cry it doesn't mean I'm not emotional," she said quickly.

I looked down at my notes, failing to make sense of them. One of the headings from my CV popped into my head just then; Excellent Communication Skills. Ha! Lorna was at the flat for quite a while, a couple of hours I think, but I don't remember the whole conversation. It turned into a bit of a counselling session really, with me moaning about how I didn't know what my role was at work, what level of authority I had. If someone did something wrong, how should I deal with it? I asked. Lorna laughed the question off and said if it was her she'd be grateful if I had a quiet word in her shell-like. I said of course it wasn't her. Lorna was clearly wondering if there was something specific, but I was cagey about concrete examples.

I remember telling her, in a pretty inarticulate way, some of my worries and niggles about how things worked at the magazine. That I worried about various people not getting on well, that I felt under pressure, that everything would be OK if I could just clone Michelle, my features writer, and there were three or four of her to help me get everything done. I probably babbled on about loads of other stuff. Maybe some of it even made sense. I definitely mentioned a few of the things that pissed me off, things I felt weren't right, though I don't know if I was coherent enough for her to understand what I meant. I mentioned, for example, how difficult it was for everyone else (well, certainly for me, I don't know if anyone else cared as much) when her and Craig, the two bosses who owned the company, fought like cat and dog. When I was talking about what you could call 'staffing issues' Lorna brought me back to basics, reminding me that my job was to write articles for the magazine.

"That's why I employed you and that's what you're good at," she said.

"But I feel like I never get enough time to do that, because I'm always making sure everyone else is... well, not exactly making sure they're doing their job properly, but..."

"I know, I know. It's hard to get anything done when people are always coming up asking you questions. I have the same problem. But I think normally you handle that well, and you do a really good job as editor."

"But how am I supposed to know you think that?"

"That's exactly what I tried to tell you last week," she said, sounding exasperated. She was referring to a night in the pub with a few people from work the weekend before, when she'd got really drunk and told the barman (several times) I was the best editor she knew.

Lorna listened to my worries for a while and then said the only thing she could liken it to was when her friend Kirsty got completely strung out before going off work long-term with stress. I was shocked by that comment; that was the sort of thing that happened to other people... wasn't it?

"But I remember her boss saying to her at the time, that it wasn't him putting all this pressure on her; she was putting it on herself. Nobody was forcing her to do all these extra hours, to stay late in the office every night."

She looked at me and let this sink in. Is that what I was doing, putting myself under pressure? But... surely, the magazine would never get done on time, would never get done properly, if I didn't do all the overtime. I was starting to doubt myself now. Maybe it was my fault I was working so hard; if I wasn't such a control freak and could learn to delegate, to trust others more, I wouldn't need to put in all the extra hours. Before the meeting, I'd thought I did overtime because my workload was too heavy. My reluctance to delegate had been mentioned before, mainly at my annual reviews. But I still secretly believed I was right to be a control freak. If other people did things properly (exactly the way I did them, for example), I wouldn't need to be controlling. People could call it OCD if they wanted, but I was just making sure things were right. The magazine would be full of mistakes if I didn't keep my beady eye on it! Eagle-eyed Ros, my workmate Lewis sometimes called me. I'd always taken it as a compliment...

"And I'll say to you what I said to Kirsty, which is that no job is worth feeling like this for, no job is more important than your health. I mean, your life is here, with Rob. Work should only be a small part of that."

I was nodding. Though my brain wasn't even close to full capacity, I got the point. Get your priorities in order, you're work-obsessed. There's more to life, all that stuff. So in the nicest possible way, Lorna basically told me to get a grip.

"If I was talking to you as a friend, I would also say I think you should try to relax a bit Ros, and, you know, don't be scared to use alcohol to help," she said, laughing a little. I thought about how often I'd been using alcohol to help me relax recently. Possibly a little too often. Maybe I should try yoga or something.

When she stood up to leave I thought for a horrible second that she was going to hug me. That would have been far too weird. Everyone at work thought of Lorna as a brilliant boss; she was great at her job, really sharp, but also good fun. Don't get me wrong, she was scary too, in a kind of force of nature, never-gets-tired way. She was always organising nights and sometimes days out, she was a good laugh, easy to talk to. But her friendliness never extended to physical contact.

Instead she said, "Well, thanks Ros. This has been really helpful."

Oh God, I thought, helpful in that at least you know your editor's gone right round the bend now.

Once she'd left I felt terrible. What the hell? My boss had just come round to my flat and told me to pull myself together. Oh God. I felt such a dick. How embarrassing! When Rob came home I told him some of what had happened, but in hindsight I don't think I was entirely honest about how awful I felt. I was too embarrassed to tell him exactly how bad it was. That evening I decided to take Lorna's advice and drink some red wine. Rob went out for a drink with a mate but I didn't feel like going, couldn't be bothered pretending to be happy. He said he'd just go out for a bit and I didn't want to be one of those nagging wives by stopping him, but the truth was I really didn't want to sit in on my own.

Once I was half-drunk I felt bereft, lonely and horrified by the way I'd come across. I phoned my sister and luckily she wasn't working. Unlucky for her though! I poured myself another glass of wine and poured out all my troubles. Sylv listened sympathetically and seemed to understand. I felt a bit better afterwards. A few weeks later Sylv told me we were on the phone for about five hours that night, which surprised me. God, Mark must think I'm a right pain in the arse! I imagined him rolling his eyes as he realised who was on the phone. Not her again...

I slept well that night, for the first time in ages, thanks to the wine and no longer having The Big Meeting to agonise over. But I didn't feel a whole lot better in the morning, despite being less tired. As well as being a bit hungover, I kept getting waves of embarrassment, blushing as I remembered crying in front of Lorna. What a loser. I lay in bed thinking about what had happened the day before, what conclusions I should draw from it. I decided I was a workaholic, had OCD and was probably drinking too much as well. Great.

I was meant to be having my hair cut that afternoon, by Ramilia, a Russian lady who was great fun. I liked her a lot, she always made me laugh, but my instinct was to curl up in bed and hide from the real world.

"I'm wondering if I should cancel my appointment with Ramilia," I said to Rob.

"Mmm, I don't know. I think it's important to keep to your routine, do what you'd normally do."

"Yeah I suppose."

So I went to the hairdressers. It didn't go brilliantly. When I got there, Ramilia (who always says exactly what she thinks in that way non-British people often do) looked aghast. I think that really is the right word.

"Ros! Oh my God, you're so thin!"

"Am I?"

If I was winning the battle with my chocolate belly, I hadn't noticed. She sat me down and offered me a cup of tea. Then she asked how Rob was and I immediately burst into tears. She quickly led me through to the back room where it was much quieter, sat me down again and gave me a tissue and a glass of water.

"What's wrong?"

"Sorry," I said, feeling stupid. "Things are a bit difficult at work."

But when I tried to explain that Rob had been having a tough time at work, I couldn't get the words out. I hadn't realised how bad I felt about that. It seems obvious in hindsight; I thought I was angry with my workmates for being lazy or manipulative or whatever, but really I was much more angry and upset about how Rob had been treated at work. I felt sorry for him, and I hated feeling sorry for Rob. It gave me a pain in my stomach.

When Ramilia had stopped me crying and asked how I wanted my hair, I rambled on for a bit, said something about making it neat. She gave me a funny look.

"But you're not making sense. You just said something about the messy look."

She was quite right. I had.

"Oh I don't know, just do whatever you think."

She usually did anyway, I thought, with the edge of a smile. Ramilia was very sympathetic in her own unique way and managed to cheer me up with her strange stories and bad jokes. Her advice for work stress was to go shopping.

"Then you can come home and get annoyed with all the crap you've bought instead. Look at this rubbish, why did I buy this stuff?" she said, making me smile. Maybe she was right, a bit of retail therapy might take my mind off the awfulness of the day before. So once my hair looked a bit better (and quite a lot shorter than I'd imagined it would be; I'm sure a hairdresser's inch is the equivalent of a baker's dozen, ie not a flipping inch at all), I went to Primark and bought some new clothes.

I got a tiny pang of guilt as I walked through the doors (and again on the way home) because it's not the most ethical choice of retail outlets. I always felt a bit guilty about spending money unnecessarily. I think that's something to do with my parents having no money at some point during the 1980s. I often thought back to one Christmas when, instead of getting us proper presents, my Mum and Dad made some kind of toy castle structure out of toilet rolls. Quite resourceful really. But I remember thinking, bloody hell, things must be pretty bad if we can't afford real presents.

Anyway, back to the future and I really didn't think an outlay of £19 was going to make much difference in the overall scheme of financial things. Also, I read a book once that implied, heavily implied, shopping unethically wasn't actually unethical, because even though the people making clothes for Primark were being paid badly and were treated quite appallingly, at least they had an actual job, as opposed to fishing round rubbish dumps for bits of plastic they could sell. I wasn't quite sure that argument would stand up against the most ethically aware of my friends, but that's how I justified it. I felt a bit spaced in the shop, went slightly hot and faint when I had to stand in the queue for a long time. That was probably something to do with the red wine and horror of the previous day, but as shopping trips went it wasn't disastrous and I went home with a few nice new tops.

On Sunday Rob and I went to T in the Park for the day, something I hadn't done for years. The only reason we were going was because my wee brother had won tickets through his work and wasn't able to go. We got a lift there with my workmate Beth, along with Beth's sister and her mate, which meant quite an early start, but I didn't sleep too badly on Saturday night. I was really looking forward to seeing Blur, one of my favourite bands. They had split up years ago but had briefly got back together at that point, so it felt like an amazing chance to see them play live. A day out was also a good distraction from all the work business.

When we got there Rob, Beth and the others started drinking (except for Beth's sister's mate, who was driving). I limited myself to one little bottle of red wine. I really didn't want to be hungover as well as embarrassed when I had to face people at work the next day. My main worry about Monday was that everyone would be laughing at me behind my back, sniggering in the staff room. What a freak, getting in such a state that Lorna had to come round to her flat! Serves her right, she was getting too big for her boots anyway. That sort of thing. I assumed everybody knew. Now though, looking back from a less uncomfortable distance, I wonder whether most of them were kind enough to feel sorry for me. Or maybe they were just relieved that the status quo was intact.

I managed to have quite a nice time at the festival, except for a few minutes waiting for Blur to arrive. We were in the pen at the front and it was getting crowded, which started to freak me out. I was scared of being squished by the big crowd. I'd been stuck in human traffic a few times at Glastonbury and found it very frightening. Because there was a delay with the band coming on, I had plenty of time to worry.

"What happens when everyone surges forward? We'll get trampled to death," I said to Rob. I knew as soon as the band turned up, that's what would happen.

"Oh it'll be fine," Rob told me confidently, with what was probably meant to be a reassuring smile. "Stop worrying will you? We'll have a brilliant view from here."

Easy for you to say, I thought bitterly, you're half-cut. I wished I'd had a couple more drinks, so that I'd be more relaxed. At least I didn't need to pee. In the end we didn't get crushed to death. I had a lovely time singing along to all the old Blur hits. We had a slight incident involving a barbed wire fence and a pair of torn leggings (I told Rob I'd buy him a new pair. Ha ha.) after taking a wrong turn on the way back to the car park. Anyway, we got home safe and sound.

I was up unusually early on Monday morning. My tummy was fluttery. I was a bit nervous and embarrassed about seeing Lorna again, wished I'd just kept my mouth closed about the whole stupid thing. I nipped quietly past the admin office on the ground floor and up the stairs into editorial. No one was there, which was unusual. Where was everybody? At 9.05am my work phone went. Lorna. Oh God. She explained where everyone was. Stephen had phoned in sick and Michelle was at a funeral. That just left Lewis, who was on holiday that week anyway.

"The meeting's still on at 9.30am, but I just thought I'd explain. Didn't want you going stir crazy by yourself up there," she said, talking to me almost the same way as normal, just a touch of breathiness in her voice.

"OK, see you at 9.30am then," I said, trying not to sound like a nutjob.

At the meeting, I stayed as quiet as possible so as not to say anything daft that would add to my humiliation. Craig had positioned himself right next to Lorna, which had never happened before at the Monday Morning Meeting. Were they trying to put on some kind of united front, after my comments about them fighting all the time? Or was I overthinking it?

In the afternoon I told Michelle a bit about my embarrassing troubles. She brought it up first actually.

"Are you OK? Lorna asked me to keep an eye on you and you've been really quiet all day."

"Oh God. What else did she say?"

"Just that you were quite stressed out and felt under pressure."

"Yeah. Well, after Lorna left I sat there thinking, right, so basically I'm a workaholic, possibly an alcoholic and I've got OCD."

"I don't think you've got OCD," Michelle said. It was only later it occurred to me she hadn't denied the other two!

"Talk about a walking cliché though, the hard-drinking overworked journalist…"

"Look, I wouldn't worry too much, if you're feeling a bit embarrassed or whatever. I think everyone goes a bit mad in here sometimes."

"Mmm, maybe. The worst thing is, I can't really remember everything I said to her."

"She mentioned something about cloning me. But I think one of me is probably enough," she said with a little smile.

The atmosphere in the office was always a bit flat in the couple of weeks after deadline. But this was worse than usual. I felt low. Stupid. Useless. It was very difficult to focus on my job. Instead of just getting on with things as usual, I questioned every little thing I was doing, which made it hard to write anything and almost impossible to finish each task. Usually I wouldn't think twice about signing work off when it was ready. When the online newsletter was ready to go out, for example, I hesitated, getting stuck, frozen. It was as if someone kept hitting the pause button. I was so unsure of myself I would take half an hour responding to a simple email. Did it sound OK and make sense? Was the tone right? Had I over-explained things? Should I check with Lorna before I hit send, copy her in or not bother her at all? I was spaced too, couldn't concentrate on the here and now. My mind was haunted by replays of the meeting. Crying in front of Lorna, failing to make a cup of tea, the look in her eyes as she left. Bloody hell. I was embarrassed not just about that but about the pre-meeting chat with my colleagues too, how I was going to improve things and all that stuff. I kept thinking everyone must think I'm such a moron. In short, I'd lost my nerve. My sense of humour had taken a battering too.

Over the next couple of weeks I got totally freaked out a few times. The first time, Rob was there and managed to reassure me. I sobbed away, telling him I was worried Lorna would sack me if I didn't get my act together. He pointed out that Lorna had given me a pay rise just a month or so ago, so she must generally be quite pleased with me. Oh yeah, that was true, I thought.

The next time I got The Fear, Rob was out playing football. So I phoned my parents. Mum was in the bath so I cried down the phone to Dad, not exactly explaining the problem very well. When I said things were weird at work and "everything was my fault" he stopped me.

"I'm sorry, Rosalind, but I just can't believe that's true," he said.

He also reminded me that Lorna was a sympathetic person. When he'd stopped me crying, by talking in a nice slow calm comforting voice, he told me this reminded him of a boss of his, who'd once written that Dad was extremely competent, yet constantly sought approval. Was that part of my problem too? My Mum was always saying, "Oh you're just like your father." Usually when I was being pernickety. Mum phoned me back later. "I just don't understand why I feel like this," I told her. "I've got everything I always wanted."

A few days after that, I started crying in front of my GP. I'd gone to see her to ask if she could give me something that would help me feel less anxious. First of all she recommended I took a couple of weeks off work. I was horrified. No way, I told her. There was far too much to do! Next she told me to lighten up, go for a haircut, have a nice long shower. Quite insulting advice on both counts, I thought indignantly. In the end she told me I wasn't "superwoman" (no, really?) and prescribed a course of antihistamines to take at night.

"These should help calm you down enough to sleep properly at least," she said, doing a double take even as she said it, as if she wasn't quite sure they'd be strong enough.

I had a similar incident when I went for a massage, totally broke down and got the watery eyes again, this time in front of Nicola, my 'holistic therapist'.

"Don't worry," she told me, when I apologised several times, "you should have seen me when I worked at Ikea. I was really angry all the time, always shouting at my workmates."

She was laughing at her old self now, but I just couldn't imagine her shouting at anyone. She was so gentle.

"That's why I left and started studying massage."

Eventually I got back on an even keel. Meandered back towards normality. Started enjoying life again. Tried not to do loads of overtime. But as my friend Linsay said, "We nearly lost Ros there for a while."

That's why it's so surprising to me that I was sectioned. It caught me off guard. I was certain I'd already learnt those lessons. Thought I'd got things in perspective. It wasn't just surprising though, it was annoying! Why hadn't I noticed myself unravelling again? I shook myself back to the here and now, remembering that I'd just lost at Scrabble. The score is 12-7 in my favour at the moment. I hardly care about the Scrabble war battles now that I'm in the lead.

Day 348 — 4th December 2011
Somewhere in the north of France

We've left Cormeilles now. The weather is awful in the north of France!

But the fantabulously great news is that the clever generator got our leisure battery right back up to 100%, nae bother! As in fully charged and working just fine and dandy. A massive relief.

I have started thinking back to my hospitalisation, perhaps because we're close to home now. Can you ever *really* get over something like that? Does it cast a shadow on your psyche forever? I suppose acceptance and some understanding of it is the best you can hope for. Even if you could make a conscious effort to forget it, you shouldn't want to, because you'd be more likely to repeat the mistakes that led you down that dark path in the first place.

I get flashbacks that make me uncomfortable every now and then, but they're not intense enough to cause anxiety or fear. I sometimes make a conscious effort to step away from those bad memories, to stop the pattern of thoughts, but I'm never worried about being overwhelmed by the past. I look to

Rob beside me and the embers of anxiety fade away as if they never existed. I'm ready to start moving on now. It feels like something that happened to me rather than something that's happening. A small emotional scar, not a huge raw open wound.

Later. We watched the Lisbeth Salander sequel, 'The Girl Who Played With Fire', tonight. The Swedish version, of course. She's such a cool heroine. Bloody violent film though. Christ, don't have nightmares eh.

I won at Scrabble, partly thanks to a seven-letter word, 'reusing'. It's now 13-7. To me. Of course.

Later still. We have just moved across the street. I was pretty much asleep when Rob suggested going, so I couldn't really be bothered. But I knew he was right; the wind was very strong and we were completely unsheltered in the first location. Luckily it was only a three-minute drive to get ourselves in a better position.

Day 349 — 5th December 2011
Saint Valery au Caux, France

Well, I've just got lots of fruit for my Christmas gift jam. I paid €27 for 12 large punnets of blueberries, but that will produce a fair number of jars. All I have to do is make it now.

I went for a jog in the pouring rain last night, which I enjoyed more than my run this morning with no rain but lots of wind. You can tell from the weather that we're getting closer to Britain. And to winter. It's hailing at the moment.

After spending ages shopping at Lidl and then Leclerc (the French equivalent of Sainsbury's), we drove off towards Saint Valery au Caux. This was going fine, until we went down a really narrow street and there was a horrible scraping noise.

"What was that?" I asked Rob. He looked in the mirror.

"Shit! That was a hub cap. Can you jump out and get it?"

As I was running down the street after the hubcap, wishing I'd worn jeans and not a shortish skirt, a huge lorry pulled up behind us. By then Rob and I had both realised that the street was too narrow for us — we were stuck. Man, it's amazing how quickly things go from hunky-dory to oh bugger, how did this happen?

With a few imprecise hand movements, I gestured to the lorry driver that we couldn't fit down the street so he would need to go back up in the direction he came from. I braced myself for a French tirade, but instead he walked the length of the street moving each of the wheelie bins out of our way. What a lovely helpful man! I love the French. Then he suggested (again through sign language) that we could get past by going up on to the pavement on one side. Actually, that's not a bad idea, I thought, keeping quiet so as not to distract Rob. The lorry driver had a pretty wide load himself, if you pardon the expression, so maybe that's the technique he always used here. We made it, but only just.

"That was *fucking* tight," Rob said.

"Yep," I said, unsuccessfully wiping hubcap grease off my fingers.

Once we'd escaped the clutches of the narrow street we had what I can see, in hindsight, was a stress-induced tiff. The whole episode was made much worse by both of us being extremely hungry.

When we got to the aire we found ourselves in a lovely wee place. Bit of a shame about the pishing rain, hailstones and strong winds. The town looked just like the Seven Sisters down the road from my childhood home on the south coast. I was so happy to be by the sea.

We played Scrabble while Rob ran the generator outside. There were only a few other motorhomes in the vicinity, and nobody too close. Even so, the upside of the noisy storm was that nobody would be disturbed by the sound of the generator purring away.

I was about to take my shot when I heard a thud coming from the back of the motorhome. I looked at Rob and he'd obviously heard it too.

"I'd better go and have a look."

Rob had put a plastic crate on top of the generator earlier on, to protect it from the rain. I assumed the noise must have been the sound of the box being blown off by the wind. But when Rob came back he was raging.

"There was some guy raking about in the back!"

"What? Honestly? Wasn't it locked then?"

"I must have forgotten to lock it when I got the generator out. For fuck's sake!"

"Bloody hell. Do you think he took anything?"

"I don't think so, I think I scared him off. But it's pitch black out there so it's quite hard to tell. You can hardly see your hand in front of your face."

"Cheeky sod. What did he look like? You definitely saw someone?"

"Definitely. I mean, if he wasn't up to something dodgy what the hell was he doing out here in the dark? There's no reason to be here in this weather."

Rob looked really shocked.

"What did he look like?" I asked again.

"He was dressed all in black and when he saw me he just walked away, totally casual, you know."

I was shocked too but Rob was really freaked out by the incident.

Understandably, considering he was the one who'd come face to face with the crim. Damn, yet again my plans to stay on the coast had been thwarted! We had to move after that of course. We just wouldn't have felt safe there. Off we went on another late-night move.

Day 350 — 6th December 2011
Criel-sur-Mer, France

Got some lovely French lip balm yesterday. I can't work out what it smells of, but I'm glad I got a two-pack because it's so nice. I kept holding it up to my nose and taking massive sniffs, over and over until Rob gave me a funny look and said,

"You're weird."

We don't think our wannabe-thief took anything, probably because Rob disturbed him. But there is so much stuff rammed in the back it's pretty hard to tell.

The weather is still awful. Despite this, Rob is standing outside chatting to the English guy from the motorhome next door. Ours are the only two motorhomes here. I am pretending to be busy doing something because, quite frankly, I can't be bothered making conversation with strangers this morning. I've worked out that sometimes I feel sociable and sometimes I don't. Profound, I know. Maybe I should just accept that, rather than guiltily hiding my person from outsiders. But enough of such inward thoughts, because today is officially Jam-Making Day! We've just had another mid-drive mishap. We were going through a little residential area when a bus came in the opposite direction. Rob pulled into somebody's drive to give the guy enough space to get past. But the driver kept pointing to us or to something on our vehicle. I couldn't work out what he was trying to tell us.

"This isn't a one-way street or something is it?"

"I don't think so," Rob said.

But as we backed out into the street again, we both heard a horrific scraping noise and looked at each other.

"What the...?"

I had a terrible image of a person, perhaps a young child or a hapless pensioner, stuck under the wheel and being dragged along for several miles. But of course it was nothing as serious or dramatic as that. I looked out my mirror and saw the problem straight away. The step on my side was down and we'd just bashed it against a lamppost.

"Rob, the step's down!"

"Shit!"

He stopped and got out to check the damage. I jumped out too. It was pretty mangled.

The step had always been one of my favourite features. You press a button just inside the door and it effortlessly moved up or down. But the really clever bit is (or was) that if you happened to forget you'd got the step down and attempted to drive off, a loud beeping alarm came on to warn you. Except in this case, for some reason the alarm hadn't done its job.

Rob pressed the button a few times, but thankfully the step wasn't so mangled that it wouldn't go up and down any more. However, it did look a bit squint and made a disconcerting squeaky whine. As if moving wasn't quite so effortless now. I wondered whether it would collapse, giving way the next time one of us stepped down a bit heavily.

Maybe it was shock, but I couldn't help thinking there was something quite funny about this. Especially the sound it was making. When I looked back down the road, there was a tiny bit of damage to someone's lawn, where the step had scraped off a line of grass as it went by. I didn't dare laugh out loud, because Rob looked really annoyed. We legged it before a disgruntled French person noticed what we'd done to their lawn.

I did try not to laugh. I also resisted the temptation to say 'Ah well', because I know this is starting to annoy Rob. I've been saying 'ah well' in response to lots of the little things that have gone wrong recently. What I mean by it is, there's no point getting all hot and bothered about this, is there? It's done now. But I'm starting to think it's the antidepressants talking. I don't think they've noticeably altered my personality, but perhaps I'm five or ten percent different. Maybe I care a bit less. Maybe I absolutely piss myself laughing less than usual too. Is that sad? That I'm less me? Or is that the whole point of these little pills, to take the edge off me? Can it be more healthy to feel less? To let it all wash over me? Am I a better version of myself now? Whatever gets you through the night... is that the right attitude? I don't know, I'm probably too repressed or mellowed out to care. Ah well.

At least the jam is made and tastes pretty damn good. We are in a lay-by type of place now (off the main road of course, so it's safe as a safe house) with the generator on.

It has brightened up a bit this afternoon. Which is a relief because the weather's been relentless lately, tonnes of hail and sleet and high winds. We're on our way to Auxi-le-Château later. Or Doullens maybe.

Much later. Well, that's three nights in a row we have had to move. At 7.15am we drove off from Criel-sur-Mer because there was such a gale blowing that we thought it might damage the vehicle. Sadly, I feel destined never to stay on the coast in our motorhome.

Day 352 — 8th December 2011
Saint-Venant, France

I lost three of four games of Scrabble today, so the score is 16-11. I think.

I feel much better after my jog along the canal this morning. I will get slim!

Can't believe we only have nine days of our trip left.

We are at Saint-Venant. We tried Doullens but there was no water and lots of weird/scary-looking people. It's really pretty here. We're surrounded by water, with a river on one side and a canal on the other. The only downside is that at this time of year the only service open to motorhomers is waste emptying. So we still haven't managed to top up our drinking water supply. Water water everywhere...

Day 353 — 9th December 2011
Cassel, France

We've had a good day. It was beautiful today, but cold. You would never guess it had been stormy last night. In fact it was so stormy, we moved the motorhome a few hundred metres to get away from any trees that might decide to shed branches and smash us to death.

Rob is rough today. We are in Cassel. I wonder if this is where Vincent Cassel, the sexy French actor, is from.

We left Saint-Venant after a run down the canal. And we finally have water in the tank, not just pouring down all around us. I went to get a water 'jeton' (token) from the local tourist office (once I'd found it) and had a lovely chat with the lady working there. She was so friendly and, best of all, said she understood my French "perfectly"! I was slightly downhearted when she answered in English, having delivered my much-practised request; 'Bonjour, je voudrais un jeton pour le camping car, s'il vous plaît'. She explained that, although I'd made myself very clear, she'd responded in English because, having lived and studied in

Southampton for a year, she recognised my accent. Such an insignificant little interaction, but a friendly chat really lifts my spirits.

I'm doing the tummy-toning machine at the moment. And I'm on to strength 48, which is progress. It's a good job, as I scoffed loads of crisps last night.

Only one week to go before it's all over.

Day 354 — 10th December 2011
Cassel, France

Bit hungover. We drank two bottles of wine between us last night. Which is a lot for us. Or for me at least.

Walked for an hour this morning, which was refreshing and helped clear the hangover cobwebs a bit. We met a very friendly ginger cat, desperate for a fuss.

I saw someone who reminded me of Tommy Sheridan today, walking past the motorhome with a yappy little dog. I find that delusion quite funny now. It is true that I once spent over an hour alone with him, but it was all perfectly innocent. As a journalism student I'd chosen Tommy as my 'celebrity interview' assignment. This was in 2002, well before his court cases, so he was only famous as the firebrand leader of the Scottish Socialist Party. I was a big fan. I loved his passion and the way he could inspire a crowd; we were all 'brothers and sisters' together. He was a rare breed, a politician who spoke like a normal person, a politician with principles! I saw him as someone who stuck up for ordinary people, who tried to protect them from nasty policies like nuclear armament and the dreaded poll tax. He'd even spent time in prison for these worthwhile causes. Risking his personal freedom for what he believed in seemed heroic, even romantic, to me. How many people, let alone politicians, would do that?

So as an idealistic 21-year-old, I was slightly nervous about meeting him. And a bit starry-eyed too. I'd never been to the Glasgow City Council chambers in George Square before and was, stupidly, surprised by how plush they were. Everything was gold or dark wood, and there were loads of massive gilt-framed oil paintings. Tommy was taller than I'd realised. He was wearing a smart navy suit with a well-ironed white shirt that showed off his tan. I noticed equally golden cufflinks and a shiny wedding ring. He gave my hand a hearty shake and led me up the stairs into a large oak-panelled room. We sat at a massive oval table and I plucked my little Dictaphone from my handbag. I was in awe of him of course, completely captivated. He struck me as genuine, down to earth and charismatic, giving off that intoxicating vibe powerful people project. I wondered whether he was aware of that. Maybe it just feels normal after a while.

Tommy was the ideal interviewee for a shy unconfident student like me. I always liked to be well-prepared and had spent many many hours finding out everything I possibly could about him. But as it turned out, I barely had to bother asking any questions at all from my extensive list – he never stopped talking! I tried my best to absorb everything, hoping the tape recorder wouldn't fuck up and scrawling some notes just in case. I wondered how the hell I would be able to squeeze all the good bits into just 1500 words. I have to admit, I was slightly distracted by his chocolatey eyes, even more so by his unbelievably hairy hands. Not his palms, I should say, just the backs of his hands. Man, he was a gorilla! A very articulate gorilla, but still. I tried not to stare and to concentrate on looking professional, wondering how recently he'd been on a sunbed. I wondered whether his wife (Gail was it?) also had a Glasgow tan. Maybe not, I think she's a redhead. Tommy was famous for his fake tan at the time. When I asked him about it, he described this vanity as his only vice. Told me he'd never fancied smoking or drinking much alcohol. I thought about the cigarette I would undoubtedly light up as soon as the interview was over, and wished I could be as pure and saintly as Tommy. Ha!

I still find it difficult to believe he lied, despite everything that was reported in the perjury case. Surely power doesn't always corrupt? That interview felt like a long time ago now. Well, it was a long time ago. I don't know how the hell my worn out brain went from that, to thinking I'd been to a swingers club with him. And then forgotten about it! It's not the sort of night out that slips your mind really, is it?

Scrabble time now. I lost really annoyingly yesterday. Can't help thinking he's about to overtake me and prompt a return of my Scrabble rage.

Day 355 — 11th December 2011
Aalter, Belgium

I ran for forty minutes this morning and did the first 25 without stopping. Nice. Despite all my jogging efforts, my waist measurement is the same as last week, ie massive. I need to try not to be such a greedy bugger I suppose. I'm guilty of overcompensating every time I run; being even greedier than normal, I mean, stupidly acting as if a slow low-intensity run in the morning justifies any amount of gluttony for the rest of the day.

This Aalter place looks pretty enough and is by a river. Or is it a canal? Well, it's definitely water anyway. The first aire we tried, the place we parked at on one of our very first nights of the trip — the one where we accidentally accessed the free electricity — was full.

Five days left!

Damn, I just lost two games of Scrabble. Bollocks. It's so annoying! 18-16 now. I'm sure he's about to overtake me.

Day 356 — 12th December 2011
Aalter, Belgium

We just got ourselves all ready to go and get GPL (as LPG's called on the continent), go to Lidl and do all those boring little chores, then decided that we didn't really need to go anywhere till tomorrow. So we played two games of Scrabble instead. Which I won. Cue smug face. Yes! We've reached a much less worrying 20-16 now. Bobert is not happy.

It's another beautiful day, but cold. Ran for forty minutes this morning, without stopping at all. Quite proud of myself. I actually felt achy this morning, which I took as a good sign; I must have properly used my muscles for once. Maybe I need to run for longer each time. I so want to get rid of this damn stomach.

Four days left.

Day 357 — 13th December 2011
Arques, France

We decided to move last night as we weren't at all sheltered and it was getting quite windy. We drove around for a while not finding anywhere, with the satnav helpfully trying to encourage us down all the narrow streets. Eventually we settled at an industrial-looking part of town near the port at Arques, around 11pm. Not pretty but adequate. A terrible storm started at 3am, so we were right to move.

"You know what?" Rob said this morning.

"What?" I answered, barely awake.

"I've just checked the forecast and I'm wondering if we should head back tonight, or tomorrow night maybe."

"Oh, get the tunnel early?"

"Yeah. I mean, you can change the booking easily enough can't you? And what's the point in hanging around here, when the weather's like this?"

"Yeah, I suppose that makes sense. Let me go online and check what happens to our ticket price if we change it."

Three minutes later it was done; we're all set to get the train back to England tomorrow night.

Day 358 — 14th December 2011
Service Station off the A303, England*

We visited the Commonwealth War Graves Cemetery at Tyne Cot today, one last outing before we went home. I didn't realise how huge it was, what an immense sight it would be. Thousands of unnamed and named soldiers are buried there. Blimey, that was one bitter, icy wind ripping through the place! The rain whipped viciously across my face. I couldn't hack it outside for long. We're now off to fill up on water with the last of our *jetons*, in the pissing rain. Last stop is a supermarket, to buy a shedload of wine and cheese, before getting the Eurotunnel tonight. I feel quite excited about going home.

***

We got to Calais in plenty of time, the motorhome slightly heavier thanks to a few kilos of lovely cheeses and ninety litres of wine. That's about as much booze as you can take back without attracting unwanted attention from the customs people. There was a terrible storm sweeping through Calais. Poor Rob got soaked adjusting the headlights; they have to be positioned differently when you're in Europe, so that you don't dazzle someone with your beam — something to do with driving on the right on the continent. Is it just me or does that sound like a euphemism? Ooh, stop dazzling me with your beam will you, I'm a married woman!

Because we were there in good time we managed to hop on an earlier train than the one we'd booked. French customs was a tiny bit scary. One of the guys, dressed head to toe in black, asked whether we spoke French. We said no rather than the usual 'un peu'; in these circumstances I didn't want any room for misunderstandings. He switched to English.

"Can you open the door please?"

I thought for a nasty moment he was going to ask Rob to step out of the vehicle. But he just put some kind of magic wand inside the cab and ran it over the steering wheel, explaining that he was checking for explosives. I relaxed once I knew what he was looking for. Moments later we were through and properly homeward bound.

* This is where we eventually spent the night, having started the day in France.

Day 359 — 15th December 2011
Somewhere in Somerset, England

We're back!

We slept in a service station off the A303 last night. Oh the glamour! It was OK, but I'm tired now because we didn't stop driving till 3am and then got up at nine.

It's strange being in Blighty again. I'd forgotten how different car number plates and road signs look in the UK. That typeface is so synonymous with Britain. Rob adjusted to driving on the left again with no problems, so far. I keep thinking we're going the wrong way round roundabouts.

We stopped in at Stonehenge this afternoon, to take a look at the famous landmark. I stayed in the motorhome because it was pissing with rain and bloody freezing. Rob did his best to take photos without getting close enough to the cordon to have to pay the extortionate entrance fee. It was over £10 each to get in. To see some flipping stones!? I don't care how old or mysterious they are, that's ridiculous.

Our next job was to find somewhere motorhome-friendly to stay overnight tonight. This is much trickier now we're back home. But after doing some research online, Rob found a pub in a handy location, the Royal Oak in Stoke St Gregory, where motorhomers were apparently welcome. When we got there the manager said we could pitch up for the night on their car park for the grand total of a fiver. Pretty reasonable, we thought. It would have been rude not to have some scran there too.

We had a couple of glasses of red wine in the van before going into the pub for an early tea. The Royal Oak looked lovely and cosy. I took it all in, the oak beams on the ceiling, the cheerful Christmas decorations, the inviting log fire and the few old man regulars. The whole scene was so British! The regulars included some ruddy-faced farmer types who looked to be permanent fixtures at the bar. They all had excellent West Country accents. I kept wanting to shout 'Ciderrrrrrrr' at them. I didn't though. That would have been rude. The barman, who was dark-haired and quite handsome despite being a bit cross-eyed, was friendly and said he'd bring our drinks over.

Sometimes good-looking people make me feel self-conscious. Not because I want anything from them, but because I think they must know they're good-looking and will probably assume that I'm attracted to them. Maybe it's unfair to assume they assume that, but I always try to go out of my way to not act as if I find them attractive, in case I make them feel uncomfortable. Which in turn makes me feel uncomfortable because I start over-thinking every little gesture and sentence and wonder whether I've gone too far, overcompensating by being a bit aloof and unfriendly. So it's hard work sometimes, interacting with them. It would be much better if I ignored their good looks completely and just relaxed and behaved normally around everyone, no matter what they looked like. Unfortunately I do tend to over-analyse things. I should work on that.

Anyway, it wasn't like this guy was Johnny Depp or anything, he was just a nice-looking guy with quite a funny eye. Hey, that sounds like a song. I still felt shy doing my best to convince him I didn't fancy him whilst still hopefully coming across as a nice, friendly person.

We both ordered fish and chips with mushy peas. It tasted pretty good, the fish and batter were fresh and the chips weren't greasy. We polished off a bottle of wine over dinner and I carried on drinking red when Rob switched to pints of lager.

We moved from our table to stools at the bar and started chatting to the barman and farmer types. The barman told us that like most people he knew, he had two jobs. He was a farmer as well as a barman. He asked us where we were from and we talked a bit about the trip we'd just been on. It felt nice not having to think about language barriers. As the wine eased my social timidity, I soon forgot I'd ever felt self-conscious around him.

My merry state had brought on a strong urge to hear some decent tunes, so I asked the barman if he had any good CDs he could play. There were slim pickings, to put it mildly. Elton John, All Saints and the Rolling Stones were about the best of the boring bunch. According to my impeccable musical taste buds, that is. I looked him steadily in the eye and said, "You know, I really thought you might have good taste in music," shaking my head in mock disappointment.

"Hey! Just remember who's pouring your drinks, Glasgow."

I laughed at the surprised look on his face. I'd gone from 'too shy to talk to anyone except Rob' to 'tipsy enough to bam* up the barman I'd only just met' in about two hours.

I really was starting to feel quite drunk. There was a not-unpleasant dizziness in my head and I seemed to be giggling a lot more than normal. I noticed the top of the bar was decked out with a load of amusing black baubles, captioned with phrases such as 'ho bloody ho', 'bah humbug' and 'I hate Christmas'. In my drunken state I thought these were the most hilarious things I'd ever seen and cheekily asked the barman if I could pinch one.

* Bam up is a Scottish term meaning wind up.

"Stop being so northern!" he said, tutting at me but smiling a bit too. I just giggled. A few minutes later he said, "Yeah, I thought that'd be the answer. Sorry, Glasgow, you can't have one. I just text the boss and he said, 'No way. They cost about four quid each'."

Oh well, I thought. Nice of him to try. Aren't people nice? I felt full of love for everyone tonight.

Later on, when I was even drunker, I thought, well, I could at least have one of the *ordinary* baubles, surely? As a wee keepsake. Nobody had said not to take one of those. Ha ha! Thinking this was an altogether *brilliant,* not to mention cunning and very clever idea, I swiped a traditional bauble and stuck it in my bag. No one saw me and I felt quite smug that I'd managed to get away with it without anyone noticing. It didn't even occur to me that I might have slipped back into the klepto habit that formed when I was under lock and key. I suppose being extremely drunk is a kind of temporary madness. At least I got away with it this time.

Soon I'd got to the point where I couldn't really manage a whole sentence. Or even half a good one. I tended to forget exactly where I was going with the thought before it came out as coherent speech, so it would just sort of fizzle out into nonsense. When I realised this, I told Rob we'd better get going pretty soon. We heartily thanked the nice barman and paid our bill. He gave us a compliments slip and a couple of mints. I scanned it and noticed he'd written, 'Thanks very much, Bill'.

"Your name's not really Bill is it?" I accidentally said this quite aggressively, as if being called Bill was some sort of crime. Only because, well, he didn't look like a Bill at all. It didn't suit him.

"No, it's just a joke, you know. Bill? As in, you've just paid your...? Never mind."

"Oh, I see! Bill! Ha ha, that's a good one!"

The barman looked at me in that slightly amused, slightly more wary way that sober people look at drunk people.

"Come on, Ros." Rob was using the not-very-subtle strategy of pulling on my arm to get me to leave.

"OK, bye barman! Bye old man regulars! Bye bye all the farmers! Enjoy your ciderrrr, ha ha!"

They said goodbye, although not quite as enthusiastically as I had, I noticed.

When we got outside the cold British air hit us.

"Ooh, isn't this great Rob? We've only got a few steps and we're home! How cool is that?"

Rob was quite giggly, which was normal for him, sober or drunk, but I could tell he was almost as merry as I was. In the pub we'd come up with the amazingly crafty plan of not ordering dessert to save money, knowing that we had plenty of lovely chocolate we could attack once back in the van. Not sure how that brilliant strategy worked out considering how much we'd just spent on booze, but there you go.

"Hmmm, let's have tea and chocolate. That'll bring us round a bit!"

So we had tea and chocolate. Lots of chocolate in fact. Too much chocolate, perhaps.

"Rob..."

"Mmm," he said, suspiciously sleepy.

"Don't feel very good. Am *so* full."

"I don't feel too good m'self."

"Oh, man..."

I tried to distract myself from feeling sick. It didn't work. For some reason my brain kept sabotaging the strategy, harking back to images of the massive portion of fish and chips I'd eaten earlier. The more I tried not to think about it, the more it came back to haunt me. Why does my mind work against me at times like this?

Soon the fish and chips literally came back to haunt me. I squatted over the toilet bowl waiting for it to be over.

Oh dear. What a dick. Why did I drink so much? Acting like some kind of stupid teenager... I'm a disgrace to the human race. At least I felt a bit better afterwards. Except for that bitter burning acidity that lingers in your throat post-sickness. Wow, that was horrible. I cleaned my teeth and conked out for the night.

Day 361 — 17th December 2011
Stoke-Sub-Hamdon, Somerset, England

Oh God. Red wine hangover. Horrendous. Head throbbing. Tongue like leather. Damn those tannins.

"Rob?"

"Mmm."

I turned to look at him and with his eyes closed and the duvet wrapped all round him, he looked so sweet and cute and lovely and cosy. Innocent almost.

Tears jumped into my eyes. I'm so grateful he's mine. OK, it's going to be one of those emotional hangovers is it?

"Rob, I've got a bastard behind the eyes," I whined.

"Mmm, me too. Go back to sleep."

I did. But I didn't feel much better when I woke up a few hours later. I dragged myself out of bed and put the kettle on. However bad the situation, tea always helps.

"I can't believe we drank so much," I said to Rob.

"I know. We never do that."

"I can't believe I actually spewed, I haven't done that for years."

I opened my handbag to work out how much money we'd spent last night and a Christmas bauble fell out and rolled down the motorhome.

"Oh God, I'd forgotten about that," I said, blushing at my kleptomania.

"Ros! I can't believe you stole that," Rob said, looking more amused than concerned by my petty thievery.

"I know. I'm terrible, Muriel," I said. "Jeez man, did I make a show of myself last night? I mean, was there anything really awful?"

"What, apart from nicking things from the bar you mean? Nah, you were quite funny really."

"Funny? Funny how?"

"Well, let's see. Oh yeah, one of the best bits was when you attempted a West Country accent. You know... in front of all the West Country people?"

"Nooooo! I didn't do that did I?" I was horrified, not just by my actions but because I didn't remember anything about that.

"Was I really bad? Did I offend anyone do you think?" I clung on to Rob for emotional support.

"No, I think you just amused people, especially the 'old man regulars', as you called them."

I cringed. I did actually remember saying that, quite loudly, on the way out.

"Oh well, if that's the worst, that's not *too* ba-"

"They might have had enough of you randomly shouting 'ciderrrr' every five minutes though..."

Oh man. What a beamer. Well, there's always one drunken bum in the bar isn't there. Last night must have been my turn. At least I'd never have to see any of them again.

As soon as Rob was sober enough to drive, I was pretty keen to leave the Royal Oak, just in case we bumped into anyone. Luckily it was only a short drive to Rob's parents' place.

I was kind of hoping we could just have a nice relaxing evening while I got over my hangover quietly, in peace. I should have known that wasn't likely. Rob's parents' house wasn't the sort of place where we normally all just curl up on the sofa watching telly.

Rosie had made a gorgeous pre-Christmas Christmas dinner for everybody, with turkey, roast potatoes, honey-coated parsnips, Brussels sprouts and more. She'd produced an amazing salmon dish for Rob and me.

"This is all wonderful, Rosie," I said as we tucked in.

I cleared my plate, except for a couple of sprouts that were a little on the undercooked side. I thanked Rosie again at the end of the meal.

"I'm so sorry about the sprouts," she said, looking at the uneaten ones on my plate.

"Don't be daft, the whole meal was amazing," I said.

She'd already apologised for the sprouts several times during the meal itself.

Actually I think most of them were fine, there were just a few a bit underdone. I couldn't understand why Rosie kept drawing our attention to that one little thing, when the whole meal had been delicious. And I thought I was a perfectionist.

I still had a headache (I couldn't even stomach a glass of wine over dinner, so they probably thought I was up the duff) and all I wanted to do was curl up in a ball and sleep for days.

That didn't happen.

Instead, we were treated to a concert by Kelly and Louise, Rosie and Barry's foster daughters, with Rosie playing a supporting actress role. It's hard to describe the content of the performance really; all I can say is that it definitely involved some singing, dancing and clapping (with which everyone was encouraged to join in). That bit was quite loud. It also had a rather surreal quality. Take, for example, the item in which Rosie fed an invisible reindeer with a real carrot. She even gave each of us a carrot with which we were to feed the non-existent reindeer.

As I dutifully fed a carrot to the thin air beside me, I turned to Rob and quietly said, "Is this really happening?"

The experience simultaneously took my mind off my hangover and made it much worse.

Day 363 — 19th December 2011
Stoke-Sub-Hamdon, Somerset, England

I popped a Christmas card in the post to the nurses and doctors at Stobhill Hospital. I'd written a little note, thanking them for looking after me so well a year ago, and telling them that Rob and I had been travelling around Europe in a motorhome for the last six months. Hopefully it would get there in time. I promised myself I would send them one every year.

Day 364 — 20th December 2011
Stoke-Sub-Hamdon, Somerset, England

Having spent a few days catching up with Rob's family, we're getting ready to leave Somerset now. Bobert's in a bad mood because he's shattered and can't be arsed driving up to Dumfries, which takes at least seven hours.

Actually it won't be a seven-hour drive if we stop somewhere on the way, but we're not sure where we're staying for the next couple of nights. I'm not entirely comfortable with this lack of arrangement. In fact I hate it.

The no-plan-plan is fine for driving aimlessly around Europe, but when you're hoping to park on people's driveways and they don't know anything about it, even though you might be doing so tomorrow night... well, that troubles me.

I know Mike, I know; *our circumstances are not always ideal.* That's life eh, so stop whinging. I think that's what he was getting at.

We have some decorations in the motorhome now, thanks to my little shopping trip yesterday. I'm pleased about this.

I've not slept too well the last few nights. Mainly due to the always full on, high-intensity nature of the Egerton household, as well as not getting any exercise and going to bed too late. And eating too many chocolates right before bed. Not a brilliant combination really.

Day 366 — 22nd December 2011
Glasgow, Scotland

I got the underground to the west end. God it was so good to be back. We were staying with friends for a couple of days before going to my parents' house in Dumfries for Christmas. I *love* Glasgow! There's always such a lively buzz here.

I still had a few wee presents to buy, but I was feeling very smug about the fact that I wouldn't be running around like an idiot on Christmas Eve this year, for the first time since I could remember. Christmas preparations are so much easier without a stressful job to worry about.

I was walking back towards Sausageroll Street (or Sauchiehall Street, as other people insist on calling it) dodging the hordes of shoppers, pondering whether or not my sister would find a Cliff Richard calendar funny, when I realised. It was exactly a year to the day since I'd been taken into hospital.

Although I was well, and happy (most of the time), I was also technically jobless and homeless, which means facing some uncertainty. But hey, there was plenty of time to sort the practical things out. Generally, I felt relaxed, hopeful and healthy. Isn't health and well-being supposed to be at the top of the life wish list? After all, without it all the other stuff can't do you much good.

As I took in my surroundings, I felt like grabbing all the people who looked grumpy and cold and harassed and telling them to make the most of the loving relationships and any other good things in their lives. To appreciate and relish the simple pleasures they might have accidentally learned to take for granted. I felt as lucky and happy as Jimmy Stewart at the end of 'It's A Wonderful Life'.

I refrained from actually grabbing anyone. I didn't want to risk getting sectioned a second time, not when I was so buoyant. My happy balloon shrivelled a bit as I thought for a minute about the thousands of people who would spend this Christmas as I did last year. I wondered how many of them would get through it, how many of them were lucky enough to have someone kind by their side. I knew I'd been lucky. But I was ready to move on. Besides, I didn't want to live in the past any more, not when there's still so much to look forward to.

Epilogue — May 2014
Dumfries, Scotland

"When we imagine we have finished our story, fate has a trick of turning the page and showing us yet another chapter." Lucy Maud Montgomery

When we got back to the UK, we spent some time in Aberdeenshire, working together on a beautiful country park. We spent some time in the south of Portugal too, mostly not working. Portugal was warmer, funnily enough, but I found the local dialects equally incomprehensible. As you'll know if you've got this far, we didn't move our lives to Scoraig. But we have managed two completely off-grid trips in the Hymer. We no longer have to frantically look for electric hook up points as we travel in Europe, thanks to a set of solar panels that Rob fitted. Not that we've idled away the last few years in the sun, you understand. I've been writing this book (the struggling author cliché appeals to me, so I'll do my best not to make any money whatsoever) and Rob has worked on a few house renovations, as well as other random projects. Whatever happens next, I'm glad we didn't jump straight back on the nine-to-five hamster wheel.

There will soon be three of us (touch wood) in our cosy little wheeled unit — I have a genetically similar bun in me oven and as far as I can tell she's rising quite nicely. Actually there will be four of us, if you count the cat, Jay. Which we do. She now has her own bespoke motorhome cat flap, which she absolutely refuses to use.

I'd love to be able to report that, despite impending sprogdom, we're still gadding about Europe in the Egerton-Nash fun-mobile, carefree and zooming along like the 'Dad's Army' title sequence. Or even that we've bought a plot of land somewhere beautifully peaceful and are currently living, free and wild, much like Tom and Barbara in 'The Good Life'. But the truth is we're living in Dumfries at the moment. The location is not the least bit romantic, exciting or bohemian, but it makes sense to stick around while we get the hang of this baby/parent thing. Maybe my experience of severe sleep deprivation will help us get to grips with a newborn humanoid. While we're almost on the subject, I should let you know that it's been well over a year since I took anti-depressants to steady my sleep ship. And my mental health is still intact (touch wood again), thanks for asking. So far, so good.

ABOUT THE AUTHOR

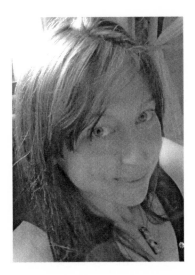

Ros, who has lived in Scotland since the age of 11, graduated from the University of Strathclyde, Glasgow, with a degree in marketing in 1998, returning to study journalism as a postgraduate student in 2001. She then spent ten years working as a writer and editor at magazines and newspapers, including the award-winning Scottish Wedding Directory, before writing 'What's Up With Ros?'

Ros lives in a motorhome with her husband Rab (or Rob, as she still insists on calling him), their daughter Zoe and their cat, Jay.

Lightning Source UK Ltd.
Milton Keynes UK
UKOW02f0902180815

257105UK00002B/91/P